The Movement for Global Mental Hea

The Movement for Global Mental Health

Critical Views from South and Southeast Asia

Edited by
William Sax and
Claudia Lang

Routledge
Taylor & Francis Group

LONDON AND NEW YORK

First published in 2021 by Amsterdam University Press Ltd.

Published 2025 by Routledge
4 Park Square, Milton Park, Abingdon, Oxon OX14 4RN
605 Third Avenue, New York, NY 10158

Routledge is an imprint of the Taylor & Francis Group, an informa business

ISBN: 9789463721622 (hbk)
ISBN: 9781041188520 (pbk)
ISBN: 9781003707004 (ebk)

NUR 860

Cover image: Death Valley National Park, United States
Photographer: Jehyun Sung/Unsplash

Cover design: Coördesign, Leiden

DOI : 10.5117/9789463721622

For Product Safety Concerns and Information please contact our EU representative:
GPSR@taylorandfrancis.com
Taylor & Francis Verlag GmbH, Kaufingerstraße 24, 80331 München, Germany

Table of Contents

Afterwords

List of Tables

1 Global Mental Health

Views from South Asia and Beyond[1]

William S. Sax and Claudia Lang

Abstract
Although the contributors to this volume are sympathetic to many of the goals of the Movement for Global Mental Health, we are also of the view that its agenda at the time of publication is based upon a number of problematic assumptions, that it may serve unacknowledged interests, and that in some respects it might even have harmful consequences. In the introduction we focus on the problematic assumptions that "mental disorders" can clearly be identified; that they are primarily of biological origin; that the world is currently facing an "epidemic" of mental disorders; that the most appropriate treatments for them normally involve psycho-pharmaceutical drugs; and that local or indigenous therapies are of little interest or importance. We also question the value of "scaling up" mental health services, as advocated by the Movement for Global Mental Health, and conclude by summarising the structure of the book, with brief comments on the various essays.

Keywords: Movement for Global Mental Health, treatment gap, treatment difference

Global mental health is something that everyone supports: Who does not want everyone on the planet to be mentally well? But what does it mean to be mentally healthy, or mentally ill? What concepts of "mind", "health", and "illness" are applied, by whom, and with what authority? What visions of global mental health have been articulated, and by

---

1   Thanks to Stefan Ecks and Laurence Kirmayer for their comments on earlier versions of this introduction.

Sax, William, and Claudia Lang (eds), *The Movement for Global Mental Health: Critical Views from South and Southeast Asia*. Taylor & Francis Group, 2021
DOI: 10.5117/9789463721622_CH01

whom? Must one choose between them, and if so, how? In recent years, one particular vision of global mental health has come to dominate the field, and its answers to these questions have become increasingly influential. The Movement for Global Mental Health (henceforth MGMH) is a worldwide assemblage of psychiatrists, psychologists, government agencies, medical doctors, public health professionals, health policy makers, private foundations, medical journals, and others "committed to collective actions that aim to close the treatment gap for people living with mental disorders worldwide, based on two fundamental principles: evidence on effective treatments and the human rights of people with mental disorders" (Patel et al. 2011). It rose to prominence in 2008 following a series of articles in one of the world's leading medical journals that culminated in a call "to scale up the coverage of services for mental disorders in all countries, but especially in low-income and middle-income countries" (Chisholm et al. 2007, 1241; for the genealogies of global mental health cf. Ecks 2016 and this volume; Lovell et al. 2019). The MGMH has no rigid hierarchical structure, and this allows it to respond to its critics quickly, flexibly, and (in our view) usually productively. The protean quality of MGMH also means that any attempt to characterise it risks immediate obsolescence.

We do not doubt that virtually all of those involved in the MGMH are committed to relieving the suffering associated with what are called "mental disorders", and ensuring equal access to mental health resources on a global level. But the contributors to this volume are also of the view that the MGMH's agenda at the time of publication is based upon a number of problematic assumptions, that it may serve unacknowledged interests, and that in some respects it might even have harmful consequences.[2] And because the MGMH has become so influential, we feel that it is important to subject these assumptions to critical scrutiny.

Problematic Assumptions

These problematic assumptions are numerous, and appear regularly in the movement's literature. In some of their recent publications, leading figures in

---

2   We have had some difficulty in deciding whether we should define the topic of this introduction as "Global Mental Health", or as the "Movement for Global Mental Health", where the latter is a subset of the former, and whose active core consists of a smaller group with a slightly more precise agenda.

the MGMH have critically re-examined and partially revised some of them. This is an example of the MGMH's dynamic, protean nature, as mentioned above. We applaud the MGMH's willingness to engage in self-criticism, and want to suggest ways in which this might be carried much further. In order to do so, we will focus in this introduction on the following problematic assumptions: the idea that "mental disorders" can clearly be identified; that they are primarily of biological origin; that the world is currently facing an "epidemic" of mental disorders; that the most appropriate treatments for them normally involve psychopharmaceutical drugs; and that local or indigenous therapies are of little interest or importance. We will take a close look at each of these assumptions, which are sometimes explicit and sometimes implicit, but are in either case pervasive in the literature associated with the MGMH.

Let us begin with the idea that "mental disorders" are clearly identifiable. This is simply not true. One can only say that psychiatry is and always has been characterised by a fundamental *lack* of agreement about the classification of mental disorders, their causes, and the best ways to treat them. (See below for our analysis of the reasons why.) Psychiatric thinking about these topics was dominated for a long time by psychoanalytic approaches, but these failed to deliver on their grandiose promises so that, beginning in the 1980s and culminating in the 2010s, psychiatry came to be dominated by materialist approaches like neuropsychiatry and genetics. But these, too, have failed to lead to any striking advances in the understanding and/or treatment of mental disorders, and there are signs that the biopsychiatric consensus is breaking down (Harrington 2019). Periodic statements by the MGMH that mental diseases are well understood – in one of their most recent publications, they write of "the convergence of evidence from diverse scientific disciplines on the nature and causes of mental health problems" (Patel et al. 2018, 1) – may therefore be read as unjustifiably optimistic assessments intended to shore up support for their program. Or they can simply be regarded as false and misleading.

Athough the MGMH makes use of a variety of disciplines, including clinical psychology and social work, and increasingly includes self-identified "service users" or "people with psychosocial disabilities", it is first and foremost a vehicle for the introduction of a comprehensive programme of mental health care based upon contemporary biomedical models and therapies, and ultimately under the direction of psychiatrists. But how, exactly, should one define the mental disorders to which such models and therapies respond? As a standard-bearer for international psychiatry, the MGMH faces the same intrinsic challenge as its apex discipline – namely, that the signs and symptoms of mental disorders are overwhelmingly behavioural and not physical, making them exceedingly difficult to measure and quantify. Psychiatry has a fundamental problem with validity,[3] because the illnesses with which it is concerned rarely have physical markers, and this complicates all of its branches: psychiatric aetiology, nosology, and therapy. As Canguilhem might have put it, those suffering from mental disorders rarely have "lesions" that can be measured, dissected, and analysed; nor are there visible aetiological agents like bacteria or viruses. Biomedicine is very good at counting and measuring such things, and its continuing refinement of the techniques of measurement has contributed much to the production of its so-called "miracles". But although many psychiatrists in the twentieth century believed that one could dissect the brain and "see" the biological causes of mental illness, and even though many psychiatrists in our own century continue to believe in similarly material (genetic or neurological) causes, such beliefs have always turned out to be largely illusory: The lesions cannot be found, much less measured, and this creates problems for psychiatry. As Wittgenstein might have put it, making a psychiatric taxonomy is like trying "to classify clouds by their shape".[4] Ian Hacking (2007) describes mental disorders as "moving targets", assembled at different scales and grounded in multiple social, historical, and political contexts.

For example, the disease entities in clinical psychiatry's "bible", the *Diagnostic and Statistical Manual* (henceforth DSM), and its international sister, the *International Classification of Diseases*, are often of contingent historical origin, with no common aetiological theory to link them (Bowker and Star 2000). In their book *Making us Crazy*, Kutchins and Kirk (2003) argued that the DSM is the result of the industry's internal lobbying for financial gain; that it contains much racial and gender bias; and that it persists as a necessary step in the remuneration of health professionals and drug companies (cf. Harrington 2019, 267-68). The absence of agreement within psychiatry on fundamental questions of aetiology explains why the DSM V and ICD-10 came to rely on what is called the "phenomenological approach", focusing on symptoms and contexts rather than aetiology. Few of the disorders listed in these manuals have measurable physical correlates, and most consist of collections of symptoms, so that they might better be

3   "Validity" refers to the degree to which a concept "correspond[s] to external reality" (Aragona 2015). See the very useful discussions of validity in psychiatry by Jablensky (2016) and Zachar (2012).

4   This observation was made by the neuropsychiatrist Jablensky (2016), referring Wittgenstein's (1975) remark that "the classifications made by philosophers and psychologists are as if one were to classify clouds by their shape."

labelled "syndromes", rather than "disorders" (Jablensky 2016). But definitions of both symptoms and syndromes change over time, according to broader collective judgments about what kinds of behaviour – and what kinds of mental suffering – are acceptable or unacceptable. As Jablensky, a leading cross-cultural psychiatric epidemiologist, puts it,

> The present diagnostic manuals, ICD and DSM, are classifications of current diagnostic concepts, and not of "natural kinds", such as people or diseases. There is little evidence that most recognized mental disorders, including the psychoses, are separated by natural boundaries. (ibid., 30; cf. Hacking 2013)

The second problematic assumption characteristic of the MGHM is that mental disorders have a material cause. Like the assumption that mental disorders can be easily identified, this idea is omnipresent in psychiatry. Because mental disorders have few measurable physical symptoms, psychiatry relies more heavily on interpretation and clinical judgment than other medical disciplines do, and thus it is often regarded as one of the least scientific branches of medicine. Many psychiatric researchers try to overcome this problem by defining the psyche and its disorders in material terms, in an (in our view, highly problematic) attempt to facilitate their quantification. This explains the ongoing, frantic search for genetic markers and neurological causes of mental disorders, which would effectively constitute the psychiatric version of Canguilhem's "lesions" (1991). If only the material causes of mental disorders could (finally!) be identified, then the disorders themselves would be more susceptible to treatment (presumably by means of psychopharmaceuticals), and the medical profession would (finally!) acknowledge psychiatry as a properly scientific discipline. But in our view, the very idea that (presumably disease-specific) drugs will be discovered, which produce their effects by reversing the particular brain abnormalities that give rise to symptoms (in more colloquial terms, drugs that "rectify a biochemical imbalance in the brain") is, as Moncrieff (2008) has convincingly shown, a myth. The relationship between neurochemical processes in the brain and psychiatric symptoms and treatments remains an unsolved puzzle, and that is why the pharmaceutical industry has largely abandoned research in psychiatry, resulting in a dearth of new psychopharmaceuticals (Dumit 2018).

A good example of psychiatrists' determination to find material causes of mental disorders is provided by the repudiation of the DSM-V, shortly before its publication, by Thomas Insel, who was then head of the US National

Institute for Mental Health (the primary funder of research in the field).[5] Insel justified his actions with the argument that the DSM concerned itself only with symptoms, whereas he wanted "causation", by which he meant neuropsychiatry (Insel 2014).

Both the dogged insistence on material explanations for mental disorders, and the increasing neglect of research into social explanations for them, is difficult to explain, since the results of neuropsychiatric and genetic research have, to date, been quite disappointing (Kendler 2013; Harrington 2019). Although some forms of mental disorder can be strongly correlated with particular processes in the brain, a correlation is not a cause. The *causes* of mental disorders are likely to be found in some combination of biological (genetic, neurological) risk factors and the particular conditions of a person's life (e.g. poverty, abuse, stress, personal tragedy, etc.). In fact, there is little evidence that behavioural disorders are caused by genetic problems or chemical disturbances in the brain, but much hard evidence of the damage done by psychopharmaceuticals used for therapeutic purposes (Moncrieff 2009). Nevertheless, the default position of contemporary psychiatry is to look for pharmaceutical solutions to behavioural disorders, and in the final analysis this is traceable to the widespread assumption that such disorders have neurological or physiological causes.

Here it must be acknowledged that leading voices in the MGMH have acknowledged these criticisms, and claim to favour a more holistic, multi-disciplinary approach to mental health than previous ones. For example, a recently published report of the Lancet Commission on Global Mental Health and Sustainable Development admits the inadequacy of "biomedically defined mental disorders" (Patel et al. 2018, 11). The report begins by noting sympathetically a set of critiques very similar to those articulated in this volume.

> [T]he biomedical framing of the treatment gap has attracted criticism from some scholars and activists championing a cultural perspective and representing people with the lived experience of mental disorders. These voices fear that a biomedical emphasis will take priority over indigenous traditions of healing and recovery, medicalise social suffering, and promote a western psychiatric framework dominated by pharmaceutical interventions. (ibid., 8)

---

5   Insel's research on communication and social attachment amongst rodents (and later, primates) had somehow qualified him for this post. Before resigning to work for Google.com, he slashed funding for research into the social causes of mental illness, in order to focus on neuropsychiatry.

In response to such criticisms, the report specifically acknowledges the "social determinants of mental health" (ibid., 14), and articulates an approach to mental health and illness in terms of the interactions among biology, inherited genetic causes, and "environment" in both its social and physical dimensions (ibid., 18 ff.). We applaud this recognition of the complex aetiology of mental illness by the MGMH, and hope that it continues. But this will not be easy, since psychiatry is the apex discipline within the MGMH, and its very location within biomedicine predisposes psychiatrists toward materialist/neurological paradigms, even in the absence of good evidence for them. This is clearly shown by a passage on "deep phenotyping" immediately following (and in our view, at odds with) the enthusiastic words regarding "the convergent approach to mental health" quoted above.

> Deep phenotyping involves the collection of observable physical and behavioural traits of an individual down to the molecular level. When anchored by a carefully constructed clinical profile, the resulting multilevel biomarker set *could* provide more precise understanding of the causes of disease, and *could* eventually produce a more accurate way to describe and classify mental health conditions than current diagnostic classification systems. In the future, deep phenotyping *could* enable precision mental health care – for example, treatments *could* be targeted on the basis of the underlying disease mechanisms, such as depression linked to immune dysfunction. (ibid., 11; emphasis ours)

Old Habits Die Hard

A third problematic assumption characteristic of the MGMH is that we are faced with a "global epidemic" of mental illness. The foundational literature of the MGMH often invokes two highly publicised studies (Desjarlais et al. 1995; WHO 2001) purporting to show that the global burden of mental disorders is significant and growing. Based upon these and similar studies, some scholars refer to a worldwide "epidemic" of mental illness; others argue that the so-called epidemic is, to a significant extent, the effect of a new metric that has come to dominate the field of health economics in recent decades: the DALY or Disability Adjusted Life Years. This measure was first used in the 1995 World Mental Health report (Desjarlais et al. 1995), and then in the 1996 Global Burden of Disease report, and purportedly revealed an "unseen burden of psychiatric disease" that had hitherto gone unperceived (Murray and Lopez 1996, 21; cf. Bemme and D'Souza 2014; Lovell et al. 2019;

also Ecks's and Das and Rao's contributions to this volume).[6] Technically, the DALY need not be a measure of productivity but only of healthy years lost by a person who is ill or disabled. Practically however, it is very often used in conjunction with "age-weighting" to distinguish between the maximally productive years of young adults and the less productive years of children or the elderly. In this sense it is a textbook example of what Foucault calls "biopower", since it measures lost economic productivity rather than human suffering. According to Li, use of the DALY persists because "the power structure of global health has changed from the political to the economic and biomedical, and power (and money) have become concentrated in the hands of a few individuals" (2014, 1; cf. also Mahajan).[7] But even if we were to accept the claim that the statistics represent a real increase in mental suffering worldwide, this would not necessarily imply that therapies and interventions to address it should be uncritically imported from the West (Mills 2014; Mills and Fernando 2014). Movements like the MGMH and organisations like the WHO are intent on medicating the symptoms of non-Western others so that they can be more economically productive, but might it not be even more important to help them address the social determinants of mental suffering, which may include such things as inequality, prejudice, and violence?

Beginning with the assumption that European definitions of mental health and illness are universal, those in the MGMH have, in the past, made the further, equally problematic assumption that mental disorders are best treated by psychiatrists or those working under their direction. And since there are precious few psychiatrists or other mental health professionals in South Asia, people there (as well as in other regions that are culturally and geographically distant from Europe and North America) are said to suffer from the "treatment gap", a phrase that is constantly invoked in the MGMH literature. By contrast, the contributors to this volume take the view that South Asians have abundant resources for maintaining mental health, so that it would be better to speak of a "treatment difference" than a "treatment

6   Anne Harrington argues that the explosion in the incidence of depression is due to the collapsing of previous distinctions into one grand category of depression when applying the widely used HAM-D scale to measure it (2019, 203-04).

7   Something similar may be happening in the MGMH's advocacy of a "balanced-care model" that is differentially applied depending on whether the location is wealthy or not, viz., "The balanced care model is an evidence-based, systematic but flexible approach to planning treatment and care for people with mental disorders" (Patel et al. 2018, 158), and argues that the provision of mental health services should distinguish between low-income, medium-income, and high-income country settings (ibid., 176).

gap". The problem is that such resources are rarely "seen" by advocates of global mental health, and when they are, they are either dismissed or, even worse, denigrated as inhumane, because they do not correspond to Western psychiatric models. This is confirmed in a recent publication by leading figures in the MGMH. They begin by significantly moderating their claims regarding the efficacy of psychopharmaceuticals:

> The effect sizes for psychological treatments typically range from moderate to large, and sideeffects are relatively rare. The strength of evidence for psychological therapies is at least as strong as for other treatment methods. Furthermore, when headtohead comparisons of efficacy have been done between pharmacological and psychological therapies (notably for mood, anxiety, and traumarelated disorders) no consistent evidence has been reported for the superiority of either in terms of attaining remission; additionally, psychological therapies seem to have a greater enduring effect than pharmacological therapies. (Patel et al. 2018, 21)

Furthermore, as an alternative to psychopharmaceuticals they enthusiastically advocate a large number of psychological therapies, citing numerous studies pointing to their efficacy. They emphasise the need to localise psycho-social treatment modalities, and suggest that the content of therapies needs substantial modification to incorporate local metaphors and beliefs, and to combine psychological skills building components with social work components. The tasks should also be adapted to ensure acceptability for people with limited literacy (e.g., completing homework in sessions). (ibid., 25).

But nearly all of the therapies mentioned originate within the disciplines of psychology and psychiatry, and none is "indigenous" in the strict sense. The overarching assumption has not changed: namely, that psychiatrists and psychologists from the resource-rich "countries of the North" (formerly known as the First World) know what is best for those living in the resource-poor "countries of the South" (formerly known as the Third and Fourth Worlds); and that the latter must be trained, cajoled, perhaps even forced to recognise this. The language in the passages cited above provides the clue: local ideas consist of "metaphors and beliefs" rather than facts or knowledge, and those suffering from mental disorders must be made to comply with the psychiatric regime by "completing their homework".

In this way, a reflexive and self-confirming loop is created and reiterated over and over in the publications and policies of the MGMH: Mental disorders are defined primarily in terms of Western psychiatric nosology, for which only biomedical, or biomedically-approved, therapies are considered. It is true that activists in the MGMH often claim that their movement is not about exporting Western therapies, but rather involves providing (and eventually up-scaling) "packages of care" developed in the countries of the Global South in a situation of scarcity (of professional psychiatric and psychological services). But these packages always place the psychiatrist at the apex of the system, and none of them include the most prominent practices and forms of treatment in such countries: namely traditional medicine, ritual, and religious healing (see Sax, this volume). The single exception in South Asia is yoga, which is deeply ironic, since recent scholarship has shown that modern postural yoga is not traditional at all, but rather a twentieth-century invention, jointly produced by Western doctors and Indian spiritual entrepreneurs (Alter 2004).

This is indeed the crux of the issue. For most of the contributors to this volume, the very definitions of terms like "mind", "mental", "mental health", "mental illness" and so on are highly variable, both culturally and historically. Moreover, language has its own powerful agency such that, for example, people who are told over and over that they are mentally ill finally come to experience themselves that way (cf. Hacking 2002), whereas at an earlier time or in a different culture some of them might have experienced themselves as "holy" or simply "different". The agency of language is even more powerful when it is associated with authoritative figures like doctors and psychiatrists (or priests and shamans) (Kirmayer 1987). The difference between "scientific" and "traditional" understandings of mental illness is very great: in effect, they represent different ontologies, and one wonders if they can ever be truly integrated, although, as Lang shows in this volume, there are increasing efforts to do so. The publications of the MGMH strongly suggest that in their view, this integration should take place, but can only do so within an epistemic hierarchy in which "religion" and "tradition" are subordinated to "science", which adjudicates all questions of truth. And how could it be otherwise? To critically examine the collusion of science and biomedicine with modern, neoliberal capital-ism (see below), or to open the door to non-scientific theories of causation, would threaten the economic, political, and scientific foundations of "modern mental health care", and cannot be seriously contemplated. To put it in other words, advocates of the MGHM do not take alterity seriously: Ontological differences are re-interpreted as "metaphorical", and the therapist is urged to learn the native metaphors, not in order to broaden his/her interpretive horizons, but merely in order to implement the therapy more effectively.

According to the proponents of the MGMH, there are two main problems in implementing mental health. First is the stigma associated with mental illness (a stigma that is, by the way, strongly associated with psychiatry and the labelling of psychological alterity as a "disease", but generally absent from traditional understandings), and second is the fact that the intended beneficiaries do not seek psychiatric help for their problems, because they have different explanatory models (Patel et al. 2018, 25). Such models must therefore be eliminated or transformed in order to provide modern, biomedically-approved therapy and in our view, this rejection of non-psychiatric ontologies of suffering is a form of epistemic violence.

> In many communities, the widely varying explanatory models of mental health and disorder (e.g., that they are equivalent to social suffering or are the result of moral weakness, or spiritual or religious misfortune) lead to low levels of self-recognition or detection by health workers. Innovative strategies for educating health workers and communities that integrate biomedical and contextually appropriate understandings and messages improve detection of common mental disorders and enhance demand for health care (ibid., 25).

With its vision focused narrowly on psychiatry, the MGMH fails to take seriously the idea that ontologies and experiences of mental health and illness might vary significantly between (and within) cultures, and that "mental health resources" include traditional approaches to mental suffering, and not just techniques developed in the West. Take schizophrenia, for example: Certainly there have been many times and places in human history where it has been neither recognised nor named. Indeed, it only came to be regarded as a universal disease with a stable cross-cultural epidemiology after the 1966 International Pilot Study of Schizophrenia (Lovell 2014). The essay by Hornbacher in this volume is relevant here, as it points not only to the important role played by anthropologists Mead and Bateson, and their research in Bali, in the historical production of "schizophrenia" as a universal psychiatric disease category, but also to more general philosophical problems associated with the history of the term.

Are not the symptoms psychiatrists associate with schizophrenia some-times considered to indicate a special, even valued state of mind? Are there non-biomedical models of mental health and illness where the category "schizophrenia" does not fit? And are such models not associated with kinds of therapy that are more culturally appropriate than those employed by psy-chiatrists? Is it not worth seriously considering the possibility that in some cases, such therapies might be more effective than psychopharmaceuticals? Anthropologists have identified numerous internally coherent models of mental health and illness amongst the world's cultures (two good examples are Laderman 1993 and Tambiah 1990, chap. V), but as Stefan Ecks points out in his essay in this volume, such questions have simply been erased from the agenda of the MGMH. Perhaps they are simply too difficult.

All human cultures, including those in Europe and North America, use ritual and religion to heal or mitigate mental suffering, but such techniques are almost never taken seriously by those in the MGMH – not because there is no evidence of their efficacy, but rather because religion and ritual are assumed to be fundamentally at odds with the modern, scientific episteme (Sax 2010, 2014, 2015; Quack and Sax 2010). Meditation and related practices are popular components of health programmes in schools, prisons, businesses and government agencies, and they are increasingly subject to scientific trials of various sorts, but similar studies of ritual healing are practically non-existent. We suspect that this is largely because methodology and class reinforce each other in determining research protocols: While it is indeed possible to measure the effects of meditation on those middle- and upper-class persons who practice it, it is much more difficult, perhaps even impossible, to obtain similar measurements of traditional forms of ritual healing with their ecstatic trances, bloody sacrifices, and oracular diagnoses (though see Snodgrass et al. 2017a and 2017b.). To find out what people actually do when they suffer "mental illness" outside the laboratory or clinic, one would have to observe them, rather than subjecting them to artificial experimental environments. In other words, one would have to proceed like an ethnographer rather than an experimental psychologist. However, such radically empirical methods are unfamiliar or unacceptable for most researchers. Moreover, the health authorities are more likely to criminalise such activities than to investigate them (Sood 2016). The best known example from South Asia was the so-called "Erwadi tragedy" of 2001, where pilgrims chained to trees and other structures near a South Indian Sufi shrine famous for mental healing perished in a fire, resulting in a series of attempts to criminalise ritual and religious healing throughout India. There is no doubt that the fire was a terrible tragedy, and that it pointed to the need for fire safety regulations in such places. But there have been tragic fires in mental hospitals, too (Barry and Kramer 2013) and these have not led to calls for the state to criminalise them.

As many of the articles in this volume make clear, South Asians do in fact have access to a variety of resources for maintaining or improving their mental health. In this sense there is not so much a "treatment gap" as there is a "treatment difference", and it may even be that the existence of a great variety of non-medical forms of therapy contributes to a high level of mental health for regions outside of Europe and North America. Relevant here are a series of robust, "gold standard" epidemiological studies by the World Health Organization, which have consistently shown that Nigerians and Indians have better rates of recovery from severe mental illness than Europeans and Americans (Hopper and Wanderling 2000; Sartorius et al., 1986). Although there is continuing debate about what these studies really show, one persuasive view is that their overarching lesson is about the importance of social bonds for recovery (Jablensky and Sartorius 2008).[8]

Although we have, in this introduction, questioned the universality of the disease categories focused upon by this well-known series of studies, still, the results give us pause. They document a markedly higher reduction of psychiatric symptoms and mental suffering in regions where psychiatry is difficult to access, than in regions where it is readily available, and this suggests that psychiatry is not necessarily the key to relieving mental disorders. At the very least it would make sense, as Halliburton (2016) argues, for those in the MGMH to first ask what they might learn from non-Europeans' approaches to mental health before rushing in with psychiatry, pharmaceuticals, and other exogenous therapies in order to "save" them. But because of the presumed universality and superiority of biomedical psychiatry, this is simply not done. Perhaps the Nigerians' and Indians' higher recovery rates have partly to do with the "treatment difference"; that is, with the fact that they live in medically plural societies, where there are numerous alternatives to psychiatry with its drug-based therapy. Unfortunately, such a hypothesis cannot be tested, since the studies did not control for which therapies were used: Some test subjects used biomedicine, others used traditional healing, still others used nothing. Nevertheless, it strikes us as highly problematic that rather than focusing on why the non-Europeans' scores are so high, the MGMH seeks instead to provide them with an exogenous disciplines – psychiatry with its armoury of drugs, and a form of counselling loosely based on cognitive behavioural therapy – both of which originate in a region with a comparatively poor record for recovery from severe mental illness.

In order to understand and evaluate non-medical techniques for promoting mental health, health professionals would have to take them seriously. They would have to *learn from* local people rather than simply indoctrinating them. But in practice, such traditions are of little or no interest to most

8   Thanks to Laurence Kirmayer for pointing this out in a personal communication.

health researchers, who regard them as unscientific and even dangerous. Neither can they be "seen" by Ministries of Health, which are not interested in them and therefore collect little or no information about them.[9] And although they are not entirely absent from the MGMH literature, they are still difficult to find there, and are certainly subordinated to psychiatry. As a result, we think it is fair to say that the MGMH necessarily rejects pluralism – the deliberate encouraging of a variety of models and approaches – with respect to mental health and illness. Instead, it carries forward what Mills (2014) calls the neocolonial "psychiatrization of the majority world" – what others criticise as a top-down, imperial project exporting Western illness categories and treatments that would ultimately replace diverse cultural environments for interpreting mental health (Watters 2010; Summerfield 2013; Mills and Fernando 2014).

And what, precisely, might be learned from these local traditions? Some of the essays in this volume provide answers to this question. Lang discusses a form of psychiatry based on Ayurveda, India's dominant indigenous medical system (cf. Halliburton 2009; Langford 2002). Ayurvedic psychiatry is a highly dynamic field that draws upon a truly ancient tradition based on classic texts, which it combines with vernacular practices and globalised psychiatric knowledge so as to know and treat distressed embodied minds. Halliburton shows how South Indian psychiatric hospitals and rehabilitation centres used "love" to aid the healing process, Mukherjee shows how the MGHM is as blind to forms of group possession as it is to any forms of non-individualised suffering. Sax and Mukherjee each write about Muslim religious healing of mental suffering, which is widespread in Europe as well as South Asia (Sax 2013). Elsewhere, Ecks (2013) has explored how, in India, non-biomedical forms of healing like Ayurveda and homeopathy are redefining notions of what it means to be mentally ill, and shown how Indian psychiatrists, finding themselves in an extremely pluralistic context, adapt their prescribing practices to local expectations. Critics suggest that global mental health discourses and initiatives have conceptualised "community" much too narrowly, merely as a method of service delivery, and that a subtler conception might help to employ resources more effectively (Campbell and Burgess 2012; Das and Rao 2012). In the same vein, Jansen et al. "propose that 'community' should be promoted as a means of harnessing collective strengths and resources to help promote mental well-being" (2015, 1). Rather than conceiving of communities as targets of psychiatric interventions, it

---

9   Cf. Ecks and Basu's 2014 discussion of "strategic ignorance" in relation to GMH strategies of "task-shifting".

might be better to think of "community" whether local, transnational or digital as another aspect of the "treatment difference"; that is, as a mental health resource, providing active participants in the therapeutic process.

A final problematic assumption is suggested by the very name of the Movement for Global Mental Health, which implicitly distinguishes mental from physical health. This dualism of mind and body may be simplistic, but it is certainly pervasive, having been institutionalised in the world's medical schools and health ministries. It is true that many MGMH programmes seek to resist this distinction by arguing that mental health is part of general health and well-being and by locating mental health treatment within primary health care, and it is also true that the comorbidity (i.e. the close relationship) of psychiatric and somatic symptoms is well known to mental health care workers everywhere. But none of these assumptions and practices implies a redefinition of the relation between mind and body, only a re-administration of it. And this should not surprise us, since there does seem to be something universal about the distinction between mind and body. Indeed, we are suspicious of the oft-repeated assertion that this "dualism" is peculiarly Western, or that it is not found in Asian or other non-Western medical systems. On the contrary, all the South Asian medical systems with which we are familiar distinguish between a locus of thought and consciousness on the one hand, and the human body on the other (Langford 2002; Lang this volume). But such distinctions are made differently in the various systems, and are never precisely parallel to those found in modern psychiatry and medicine, and in our view, any therapeutic regime should at least be aware of the differences among them. Ideally, each system should be willing to learn from the other. Perhaps a greater awareness of the ways that physical injury or disease can lead to mental disorder (and vice versa) would be useful for local healers, and one wonders whether a serious investigation of non-psychiatric therapies might fruitfully lead us away from the contemporary reduction of mind to brain.

In sum, the MGMH has in recent years begun to question some of its earlier assumptions that we regard as highly problematic; for example, that mental illness is better explained in terms of neurology than as a result of social factors like poverty, prejudice, stigma, pressures of consumerism, addiction, family breakdown, relationship difficulties, unemployment, etc.; and that the default modality of treatment is the administration of psychopharmaceuticals. In recent publications, both of these assumptions have been revised, and we heartily applaud these refinements and improvements. Nevertheless, a significant number of problematic assumptions continue to inform the agenda of the MGMH: that the paradigms of biomedical psychiatry are universally true, and unquestionably superior to those of non-biomedical systems; that non-biomedical resources for mental health are scarcely worth being investigated; and that the world faces an "epidemic" of "mental illness". We do not claim that all of these assumptions are false; we do however think that it is important to acknowledge their existence, and to note how profoundly they influence the agenda of the MGMH.

Unacknowledged Interests

In addition to these unexamined assumptions, the MGMH may well be unduly influenced by a number of unacknowledged interests. One of these is the pharmaceutical industry. Harrington for example argues that the dominance of biological psychiatry has to do with the fact that by the late 1980s, "a critical mass of clinicians and researchers had aligned their professional interests with the commercial interests of the pharmaceutical industry" (2019, 249). A forerunner program of the MGMH, the Nations for Mental Health, was partly funded by two large pharmaceutical companies (World Health Organization 2002). Earlier agendas of the MGMH (e.g. Patel et al. 2011) focused much more heavily on the use of psychopharmaceuticals. Such pharmaceuticalisation creates markets for the pharmaceutical industry, either by depoliticising and silencing social inequality, marginalisation, and suffering or by providing an idiom of critique and a powerful tool for mobilising care and social inclusion (Kitanaka 2012; Lang 2019). But not only are funding and financing streams difficult to track (cf. Erikson 2015); the pharma industry's interests are rather ambiguous and difficult to characterise. "Big Pharma" has been unable to develop any new, reliable drugs for quite some time (Dumit 2018; Harrington 2019). Perhaps this has something to do with the fact that the social environment really does play an important role in the aetiology of what is called "mental illness", which cannot be reduced to "brain disease". Kirmayer and Gold ask if such research has been largely unsuccessful because of its valorisation of the brain and with it the creation of a psychiatric discipline that is both "mindless and uncultured" (2012, 308). In India the "Big Pharma" companies' patents have mostly expired, and the market for psychopharmaceuticals is predominantly generic, so that such companies doesn't have much of an interest in them. The result is that nowadays it is the smaller regional companies that push psychopharmaceuticals, often by means of what is called "outreach" or "patient education" (Ecks 2018; cf. Applebaum 2015).

Psychiatric training in India overemphasises the role of psychopharmaceuticals, so that pharmaceutical representatives have an enormous influence on South Asian doctors' prescribing patterns. Moreover, to the extent that psychopharmaceutical interventions moderate the symptoms of mental disorders, they are truly needed by poor people in South Asia and elsewhere, who may well respond quite positively to the "psychopharmaceuticalisation" of their mental health. The reason is simple: if the poorest don't work, then they don't eat (and nor do their children). That is why drugs that relieve their symptoms, thus allowing them to work, are likely to be enthusiastically received, even if the duration and dosage of those drugs is observed only in the breach (Han 2012; Barua and Pandav 2011; Ecks and Basu 2014). This is one of the many ways in which the worldwide system of consumer capitalism creates its modern subjects.

Another way involves the use of digital technology for diagnosis and treatment. Despite the growing literature pointing to the deleterious effects of modern communications technology on mental health, the members of the Lancet commission on global mental health and sustainable development (Fairburn and Patel 2016; Patel et al. 2018) have an unbridled enthusiasm for it. Traditional healing methods may be ignored by the MGMH, but there is an exaggerated faith in the capacity of technological "fixes" to address mental health problems. Such fixes are much more business-friendly than social interventions, and the medicalisation of mental health promoted by the MGMH serves the interests of those manufacturing software for mental health apps, tablets and mobile phones for health workers etc. Despite our intuition that the physical presence of the therapist is important for mental health therapy, and the growing evidence that social media is strongly associated with mental pathology (Hunt et al. 2018; Kross et al. 2013; Steers et al. 2014; Twenge et al. 2017), the MGMH seeks (at least partly) to abolish the former and replace it with the latter:

> The nonspecialist healthcare provider should ideally work within a collaborative care framework with access to a specialist provider who can be remotely located, participates in training, oversees quality, and provides guidance or referral options for complex clinical presentations [...] Several innovative strategies can facilitate dissemination of psychosocial therapies. First, a major bottleneck to task sharing is the reliance on traditional facetoface methods for training and on experts for supervision. These barriers are being addressed through online training. [...] Technology applications include mobile and online programmes for illness self-management and relapse prevention, SMS text messaging for promoting

medication and treatment adherence, and smartphone applications for tracking and monitoring symptoms (e.g., moodgym, Living Life, and 7 cups). Opportunities could also be available to track highrisk situations with wearable sensors or smartphonebased location, time, or activity data and to send realtime alerts to patients or designated caregivers. Additionally, social media offers peertopeer networking combined with individually tailored therapeutic interventions. Telepsychiatry applications such as online videoconferencing can allow patients to connect with mental health providers for clinical consultations for diagnosis, followup care, or longterm support. Websites and mobile applications can also be used to deliver evidencebased treatments (e.g., those to reduce alcohol consumption, or cognitive behavioural therapies) [...] (Patel et al. 2018, 22)

MGMH proponents advocate the use of digital technologies as technical fixes to manage the presumed gaps in training, diagnosing, treating and governing mental health. Here they are in line not only with the emphasis on technological fixes in global health more generally (Li 2011; Geissler 2013) but also with the increasingly use of online technologies and techniques for managing mental distress (Fullagar et al. 2017; Lupton 2017; Ruckenstein and Schüll 2017) that paradoxically decentre the hegemony of the psychiatrist by expanding the psy-ing gaze beyond the clinic. Not only must the ontological assumptions of the suffering subjects be brought into line with those of the psychiatrists and psychologists or their digital proxy, they must also be trained to conform to a modern, neoliberal and consumerist model of rational agency that makes extensive use of commercially-available technology. And all of this takes place against the background of the psy-experts with their disciplinary powers as agents of the state. Why else would these kinds of consumer-led initiatives be praised as "effective under some circumstances in reducing compulsory admission to psychiatric hospital" (Patel et al. 2018, 22)?

Harmful Consequences

In addition to the unexamined assumptions discussed above, and along with the danger of serving unacknowledged interests, we also think that the implementation of the agenda of the MGMH may run the risk of causing harm.

In its earlier versions (e.g. Patel and Prince 2012) the MGMH assumed that the aetiology of mental disorders could best be accounted for by theories of biological causation, so that psychopharmaceuticals were the "default" mode treatment. These paired assumptions allowed those in the MGMH to make two – not necessarily consistent – claims at once. First of all, they could make a moral case for the introduction of pharmaceuticals, claiming that sceptics effectively block the human rights of those suffering from mental disorders. Second, they could at the same time prevent a serious discussion of the moral and ethical problems faced by psychiatry. There are several prominent examples of how such rhetoric was employed, perhaps the most notorious being the photograph accompanying an article by Insel, Patel, and other leading advocates of GMH in the 7 July 2011 issue of *Nature* magazine, entitled "Grand Challenges in Global Mental Health". The photo is of a small girl chained to a tree, and this image is meant to represent the traditional healing of mental disorders, as if this had to do primarily with repression rather than the relief of suffering. But what about the well-known concept of chemical incarceration (Fabris 2011)? Is a heavily sedated patient in a psychiatric ward more free than the pilgrim Sax met at the healing shrine of Balaji in north India, who had to walk slowly because of the chains on his feet, which he said were there "for his own safety"? What about the reported violations of human rights in Indian mental hospitals (National Human Rights Commission 2012)? Perhaps most disturbing are the recurring tropes used to justify certain types of human rights violations by psychiatrists in India, for example, the idea that Indians, like people from the Global South generally, are childlike and need the patronizing care of the psychiatrist. Nandy calls this "a homology between childhood and the state of being colonized" (ibid., 97). The final article in this volume, by "Anonymous", gives a highly personal account of such an experience from the point of view of a victim.

By defining mental disorders as forms of brain disease, these earlier discussions placed neuropsychological models at the centre of the paradigm, and relegated discussion of the sociocultural causation of mental disorders to second place. This had the effect of "depoliticising" mental suffering by failing to address various forms of social structural inequality and violence that contribute to it. One glaring example is farmers' suicides in India. Despite clear evidence that the "epidemic" of farmer suicides is caused by political economic factors, the Indian state looked frantically for genetic causes (Arya 2007 cited in Aggarwal 2008, 291; Mills 2014, 37), thus managing to avoid grappling with the difficult political issues involved. And although many psychiatric studies acknowledge the role of political economic factors in farmer suicides, they tend to limit the role of psychiatry to the mitigation of the resulting suffering, not the elimination of its causes, for example by focusing on restricting the availability of pesticides (a common means of suicide) rather than confronting the multinational companies whose agricultural policies led to the suicides in the first place. Such a depoliticisation of mental illness has happened elsewhere as well: Scheper-Hughes for example showed how hunger in one region of Brazil "became so normalized that it was no longer a sign of nutritional deprivation but a mental pathology – 'del deliriumirio de foe', hunger madness – to be managed by tranquilizers and sleeping pills imported from the United States" (1992, 41). Here too, the essay by "Anonymous" seeks to show how contemporary psychiatry in India is deeply gendered, with women risking the imputation of mental illness if they fail to conform to the roles expected of them.

Leading figures in the MGHM have, however, significantly revised this approach in more recent discussions of the aetiology of mental disorders. Exemplary are the discussion of the social determinants of depression by Patel et al. (2009) and Patel and Thornicroft (2009), and of the "social determinants of mental health" found in Patel et al. 2018, which includes a lengthy and persuasive section on how poverty, gender inequality, forms of racism and other social factors contribute to mental illness. Once again, we enthusiastically support this acknowledgement of the complexity of causal factors in the arising of mental suffering, which is not only consistent with the best scientific evidence, but also helps to relocate the causes of mental illness where they belong: in the interplay between "biology" and "society".

"Scaling Up"

Like global health more generally, the MGMH promotes research on the effectiveness of its interventions, and this is linked to the "scalability" of its projects (Adams 2016). Testing interventions in randomised control trials (RCTs) and scaling up these "evidence-based" interventions in low-resource setting have been central activities for the MGMH since its beginnings. In 2009 for example, Patel, Goel, and Desai (2009) called for "[s]caling up services for mental and neurological disorders in low-resource settings." The authors acknowledged several times that there was little evidence for the efficacy of Western psychotherapy at the scale of the Indian village where they were working, and particularly with the "technically simple and affordable treatments delivered by non-specialist health workers" that they advocated. They also accepted "the need for evidence to assess the impact of scaled-up interventions." But this did not lead them to re-think their programme; instead, they simply pushed ahead with a plan to create a large number of parallel units with identical operative assumptions, so that these could be "scaled up" when necessary, in the form of "a basic, evidence-based package of services for core mental disorders." In the meantime, numerous research projects by NGOs that are part of the MGMH network have (no surprise here!) been able to generate the required evidence based on randomised trials for the claimed efficacy of different kinds of psychosocial and other interventions that the MGMH hopes to "scale up" (e.g. Dias et al. 2019; Patel et al. 2010). Proponents of the MGMH attempt to combine the standardisation inherent in attempts to "scale up" with localisation by means of what Bemme (2019) calls "contingent universals" – that is, processes of constant learning and change in local contexts. But we contend that even if they do manage some sort of combination of this kind, their understanding of local context is limited and includes neither larger structural processes nor already existing forms of treatment and care.

Plans to "scale up" global mental health services have more recently been linked to the Sustainable Development Goals agenda: Patel et al. write that their goal "is to reframe global mental health within the paradigm of sustainable development" (2018, 4), and conclude their review by systematically linking mental health to each of the SDGs. At the end of the article they summarise their points: mental health is a global public good; the unique outcome of biological, environmental and developmental factors across the life course; a fundamental human right; and an essential part of health care requiring public and policy action, especially the scaling up of mental health assessment and treatment plans. All of this requires, so they argue, a comprehensive global monitoring system (ibid., 9).

Here lies yet another unforeseen, but potentially problematic, result of the MGMH agenda. As anthropologist Anna Tsing has pointed out,

> (s)calability is, indeed, a triumph of precision design, not just in computers but in business, development, the "conquest" of nature, and, more generally, world making. It is a form of design that has a long history of dividing winners and losers. Yet it disguises such divisions by blocking our ability to notice the heterogeneity of the world; by its design, scalability allows us to see only uniform blocks, ready for further expansion. (2012, 505)

Tsing is worried about "the exclusion of biological and cultural diversity from scalable designs" and she writes that:

> most modern science demands scalability, the ability to make one's research framework apply to greater scales without budging the frame

[...] Scalability is possible only if project elements do not form transformative relationships that might change the project as elements are added.
But transformative relationships are the medium for the emergence of
diversity. Scalability projects banish meaningful diversity, which is to
say, diversity that might change things. (ibid., 522).

"Scaling up" can only occur when the specifically creative aspects of social
life are deliberately ignored or defined as irrelevant. One might say that those
who promote scaling-up projects repress this creativity in order to empower
themselves. Tsing argues that the kind of knowledge produced at the macro
scale cannot see nonscalability, because of the constitutive scalability of its
own practices.[10] According to Tsing, the problems of diversity, and of living
together with others, require other modes of knowledge.

Perhaps this is also true of therapy for mental disorders. On the macro
scale, an assemblage of psychiatrists, universities, clinics, journals, hospitals,
experiments, and professional associations works to ensure that practices
relating to the diagnosis and treatment of mental disorders are standardised,
and that their efficacy is evaluated according to universal criteria, purified
of their social and historical context: a classic example of what Latour calls
"the work of purification". As is the case for global health more generally
(Reubi 2018), such activity tends to be regulated in terms of neoliberal
assumptions and managerial techniques (see e.g. Patel et al. 2018), which are
quite compatible with modern technology, re-education (replacing religious
paradigms with "scientific" ones), and comprehensive monitoring systems
to ensure compliance, but particularly unsuitable for traditional systems of
healing, whose efficacy has hardly been studied, but most probably lies in its
context-sensitivity, its cultural appropriateness, and its political economic
embeddedness (for example, traditional healers often refuse cash payment).

Meanwhile, at the "micro" end of the spectrum are thousands of isolated
traditions of ritual healing that attempt, through myriad techniques and a
veritable Babel of idioms, to re-integrate afflicted persons with their families,
communities, and cosmologies. They do so in terms of specific contexts,
which are, by definition, local and small scale. Most traditional healing is
what Tsing calls "nonscalable"; it resists the normalising practices of the
state and of biomedicine – and so it must, or else lose the very context-
sensitivity that defines it. The MGMH is blind to these local traditions
everywhere, not just in South Asia, and one of the purposes of this volume
is to remind us of this, while at the same time also suggesting that these

---

10   This is what Sax has referred to elsewhere (2014) as "structural blindness".

locally-embedded traditions may in some cases provide reasonable local alternatives to psychiatry with its predominantly psychopharmaceutical therapies, and its lay counselling based on models developed in Europe and North America.

For whatever reasons, schizophrenia, depression, and other common mental disorders are no longer limited to the industrialised, capitalist "West". Instead, they are increasingly global idioms in which people express their (and their family members') troubles, for which neuroscientists develop methods of measuring and testing, about which journalists write and report, and concerning which governments develop programmes and policies. The whole process is a perfect example of what Hacking (2007) calls the "looping effect", a kind of extra-linguistic iteration where a new disease is invented, research reconfirms its existence, people begin to receive the corresponding diagnoses, more research is done, papers published, and diagnoses made, until finally people have internalised an illness category to which they previously had no access.

Perhaps, with this volume, we can set in motion a few "loops" of our own, by suggesting that "mind" cannot be reduced to "brain", that the experience of mental health and illness is located in particular historical and cultural contexts, that effective therapies for mental suffering sometimes arise in such contexts, and that a truly pluralistic model of mental health care, in which many alternatives are available, is something worth pursuing.

Structure of the Book

In this book we have attempted to assemble a number of voices from South and Southeast Asia, each of which take a critical look at the MGMH. The volume's strength lies in its multivocality, with voices from anthropology, history, public health, psychiatry, and service users. Plurality is more important to the editors than doctrinal homogeneity, and we do not agree with every voice expressed in this volume. Following this introduction are two essays focusing on historical themes. In "Mental Ills for All: Genealogies of Global Mental Health", anthropologist Stefan Ecks writes about the recent History of the Movement for Global Mental Health and its three "pillars": economics, epidemiology, and the "scaling up" of mental health services. In "Schizoid Balinese? Anthropology's Double Bind: Radical Alterity and Its Consequences for Schizophrenia", anthropologist Annette Hornbacher reviews the many conceptual and empirical problems with the disease entity "schizophrenia", and also tells the story – unknown until now – of the influence of Gregory Bateson's joint fieldwork with Margaret Mead in Bali on his famous "Double Bind" theory of schizophrenic aetiology. The research was funded by the American "Committee for Research in Dementia Praecox" in the 1930s, and might be seen as one of the earliest forays in Global Mental Health. The second section of the book has three articles critiquing the Movement for Global Mental Health. In "Misdiagnosis: Global Mental Health, Social Determinants of Health and Beyond", psychiatrist Anindya Das and public health physician Mohan Rao use the "social determinants of health" approach to argue that the MGMH has taken insufficient account of economic and political realities of India, and that it embodies a thoroughly Western discourse that is not appropriate to India. In "Jinns and the Proletarian Mumin Subject: Exploring the Limits of Global Mental Health in Bangladesh", historian Projit Bihari Mukharji analyses cases of "mass possession" that illustrate the "ontopolitical confrontation between mental health professionals" on the one hand, and local models of explanation in relation to "fundamental assumptions regarding the nature of the suffering subject" on the other.

The third section of the book explores alternatives to modern psychiatry with its drug-based therapies, and challenges the MGMH's notion of a treatment gap. In "The House of Love and the Mental Hospital: Zones of Care and Recovery in South India", anthropologist Murphy Halliburton provides an inspiring ethnography of one particular clinic in South India, and discusses the "role of love and family involvement" in mental health care, suggesting that this local, enhanced version of psychiatry provides an alternative to conventional care. In "Ayurvedic Psychiatry and the Moral Physiology of Depression in Kerala", anthropologist Claudia Lang discusses in detail one of the many "highly dynamic indigenous medical fields addressing mental health problems" that are typically ignored by proponents of global mental health. She is however optimistic that such local forms of medical knowledge might still be included in MGMH's agenda, as recent publications (e.g. Patel et al. 2018) testify. In "Global Mental Therapy", anthropologist William Sax asks why it is that even though, worldwide and throughout history, rituals are the most common treatment for mental distress, they are nevertheless systematically ignored by MGMH. He also makes some tentative suggestions about how rituals "work" to address mental disorders. The book concludes with two separate Afterwords. In the first of these, Johannes Quack focuses on the themes of "love" and "justice" that appear throughout the volume, and shows that they address different, though related, concerns. He also urges the contributors to think more carefully about what they might learn from psychiatrists about mental health. In the second Afterword, "Anonymous" offers a poetic memoir of her treatment in a psychiatric institution in India. She recounts her efforts to make sense of her institutionalisation, and challenges the MGMH with a feminist critique of psychiatry.

References

Adams, Vincanne. 2016. *Metrics. What Counts in Global Health*, Durham: Duke University Press.

Aggarwal, Neal. 2008. "Editorial: Farmer Suicides in India: The Role of Psychiatry and Anthropology." *International Journal of Social Psychiatry* 54 (4): 291-92.

Alter, Joseph S. 2004. *Yoga in Modern India: The Body between Science and Philosophy*. Princeton: Princeton University Press.

Applebaum, Kalman. 2015. "Solving Global Mental Health As a Delivery Problem: Toward a Critical Epistemology of the Solution." In *Re-Visioning Psychiatry: Cultural Phenomenology, Critical Neuroscience, and Global Mental Health*, edited by Lawrence J. Kirmayer, Robert Lemelson, and Constance Cummings, 544-74. New York: Cambridge University Press.

Aragona, Massimiliano. 2015. "Rethinking Received Views on the History of Psychiatric Nosology: Minor Shifts, Major Continuities." In *Alternative Perspectives on Psychiatric Validation,* edited by Peter Zachar, Peter Drozdstoj St. Stoyanov, Massimiliano Aragona, and Assen Jablensky, 27-46. Oxford: Oxford University Press.

Arya, Shishir. 2007. "Government to Study DNA Links to Suicides." *The Times of India*, 27 September 2007.

Banerjee, Madhulika. 2009. *Power, Knowledge, Medicine. Ayurvedic Pharmaceuticals at Home and in the World*. Hyderabad: Orient BlackSwan.

Barua, Nupur, and Chandrakant S. Pandav. 2011. "The Allure of the Private Practitioner: Is This the Only Alternative for the Urban Poor in India?" *Indian Journal of Public Health* 55 (2): 107-114.

Barry, Ellen, and Andrew E. Kramer. 2013. "Fire in Russian Psychiatric Hospital That Killed 38 Stirs Anger Over State's Neglect." *New York Times*, 26 April 2013.

Bemme, Doerte. 2019. "Finding 'What Works': Theory of Change, Contingent Universals, and Virtuous Failure in Global Mental Health. Culture, Medicine and Psychiatry." *Cultural Medical Psychiatry* 43 (4): 574-95.

Bemme, Doerte, and Nicole A. D'Souza. 2014. "Global Mental Health and Its Discontents: An Inquiry into the Making of Global and Local Scale." *Transcultural Psychiatry* 51 (6): 850-74.

Campbell, Cathrine, and Rochelle Burgess. 2012. "The Role of Communities in Advancing the Goals of the Movement for Global Mental Health." *Transcultural Psychiatry* 49 (3-4): 379-95.

Canguilhem, George. 1991. *The Normal and the Pathological*. New York: Zone Books.

Chisholm, Dan, Alan J. Flisher, Crick Lund, Vikram Patel, Shekhar Saxena, Graham Thornicroft, and Mark Tomlinson [Lancet Global Mental Health Group]. 2007. "Scale Up Services for Mental Disorders: A Call for Action." *Lancet* 370 (9594): 1241-52.

Das, Anindya, and Mohan Rao. 2012. "Universal Mental Health: Re-evaluating the Call for Global Mental Health." *Critical Public Health* 22 (4): 383-89.

Desjarlais, Robert, Leon Eisenberg, Byron Good, and Arthur Kleinman. 1995. *World Mental Health: Problems and Priorities in Low-Income Countries*. Oxford: Oxford University Press.

Dias, Amit, Frederic Azariah, Stewart J. Anderson, Miriam Sequeira, Alex Cohen, Jennifer Q. Morse, Pim Cuijpers, Vikram Patel, and Charles F. Reynold. 2019. "Effect of a Lay Counselor Intervention on Prevention of Major Depression in Older Adults Living in Low- and Middle-Income Countries. A Randomized Clinical Trial." *Jama Psychiatry* 76 (1): 13-20.

Dumit, Joseph. 2018. "The Infernal Alternatives of Corporate Pharmaceutical Research: Abandoning Psychiatry." *Medical Anthropology* 37(1): 59-74.

Ecks, Stefan. 2013. *Eating Drugs. Psychopharmaceutical Pluralism in South Asia*. New York and London: New York University Press.

—. 2016. "Commentary: Ethnographic Critiques of Global Mental Health." *Transcultural Psychiatry* 53 (6): 804-08.

Ecks, Stefan, and Soumita Basu. 2014. "'We Always Live in Fear': Antidepressant Prescriptions by Unlicensed Doctors in India." *Culture, Medicine, and Psychiatry* 38 (2): 197-216.

Ecks, Stefan. 2018. "Biocommensurations." *Anthropology News* 59 (3): 162-165.

Erikson, Susan. 2015. "Secrets from Whom? Following the Money in Global Health Finance." *Current Anthropology* 56 (12): S306-S316.

Fabris, Erick. 2011. *Tranquil Prisons: Chemical Incarceration under Community Treatment Orders*. Toronto: University of Toronto Press.

Fairburn, Christopher G., and Vikram Patel. 2016. "The Impact of Digital Technology on Psychological Treatments and Their Dissemination." *Behaviour Research and Therapy* 88:19-25.

Fullagar, Christine, Emma Rich, Jessica Francombe-Webb, and Antonio Maturo. 2017. "Digital Ecologies of Youth Mental Health: Apps, Therapeutic Publics and Pedagogy as Affective Arrangements." *Social Sciences* 6 (4): 135.

Geissler, Paul W. 2013. "Public Secrets in Public Health: Knowing Not to Know While Making Scientific Knowledge." *American Ethnologist* 40 (1): 13-34.

Hacking, Ian. 2002. "Making up People." In *Historical Ontology*, Chapter 2. Cambridge: Harvard University Press.

—. 2007. "Kinds of People. Moving Targets." *Proceedings of the British Academy* 151:285-318.

—. 2013. "Lost in the Forest." Review of *DSM-5: Diagnostic and Statistical Manual of Mental Disorders, Fifth Edition*, by the American Psychiatric Association. *London Review of Books* 35 (15): 7-8.

Halliburton, Murphy. 2009. *Mudpacks & Prozac. Experiencing Ayurvedic, Biomedical & Religious Healing*. Walnut Creek, CA: Left Coast Press.

—. 2016. "Snehaveedu: A Zone of Care and Recovery in South India." Paper presented at the AROGYAM Conference on Anthropology and Global Health. Attard, Malta, December 2016.

Han, Clara. 2012. *Life in Debt: Times of Care and Violence in Neoliberal Chile*. Berkeley and Los Angeles: University of California Press.

Harrington, Anne. 2019. *Mind Fixers: Psychiatry's Troubled Search for the Biology of Mental Illness*. New York; London: W. W. Norton and Company.

Hopper, Kim, and Joseph Wanderling. 2000. "Revisiting the Developed versus Developing Country Distinction in Course and Outcome in Schizophrenia: Results from Isos, the Who Collaborative Followup Project." *Schizophrenia Bulletin* 26 (4): 835-46.

Horton, Richard. 2007. "Launching a New Movement for Mental Health." *The Lancet* 370 (9590): 806.

Hunt, Melissa G., Rachel Marx, Courtney Lipson, and Jordyn Young. 2018. "No More FOMO: Limiting Social Media Decreases Loneliness and Depression." *Journal of Social and Clinical Psychology* 37 (10): 751-68.

Insel, Thomas R. 2014. "The NIMH Research Domain Criteria (RDoC) Project: Precision Medicine for Psychiatry." *American Journal of Psychiatry* 171 (4): 395-97.

Jablensky, Assen, and Norman Sartorius. 2008. "What Did the Who Studies Really Find?" *Schizophrenia Bulletin* 34 (2): 253-55.

Jablensky, Assen. 2016. "Psychiatric Classifications: Validity and Utility." *World Psychiatry* 15 (1): 26-31. *PMC*. Web. Accessed 20 May 2018.

Jansen, Stefan, Ross White, Jemma Hogwood, Angela Jansen, Darius Gishoma, Donatilla Mukamana, and Annemiek Richters. 2015. "The 'Treatment Gap' in Global Mental Health Reconsidered: Sociotherapy for Collective Trauma in Rwanda." *European Journal of Psychotraumatology* 6 (1): 28706.

Kendler, Kenneth S. 2013. "What Psychiatric Genetics Has Taught Us about the Nature of Psychiatric Illness and What Is Left to Learn." *Molecular Psychiatry* 18: 1058-66.

Kirmayer, Laurence J. 1987. "Languages of Suffering Healing: Alexithymia as a Social and Cultural Process." *Transcultural Psychiatric Research Review* 24 (2):119-36.

Kirmayer, Laurence, and Ian J. Gold. 2011. "Re-Socializing Psychiatry." In *Critical Neuroscience: A Handbook of the Social and Cultural Contexts of Neuroscience*, edited by Suparna Choudhury, and Jan Slaby, 307-30. Oxford, UK: Wiley-Blackwell.

Kross, Ethan, Phillippe Verduyn, Emre Demiralp, Jiyoung Park, David Seungjae Lee, Natalie Lin, Holly Shablack, John Jonides, and Oscar Ybarra. 2013. "Facebook

Use Predicts Declines in Subjective Well-Being in Young Adults." *PLoS One* 8 (8): e69841. https://doi.org/10.1371/journal.pone.0069841.

Kutchins, Herb, and Stuart A. Kirk. 2003. *Making Us Crazy*. New York: Simon and Schuster.

Laderman, Carol. 1993. *Taming the Wind of Desire: Psychology, Medicine, and Aesthetics in Malay Shamanistic Performance*. Berkeley: University of California Press.

Lang, Claudia. 2019. "Inspecting Mental Health: Depression, Surveillance and Care in Kerala, South India." *Culture, Medicine and Psychiatry* 43:596-612.

Langford, Jean M. 2002. *Fluent Bodies. Ayurvedic Remedies for Postcolonial Imbalance*. Durham: Duke University Press.

Li, Tania Murray. 2011. *Adventures in Aidland: The Anthropology of Professionals in International Development*. New York and Oxford: Berghahn.

Li, Veronica. 2014. "The Rise, Critique and Persistence of the DALY in Global Health." *The Journal of Global Health*, 1 April 2014.

Lovell, Anne. 2014. "The World Health Organization and the Contested Beginnings of Psychiatric Epidemiology as an International Discipline: One Rope, Many Strands." *International Journal of Epidemiology* 43 (suppl. 1): i6-i18.

Lovell, Anne, Ursula Read, and Claudia Lang. 2019. "Genealogies and Anthropologies of Global Mental Health." *Culture, Medicine & Psychiatry* 43:519-47.

Lupton, Deborah. 2017. *Digital Health: Critical Approaches to Health*. London: Routledge.

Mahajan, Manjari. 2019. "The IHME in the Shifting Landscape of Global Health Metrics." *Global Health Policy* 10 (suppl. 1): 110-20.

Mills, China. 2014. *Decolonizing Global Mental Health: The Psychiatrization of the Majority World*. Hove and New York: Routledge.

Mills, China, and Suman Fernando. 2014. "Globalising Mental Health or Pathologising the Global South? Mapping the Ethics, Theory and Practice of Global Mental Health." *Disability and the Global South* 1 (2): 188-202.

Moncrieff, Joanna. 2008. *The Myth of the Chemical Cure: A Critique of Psychiatric Drug Treatment*. London: Palgrave Macmillan.

Murray, Christopher J., and Alan D. Lopez. 1996. *Global Burden of Disease. Volume 1*. Cambridge, MA: Harvard University Press.

National Human Rights Commission. 2012. *Care and Treatment in Mental Health Institutions*. New Delhi.

Patel, Vikram, and Graham Thornicroft. 2009. "Packages of Care for Mental, Neurological, and Substance Use Disorders in Low- and Middle-income Countries: PLoS Medicine Series." *PLoS Medicine* 6 (10).

Patel, Vikram, Gregory Simon, Neerja Chowdhary, Sylvia Kaaya, and Ricardo Araya. 2009. "Packages of Care for Depression in Low- and Middle-income Countries." *PLoS Medicine* 6 (10).

Patel, Vikram, Digvijay Singh Goel, and Desai, Rajnanda. 2009. "Scaling up Services for Mental and Neurological Disorders in Low-Resource Settings." *International Health* 1 (1): 37-44.

Patel, Vikram, Helen A. Weiss, Neerja Chowdhary, Smita Naik, Sulochana Pednekar, Sudipto Chatterjee, Mary J. De Silva, et al. 2010. "Effectiveness of an Intervention Led by Lay Health Counsellors for Depressive and Anxiety Disorders in Primary Care in GOA, India (MANAS): A Cluster Randomised Controlled Trial." *The Lancet* 376 (9758): 2086-95.

Patel, Vikram, and Martin Prince. 2010. "Global Mental Health: A New Global Health Field Comes of Age." *Journal of the American Medical Association* 303 (19): 1976-77.

Patel, Vikram, Pamela Y. Collins, John Copeland, Ritsuko Kakuma, Sylvester Katontoka, Jagannath Lamichhane, Smita Naik, and Sarah Skeen. 2011. "The Movement for Global Mental Health." *The British Journal of Psychiatry* 198 (2): 88-90. http://doi.org/10.1192/bjp.bp.109.074518.

Patel, Vikram, Shekhar Saxena, Crick Lund, Graham Thornicroft, Florence Baingana, Paul Bolton, Dan Chisholm, Pamela Y. Collins, et al. 2018. "The Lancet Commission on Global Mental Health and Sustainable Development." *The Lancet* 392 (10157): 1553-98.

Quack, Johannes, and William S. Sax. 2010. "Introduction: The Efficacy of Rituals." *The Journal of Ritual Studies* 24 (1): 5-12.

Reubi, David. 2018. "Epidemiological accountability: philanthropists, global health and the audit of saving lives." *Economy and Society* 47 (1): 83-110.

Ruckenstein, Minna, and Natasha Dow Schüll. 2017. "The Datafication of Health." *Annual Review of Anthropology* 46: 261-278.

Sartorius, Norman, Assen Jablensky, Ailsa Korten, G. Ernberg, M. Anker, J. E. Cooper, and R. Day. 1986. "Early Manifestations and First-Contact Incidence of Schizophrenia in Different Cultures: A Preliminary Report on the Initial Evaluation Phase of the WHO Collaborative Study on Determinants of Outcome of Severe Mental Disorders." *Psychological Medicine* 16 (4): 909-28.

Sax, William S. 2010. "Ritual and the Problem of Efficacy." In The Problem of Ritual Efficacy, edited by Johannes Quack, William Sax and Jan Weinhold. New York: Oxford University Press, pp. 3-16

—. 2013. "The Reality of 21st Century Islamic Healing – an Interview with a Muslim Healer. *Curare* 36 (3): 168-71.

—. 2014. "Ritual Healing and Mental Health in India." *Transcultural Psychiatry* 51 (3): 829-49.

—. 2015. "The Law of Possession: Ritual, Healing, and the Secular State." In *The Law of Possession: Ritual, Healing, and the Secular State, edited by William S. Sax and Helene Basu*, pp. 1-27. Oxford: Oxford University Press.

Scheper-Hughes, Nancy. 1992. *Death Without Weeping: The Violence of Everyday Life in Brazil*. Berkeley: University of California Press.

Snodgrass, Jeffrey G., David E. Most, and Chakrapani Upadhyay. 2017a. "Religious Ritual Is Good Medicine for Indigenous Indian Conservation Refugees: Implications for Global Mental Health." *Current Anthropology* 58 (2): 257-284.

Snodgrass, Jeffrey G., David E Most, Chakrapani Upadhyay, Ann Grodzins Gold, Devon Hinton, Martin Lang, Richard Sosis, et al. 2017b. "A Ritual Therapeutics Paradigm Requires Better Specification of Causal Pathways: Implications for Global Mental Health." *Current Anthropology* 58 (2).

Sood, Anubha. 2016. "The Global Mental Health Movement and Its Impact on Traditional Healing in India: A Case Study of the Balaji Temple in Rajasthan." *Transcultural Psychiatry* 53 (6): 766-82.

Steers, Mai-Ly N., Robert E. Wickham, and Linda K. Acitelli. 2014. "Seeing Everyone Else's High-Light Reels: How Facebook Usage Is Linked to Depressive Symptoms." *Journal of Social and Clinical Psychology* 33 (8): 701-31. https://doi.org/10.1521/jscp.2014.33.8.701.

Summerfield, Derek. 2013. "'Global Mental Health' Is an Oxymoron and Medical Imperialism." *British Medical Journal* 346:f3509.

Tambiah, Stanley J. 1990. *Magic, Science and Religion and the Scope of Rationality*. Cambridge: Cambridge University Press.

Tsing, Anna. 2012. "On Nonscalability: The Living World Is Not Amenable to Precision-Nested Scales." *Common Knowledge* 18 (3): 505-24.

Twenge, Jean M., Thomas E. Joiner, Megan L. Rogers, and Gabrielle N. Martin. 2017. "Increases in Depressive Symptoms, Suicide-Related Outcomes, and Suicide Rates among U.S. Adolescents after 2010 and Links to Increased New Media Screen Time." *Clinical Psychological Science* 6: 3-17.

Watters, Ethan. 2010. *Crazy like Us: The Globalization of the American Psyche*. New York: Simon and Schuster.

Wittgenstein, Ludwig. 1975. *Philosophical Remarks*. Chicago: University of Chicago Press.

World Health Organization. 2001. *World Health Report 2001. Mental Health: New Understanding, New Hope*. Geneva: WHO.

—. 2002. *Nations for Mental Health. Final Report*. Geneva: WHO.

Wu, Harry Yi-Jui (in press). *Folie a Million. Mental Disorders in the Age of World Citizenship, Experts and Technology*.

Zachar, Peter 2012. "Progress and Calibration of Scientific Constructs: The Role of Comparative Validity." In *Philosophical Issues in Psychiatry II: Nosology*, edited by Kenneth S. Kendler, and Josef Parnas, 21-34. Oxford: Oxford University Press.

About the Authors

WILLIAM S. ("BO") SAX studied at Banaras Hindu University, the University of Wisconsin, and the University of Washington (Seattle), and the University of Chicago, where he earned his PhD in Anthropology in 1987. From 1987 to 1989 he was lecturer in Anthropology at Harvard University, and post-doctoral fellow in the Harvard Academy. After that, he taught Hinduism in the Department of Philosophy and Religious studies at the University of Canterbury in Christchurch, New Zealand, for eleven years. In 2000 he took up the Chair of Anthropology at the South Asia Institute in Heidelberg. He has published extensively on pilgrimage, gender, theatre, aesthetics, ritual healing, and medical anthropology. His major works (all published by Oxford University Press, New York) include *Mountain Goddess: Gender and Politics in a Central Himalayan Pilgrimage* (1991); *The Gods at Play: Lila in South Asia* (1995); *Dancing the Self: Personhood and Performance in the Pandav Lila of Garhwal* (2002); *God of Justice: Ritual Healing and Social Justice in the Central Himalayas* (2008); *The Problem of Ritual Efficacy* (with Johannes Quack and Jan Weinhold, 2010); and *The Law of Possession: Ritual, Healing, and the Secular State* (with Heléne Basu, 2015). He is currently working on a book about archaic polities in the Western Himalayas, tentatively entitled *In the Valley of the Kauravas: From Subject to Citizen in the Western Himalayas*. His 1991 book *Mountain Goddess* has been translated into Hindi under the title *Himalaya ki Nanda Devi* (Dehra Dun: Wimsar).

CLAUDIA LANG is an associate professor (Heisenberg) of anthropology at University of Leipzig and research partner at the Max-Planck-Institute of Anthropology in Halle. Before, she was a postdoc at the ERC project "GLOBHELATH: From International Public Health to Global Health" in Paris, France. She works on the anthropology of health in India and has published on various topics, including traditional medicine, mental health, psychiatry, religion and ritual, health governance, and subjectivities. She is currently working on the digitization and proliferation of mental health and global psy in India's megacities, and on memories, traces, and genealogies of primary health care in Kerala. Her most recent publications include *Depression in Kerala: Ayurveda and Mental Health Care in India's 21st century* (2018) and a co-edited special issue of *Culture, Medicine and Psychiatry*, "Genealogies and Anthropologies of Global Mental Health" (2019).

Critical Histories

2 Mental Ills for All

Genealogies of the Movement for Global Mental Health

Stefan Ecks

Abstract

MGMH was created by reassembling psychiatric epidemiology, health economics, health systems research, evidence-based therapeutics, lay awareness, human rights, and sustainable development into an set of policy instruments. I retrace the emergence and crisis of three "pillars" of MGMH: epidemiology, economics of minds and moods, and the gap in treatment provision. I argue that MGMH remains limited by its strategic ignorance of flaws in the data, of paradoxical relations between economic development and health improvement, and of how people actually seek help in low income countries. I conclude by arguing that MGMH policies are bound to fail if they fail to reckon with the contradictions in its approach.

Keywords: psychiatric epidemiology, economics of mental health, mental health treatment gap

Globalising Mental Illness

In May 2018, a report announced that diagnoses of depression are rising dramatically in the US (BlueCross BlueShield 2018). Between 2013 and 2016, rates increased by 63 per cent among adolescents and 47 per cent among millennials. The highest rates were found in the richest states of the Pacific Northwest and New England. The rise of mental disorders is said to be a global phenomenon, striking rich and poor countries alike. In October 2018, a report by *The Lancet* Commission on Global Mental Health and Sustainable Development (Patel et al. 2018) announced that low and middle income

Sax, William, and Claudia Lang (eds), *The Movement for Global Mental Health: Critical Views from South and Southeast Asia.* Taylor & Francis Group, 2021
DOI: 10.5117/9789463721622_CH02

countries needed to take "urgent action" to "fully implement" psychiatric diagnostics and therapies developed in the US and Europe – as if these interventions had lowered rates of suffering in the countries they came from. The global "scaling up" of interventions seems to scale up the suffering as well. This is the one of the key paradoxes of mental health in the world today.

"Global Mental Health" (GMH) is an interdisciplinary field of research, policy, and advocacy that seeks equal access to basic mental health care for everyone in the world. My own discipline, medical anthropology, has been part of GMH from early on. The anthropologists were among the most globally oriented co-constituents of GMH. Yet anthropologists engaging with GMH also struggle with a range of value conflicts, especially when it comes to psychiatrists saying their diagnostics are universal and their therapies effective irrespective of cultural context.

In theory, the "global" in GMH means that people from all parts of the world are included: "all countries can be thought of as developing countries in the context of mental health" (Patel et al. 2018, 1). In practice, GMH focuses on lower and middle-income countries, where the gap is deepest between what GMH advocates think should be done and what is actually done. Although GMH is described as a "global" collaboration, all its leading proponents are based in Euro-American elite institutions. The same elite bias applies to the "Movement for Global Mental Health" (MGMH) which is GMH's civil society and advocacy spin-off. The MGMH's advisory board consists of the same researchers who run GMH. GMH has a growing influence on national mental health policies, especially in countries with weak national health sectors and a strong international donor presence.

MGMH is about two decades old. The current meaning of "global mental health" emerged in the 2000s. Until that time, a more common term was "world" mental health. Neither the World Development Report (World Bank 1993), the influential book *World Mental Health* (Desjarlais et al. 1995), nor the World Health Report 2001 (World Health Organization 2001) contain the phrase "global mental health." Until the 2000s, "global mental health" was used to describe a population's overall stress levels (Cohen, Patel and Minas 2014). Replacing "world" or "international" came with a wider shift in health policy to "global" concerns. Changing the name from "world" to "global" inserts MGMH into the global health assemblage.

"MGMH" became the dominant discourse upon publication of a series of articles in *The Lancet* in 2007. "No health without mental health", the first article in the series (Prince et al. 2007), argued for a refocusing of "health" around "mental" health. Better mental health would reduce all other health problems (including infectious diseases) and all other social problems (including gender inequalities and poverty). Mental health should become central in "all aspects of health and social policy, health-system planning, and delivery of primary and secondary general health care" (Prince et al. 2007). A year later, WHO (2008) published the *World Mental Health Gap Action Programme*. Other key reports were the *Grand Challenges in Global Mental Health* programme by the US National Institute of Mental Health (Collins et al. 2011) and the WHO's *Mental Health Action Plan* (2013). The latest phase integrates mental health into the Sustainable Development Goals (SDG), so that good mental health is defined as an integral aspect of social and economic development (Patel et al. 2018).

MGMH is the latest moment in the global history of Euro-American psychiatry, which began in the nineteenth century. MGMH emerged when psychiatry teamed up with public health and health economics to scale up its impact beyond richer countries. MGMH is an assemblage of disparate concerns, methods, institutions, actors, and infrastructures, each with its own genealogy. It contains an epidemiology of who is suffering and at what rates. The relation to health economics has been fundamental to its rise: What are the impacts of poor mental health on economic growth, and how does economic growth impact on mental health? Therapies proposed by MGMH are derived from "best practices" in the psy-sciences: psychiatry (mostly psychotropics), clinical psychology, and counselling. An area where MGMH contributes to what has already been established is the trialling of psychosocial interventions for larger groups. Education is another field of MGMH, both in terms of "spreading awareness and reducing stigma", as well as the insertion of mental health into educational settings. MGMH employs methods from health systems analysis to assess what kinds of service provisions are in place in the community, primary, secondary, and tertiary levels. Finally, MGMH defines itself as human rights advocacy. This includes lobbying governments for legal safeguards for people with mental health problems. In the following, I will focus on three pillars of MGMH: epidemiology, economics, and service provision. In each section, I attempt to trace where this concern emerged, and to chart where it might be heading.

First Pillar: Epidemiology

The first pillar of MGMH is epidemiology. To make mental health a global project, it was necessary to show that mental disorders could be found in all countries of the world. Preferably, prevalence rates should be similar because this would validate both universal neurobiological disease aetiologies and the cross-cultural reliability of the symptom classifications.

Even after decades of epidemiological work, the worldwide data remain disputed. For example, rates of depression vary dramatically between countries. Bromet et al. (2011) found that the highest scoring countries could have rates of depression that were 33 times higher than those of the lowest scoring countries. Even for studies that aimed at a high standardisation of methods used, twelve-month prevalence of depression in high-income countries ranged from just 2.2 per cent in Japan to 10.4 in Brazil. Too much variance is troubling: either the data are wrong, or the methods are wrong, or assumptions of universal biological aetiology are wrong. A fourth possibility, that of mental disorders are co-constituted by local economic, social, and environmental contexts that they become "local biologies" (Lock 2001) is not considered in MGMH.

MGMH advocates – influenced by Lancet MGMH Commission members such as Arthur Kleinman – say that the field emerged from a confluence of a medical "etic" approach that treated mental disorders as scientifically as other medical conditions; and an "emic" approach taken by anthropologists "who analysed mental disorders as shaped by social and cultural forces" (Patel et al. 2018, 4). It is debatable how important the emic perspective ever was, but it is clear that MGMH, in its current formulation, is an etic project that considers local definitions of mental health as irrelevant for the MGMH project. The only importance accorded to local meanings is that they produce "stigma" and act as "barriers to care" that needs to be overcome. The question of whether the diagnostics and treatments of western psychiatry are applicable to other cultures is not even raised. The global spread of interventions becomes a matter of "scaling up" the standardised interventions. The perspective of "activists championing a cultural perspective" who fear that MGMH is "a western psychiatric framework dominated by pharmaceutical interventions" (ibid., 8) is strategically mentioned, but not taken seriously. Worse, a "cultural perspective" got blacklisted as one of six "threats to global mental health" (ibid., 7).

The quantification of mental disorders began in the mental asylums of the nineteenth century. One of the first instances of psychiatric epidemiology was in 1844 when the Association of Superintendents of American Asylums – the precursor of the American Psychiatric Association – compiled statistics of what US asylum inmates were suffering from (Solomon 1958; Horwitz and Grob 2011; Hacking 2013). The first larger studies in psychiatric epidemiology came from social scientists, such as Durkheim highly influential study suicide (1897) or Faris and Dunham's (1939) study of mental disorders in a Chicago neighbourhood. Psychiatric epidemiology took much longer to establish itself than the epidemiology of other (physical) conditions (Lovell 2014).

Currently the leading framework for epidemiological quantification is the Global Burden of Disease (GBD), which started as a collaboration between the World Bank, the World Health Organization, and Harvard University in the 1990s. In 2000, GBD estimated that psychiatric disorders contribute 14 per cent to the total burden of disease in the world, and that major depressive disorder ranks as the fourth major cause of disease globally. The World Health Report 2001 – the WHO's first ever dedicated to mental illness – predicted that depression would become "the world's second leading health problem" after heart disease by 2020 (WHO 2001, 65). Nearly every research article on global mental health begins with dire figures on global disease "burdens". The need for more research, the need for new treatments, and the need for better services are based on the burden calculations.

GBD introduced a new metric to measure the global impact of mental illnesses: the disability-adjusted life year (DALY). DALYs measure disease burdens as the number of years lost due to ill-health, disability and early death. First developed by Harvard University for the World Bank in 1990, the World Health Organization adopted the method in 2000. Previously, health liabilities were expressed using only year of life lost without taking disability into account. The 1990 *Global Burden of Disease* study was the first publication to use this method. The introduction of DALYs produced surprising insights into population health. For example, it came as shock that five of the ten leading causes of disability were psychiatric conditions. Like no methodological innovation before or since, DALYs made mental health a global concern.

Nevertheless, doubts remain about the quality of the GBD data and about the validity of the disease categories. Critical evaluations of how global burdens of mental disorders are calculated find that the amalgamation of disparate studies suffers from many problems. The individual studies compiled are of uneven quality and representativeness. When global statistics are put together from separate small studies, the specificities and limitations of the individual studies are brushed aside. Brhlikova, Pollock and Manners (2011, 25) found that most studies used in global burden calculations "exhibit significant shortcomings and limitations with respect to study design and analysis and compliance with GBDep inclusion criteria" and that the "poor quality" of the data make many conclusions questionable.

An additional problem with the epidemiology informing MGMH comes from a long-standing suspicion that psychiatric epidemiology cannot extrapolate the results of clinical studies to the population at large (Shorter 2013). The number of people found to suffer from major depressive disorder within the definition of DSM in clinical settings could not and should not be used to make claims about urgent and unmet needs in the population. Vikram Patel (2014), the most prominent proponent of MGMH, has even called for the abandoning of global burden statistics because they produce a "credibility gap" for psychiatric research (Patel 2014, 18). It was evident that large numbers of people in any country could be said to be "distressed" in the sense of being sad or fearful of the future, yet they were not psychiatrically "disordered". Epidemiological claims about the burden of depression that immense as well as specific ultimately undermine trust in psychiatry: "[O]nly a small fraction of the global population truly believes any of the astonishingly large figures that these surveys throw up. Those figures simply lack face validity because they conflate emotional distress with mental disorders" (ibid.). If the epidemiology of global mental disorders is in doubt, the whole MGMH project is in doubt, too.

Even worse for the epidemiology is the crumbling faith in symptoms-based diagnosis, which is used in the American Psychiatric Associations' *Diagnostic and Statistical Manual* as well as in the WHO's *International Classification of Diseases*. DSM is currently in its fifth edition, and ICD in its eleventh. Psychiatric epidemiology only took off in the 1980s, when DSM-III classifications were structured enough to be applied in community surveys. DSM has been the key source for psychiatric epidemiology since that time (Bromet and Susser 2006, 9). Prior research had been hampered by a lack of consensus about how to classify the disorders to be counted (Eisenberg 2010, 94).

A revolt within psychiatry against DSM and symptoms-based diagnosis has been brewing since the 1990s. The biopsychiatric faction that privileges biomarkers over reported symptoms won the upper hand in the 2010s. Biopsychiatric doubts about the validity of symptoms as true phenotypes of organic problems have been voiced since the 1980s. Doubts about the validity of DSM categories have deepened ever more when the symptoms were not found to be commensurate with biomarkers (Ecks 2018). When revisions of DSM-IV got underway, many demanded a shift towards a fully neurobiological and genetic psychiatry. The DSM-V Revision Agenda, jointly published by NIMH and APA (Kupfer, First and Regier 2002, xix) declared that merely reshuffling and refining symptom classifications would never uncover the biological mechanisms that cause the symptoms.

The disillusionment with DSM turned into a full paradigm shift when the US National Institute of Mental Health (NIMH) declared that it was turning its research strategy away from DSM and towards a new framework called RDoC (Research Domain Criteria). RDoC has been part of the NIMH's strategic plan since 2008 (Cuthbert 2014), but an open opposition to DSM had not been declared until 2013. RDoC has been described as "the latest chapter in psychiatry's ongoing story of the search for a holy grail of biological etiology" (Geppert 2017). The inability of DSM-5 to integrate symptom classifications with biological and genetic research findings pushed RDoC up the NIMH's agenda (Romelli, Frigerio and Colombo 2015). The NIMH turned against DSM a few weeks before the fifth edition was published. Thomas Insel, then the director of the NIMH, ridiculed the DSM approach to disease classification as an intuitive art: "The weakness [of DSM] is its lack of validity. Unlike our definitions of ischemic heart disease, lymphoma, or AIDS, the DSM diagnoses are based on a consensus about clusters of clinical symptoms, not any objective laboratory measure" (Insel 2013). Since DSM could never move beyond mere opinions, the NIMH "will be re-orienting its research away from DSM categories". Instead of outward symptoms, the new classificatory system should be based on measurable biomarkers (Fu and Costafreda 2013).

Insel's attack on DSM caused a stir beyond the research field. In response to the outcry caused by his critique of DSM, Insel co-authored a press release with J.A. Lieberman, President-elect of the APA, that supported the DSM as "the key resource for delivering the best available care". Patients and insurance companies could be "confident that effective treatments are available" (Insel and Lieberman 2013). Superficially it appeared as if the NIMH had retreated, but this is not what happened. Insel just said that the "best available care" may be based on DSM today, but that did not mean that it would be based on DSM tomorrow. Some NIMH statements about the relation between DSM and RDoC published since 2013 tend to portray the two frameworks as complementary, not competing (Lupien et al. 2017, 8), but it is difficult to see how these approaches could ever overlap.

These controversies at the heart of research-based psychiatry are hardly ever discussed in relation to MGMH, although they make a fundamental difference to the ground upon which MGMH is standing. One of the direct engagements with the diagnostic crisis within MGMH has been the question whether DSM-style categories "really do overlap with the main issues that global mental health must address" (Stein, Lund and Nesse 2013). Some authors point to other indicators of mental health issues in the population, such as social inequality. In any case, no diagnostic alternative to symptoms-based diagnosis in the style of DSM and ICD exists as yet. Recent moves towards a "dimensional" approach that is more sensitive to shades of severity (Patel et al. 2018) does not solve any of the fundamental problems of validity and reliability of symptom classifications.

A few indirect engagements with the problem of DSM/ICD diagnostics can be found in recent MGMH-related publications. In the new MGMH manifesto by The Lancet Commission (Patel et al. 2018, 11), the DSM/RDoC dispute is mentioned in relation to a "staging" approach to be developed in MGMH. In the future, RDoC-style research might allow "deep phenotyping", meaning that individual patients' risks could be assessed on multiple biological levels. Eventually, this could make inventions more targeted, for example, by looking for markers of inflammation in cases of depression. But deep phenotyping has no immediate for therapy, neither in rich nor poor countries.

The Lancet Commission recognises that DSM/ICD diagnostics have "limitations" because they can be "simplistic", "not always helpful", and "reductionist" (Patel et al. 2018). While the Commission "does not advocate for the abolition of classification systems" (ibid., 11), it recommends greater attention to the fact that mental disorders develop gradually. During the "prodromal" stages, signs of coming disorder are not distinct enough to be caught by symptoms-based classifications. In most cases, "non-specific psychological distress" – argued to be the most common manifestation of mental problems in large populations – does not need a diagnostic label but it still needs a full-fledged intervention: "The staging model [...] recognises opportunities for intervention at all stages" (ibid., 12). It is ironic that MGMH went from a critique of the tendency of DSM/ICD to overmedicalise popula- tions to an even *more* medicalising vision of everyone being prodromally disordered. The newly proposed "staging model" solves nothing. MGMH epidemiology is still built on the same quicksand as in the 1980s.

Second Pillar: Economics

DALYs allow a new way of measuring economic impacts of mental illnesses. MGMH would not have emerged without the economic burden argument. Mental health became a priority because worsening mental health indicators are dragging down whole economies.

The first studies on the mental/economic nexus stem from the early 1990s. In 1992, Rice et al. brought US national survey data together with a "newly developed methodology for calculating costs", and arrived at a staggering figure of an annual loss to the US economy of US$104 *billion*. US$43 billion were spent on treatments, US$47 billion were lost because morbidity reduced productivity, and US$9 billion were lost because of premature death. One key finding was that there are direct and indirect costs of rising mental illnesses. The direct costs (including medications and clinical treatments) are already huge, but the indirect costs due to reduced productivity, higher rates of social benefit payments, higher rates of incarceration and higher rates of homelessness, were just as draining. Economic burdens continue to be calculated in this way (Insel 2008). Economic cost calculations are now included in public health research and policy development in the Global North. For example, in the UK, the NHS recognises mental health problems as the largest single cause of disability in the country, making it not only a quarter of the national burden of ill health, but also the leading cause of illness-related work absence. It is estimated that mental health problems cost the country £100 billion each year – including the costs to individuals and society of treating preventable illness, the impact on quality of life, lost working days, and lost income.

All the initial research focused on rich countries, whereas a scarcity of data hampered extending this perspective to poorer countries. From early on, however, causal relations between mental ill health and loss of economic wealth were seen in poorer countries. Patel and Kleinman argued that mental ill health and lower economic wealth are typical of people with low levels of education. There was, they argue, a "vicious circle of poverty and mental disorder" (2003, 612), with one dragging down the other. Mental health interventions should, therefore, also include financial aid interventions, such as microcredit schemes.

The mental health/economics nexus took a while to get onto the political agenda. It was only in 2014 that "mental health became a hot topic" among the world's political leaders (Insel 2014). Economic growth depended on good mental health, especially because of the increasing importance of the tertiary service sector. Mood disorders were particularly rampant in this sector. Echoing the MGMH motto that there could be no health without mental health, Insel said that governments had finally realised that there could be "no wealth without mental health". Insel's argument about mental health and a transition towards the service sector has hardly been explored yet. If this holds, it would mean that mental disorders are going to increase rapidly over the coming decades. Economic globalisation is not the solution: It is the *problem*.

By contrast, MGMH scholars are optimistic that global economic growth reduces mental illnesses. Poverty makes you depressed, and wealth lifts up your mood. Economic growth becomes the engine of growth in population mental health. The "vicious cycle" model is a major component of the WHO Report 2001: poverty led to a higher prevalence of mental disorders. Higher prevalence, lack of care, and more severe course of disease had negative economic consequences. To turn this situation into a virtuous cycle, the WHO Report advocated investments in psychiatric drugs as investments in economic growth. Investments in drugs as first-line treatments became investments in global economic growth, and growth became a cure for mental illnesses. But maybe the true return on the economic investment is a *worsening* of mental health.

In the 2010s, WHO and World Bank continued to propagate the "vicious cycle" model. Much of their research focused on depression and anxiety because they are the most common and most draining. WHO/WB now put the cost of depression and anxiety at US$1 trillion per year worldwide (Chisholm 2016). All attempts at explaining the relations between mental health of a population and economic processes are fraught with unproven assumptions.

The "vicious cycle" model subscribes to a pro-capitalist approach that holds that material wealth leads to mental health. The next question is whether interventions should focus either on mental health or material wealth. Either investment in economic growth is prioritised to enhance mental health, or money is spent on targeted mental health interventions that improve economic growth. Lund et al. (2011) compared these two possibilities and concluded that targeted interventions are more powerful than broader economic growth: "We found that the mental health effect of poverty alleviation interventions was inconclusive [...] By contrast, mental health interventions were associated with improved economic outcomes in all studies, although the difference was not statistically significant in every study" (ibid., 1502) This study "supports the call to scale up mental health care, not only as a public health and human rights priority, but also as a development priority" (ibid., 1513).

But the causal links between mental health and material wealth remain murky. Lund et al. observe that the "vicious cycle" hypothesis was "fairly robust" (ibid., 1502) in rich countries, but less so in poorer countries. They describe two kinds of causation models, the "social causation hypothesis" and the "social drift hypothesis". The social causation model assumes that poverty increases stress, social exclusion, lessened social capital, bad diet, violence, and trauma. In turn, the social drift model assumes that people who are already distressed are at a higher risk of falling into, or remaining in, poverty, because of higher health expenditures, reduced productivity, and unemployment. The main problem identified by Lund and colleagues is that there are hardly any "robust" studies on the topic. Despite screening 13,000 articles, the authors found only fourteen that met their inclusion criteria.

Out of more than 1,500 randomised trials identified in the 2007 *Lancet* series on mental health, "only four measured economic status outcomes". The entire discipline was, therefore, "in its infancy" (ibid., 1508, 1513). There is a total disconnect between the high confidence levels of MGMH policy statements about economic growth and better mental health on the one hand, and reliable evidence on what these connections might be on the other.

A study featured on the World Bank's web page on mental health estimates productivity losses due to all "mental, neurologic, and substance use" (MNS) disorders at US\$ 8.5 trillion in 2010. This is expected to double by 2030, "if a concerted response is not mounted" (Chisholm et al. 2016, 416). These calculations work with two kinds of value, the "intrinsic" value of having good mental health, and the "instrumental" value of working productively, as well as being able to "form and maintain relationships, [...] pursue leisure interests, and to make decisions in everyday life" (ibid., 416). The treatments considered are: six months of continuous antidepressant treatment with fluoxetine (aka Prozac), regular visits to out-patient and primary care services for medications and psychosocial treatments; and, for a few severe cases, hospital admissions of up to fourteen days. Overhead costs like administration are also factored in. The global treatment gap stood at 72 per cent in high-income countries and at 93 per cent in low-income countries. Only 7 per cent of people in poor countries received treatment for depression (ibid., 418). These figures on treatment gaps leave out entirely what is provided outside the formal public sector (a fatal weakness of the methodology that I will return to in the next section). If treatments were scaled up, the returns on investment were 5.7:1, meaning that for every US\$ spent on treatments, an overall economic return of US\$5.70 could be realised (ibid., 422). This sounds impressive, until the return on investment ratios are compared to most other health interventions. For malaria, for example, the benefit to cost ratio is 40:1 (ibid., 422). Yet the evidence on economic returns is extremely weak. Citing Lund et al. (2011), Chisholm et al. repeat that "the evidence base for the mental health effect of interventions targeted at the poor remains insubstantial" (2016, 422). Any simplistic argument about "economic wealth increases mental health" does not stand up to scrutiny.

Another hypothesis is that greater material wealth puts mental health at risk. Mental disorders, especially mood disorders, are correlated with modernity's increasing social isolation, competitiveness, secularisation, materialism, unhealthy diets, and sedentary lifestyles. Reviewing the evidence on modernisation/depression links, the US physician Hidaka (2012, 211) concludes that "more money does not lead to more happiness". Instead, "economic and marketing forces of modern society have engineered an environment promoting decisions that maximise consumption at the long-term cost of well-being". Modernity's "overfed, malnourished, sedentary, sunlight-deficient, sleep-deprived, competitive, inequitable and socially-isolating environment" is toxic for the mind. This hypothesis of modernity's toxic influences is never seriously considered in MGMH publications.

A related hypothesis focuses on relative wealth changes, rather than absolute wealth levels. In this view, socioeconomic change in and of itself tends to be detrimental to mental health. This is especially so when people are torn from long-standing social networks and are confronted with more competition and higher aspirations (Heaton 2013). In this vein, Bhugra and Mastrogianni (2004) argue against money producing better mental health: "We have entered the brave new world of globalisation [...] Societies alter rapidly through urbanization, acculturation, modernization, and social and cultural change. The quality of life in many countries is affected by economic disintegration, unequal distribution of collective wealth, social disruption, political repression, migration and even war [...] Global economic forces have weakened poor countries and communities on the one hand, and reinforced the economic status of wealthy countries on the other" (2004, 10).

This line of argument used to be prominent in WHO publications prior to the era of DALYs, but can still be heard post-1990s. For example, in the *Mental Health Action Plan 2013-2020*, WHO acknowledges a link between the downsides of capitalism and the mental health of populations. The 2007 financial crisis has had a particularly detrimental effect: "The current global financial crisis provides a powerful example of a macroeconomic factor leading to [...] higher rates of mental disorders and suicide as well as the emergence of new vulnerable groups [...] In many societies, mental disorders related to marginalization and impoverishment [...] and overwork and stress are of growing concern" (WHO 2013, 7).

Versions of this theory have been disappearing and reappearing over the past decades. For example, it is plausible, and evidenced by WHO studies, that schizophrenia patients have a much better prognosis in poorer countries rather than in richer countries (Halliburton, this volume). The WHO's own research on better recovery in poorer countries is never mentioned in MGMH publications because it contradicts the "material wealth is mental health" model.

Where the older argument converges with MGMH is that economic decline, especially if it is rapid and sudden, is bad for mental health. When people move quickly from relative wealth to relative poverty, mental health suffers (Lorant et al. 2007). But in contexts where people move slowly from relative poverty to relative wealth, it is not clear that the opposite effect, of improving mental health, occurs.

Missing from the MGMH discourse on the economics of mental health is an engagement with *relative* gains or losses. The importance of change *relative* to the past and *relative* to social others has been highlighted by critical health economists such as Wilkinson (2002), Wilkinson and Pickett (2010), and Marmot (2005) two decades. Similarly, MGMH does not consider the "mental ills of marginality" (cf. Ecks and Sax 2005). Socioeconomic marginalisation has negative health effects (Marmot 2005). People at the margins suffer more from stigmatisation, poverty, low education, and limited access to health services. Marginalisation can make existing sickness worse, and it can push people into sickness. Marginalisation is always relational: who is on the margins and who is in the centre depends on the relations between them. For economic wealth, marginalisation is not about absolute levels (of income, wealth, etc.) but about relative levels: where do others stand, and how things are valued locally. Being economically marginalised is not an absolute state but relative to the whole (global) economy. Links between economic change and mental health can only be grasped by focusing on relative and changing status. When WHO argues that the global financial crisis has increased the incidence of mental illnesses, then the explanation for this must lie in relative changes to multiple people and groups. Any model that treats economic wealth in a static and absolute way is going to fail.

A relational way of studying the mental/economic nexus exists even within the WHO. For example, in 2009, a WHO Report on *Mental Health, Resilience and Inequality* (Friedli 2009) took the idea of relational status to mental health. The report argued that mental ill health cannot be reduced to absolute wealth levels but has to be seen as relative. This report not only argued that "higher national levels of income inequality are linked to a higher prevalence of mental illness", but even more worryingly, "as countries get richer, rates of mental illness increase" (Friedli 2009, 35). Similarly, Wilkinson and Pickett (2010) highlight inequality as source of mental illness, as "differences in inequality tally with more than threefold differences in the percentage of people with mental illness in different countries" (2010, 67).

A relational approach is sometimes mentioned in MGMH, but is lost in the drive to scale up services. In The Lancet Commission Report, marginalisation and relative socioeconomic status is taken in an absolute sense: "structural inequities [...] can have a negative effect on mental health and wellbeing" (Patel et al. 2018, 11). Inequality "erodes social capital" and "amplifies social comparisons and status anxiety" (ibid., 15), but a deeper analysis is missing. In every way, mental health is an outlier among different medical conditions. With all other illnesses, the more money is spent them, the more they are reduced. But with mental illnesses, more money spent on fighting them does not consistently reduce them. Without a relational approach to studying wealth and mental health, this paradox will never be resolved.

Third Pillar: Scaling up Services

Closing the treatment gap motivates all MGMH work. Their epidemiology shows that people are in need. Their economic modelling shows that people in need are unproductive. Their health systems analysis shows that those in need are not being helped. The treatment gap notion could only emerge from the epidemiology, and the epidemiology could only emerge from standardised diagnostic criteria. In turn, interventions are justified as cost-effective. Economic losses from mental disorders are made calculable like other economic liabilities, and the expected returns on investment into different therapies and approaches can be assessed by measures of return of investment.

One of the first moments of discovering treatment gaps was in the US in the 1980s, when the NIHM conducted a study of the prevalence of mental disorders based on DSM-III criteria. The study discovered that mental disorders were highly prevalent (20 per cent annually), and that only a minority of people with problems received care: "The message was unambiguous: the magnitude of the need for treatment is such that the only possible public health solution is to enhance the capacity of the primary health-care system to provide mental health treatment" (Eisenberg 2010, 94). The rise of depression to the most common mental disorder is part of the diagnostic criteria changes introduced in DSM-III. It expanded the definition of depressive disorder by merging severe melancholia with milder symptoms of nervous disorders. DSM-III laid the foundations of the global depression epidemic (Horwitz and Wakefield 2008; Shorter 2013).

The discovery of high prevalence rates in the general population, along with discovering a treatment gap, were both proffered by psychiatric deinstitutionalisation. There used to be millions of psychiatric hospital beds in the Global North in the first half of the twentieth century and numbers were expected to rise even further in the 1950s. But instead of increases, asylum and hospital-based care was scaled back dramatically, a process that began in the 1950s and continued until the 1980s. Deinstitutionalisation is a complex phenomenon that came about by the confluence of changing national health care provisioning (associated with privatisation of health care) as well as the availability of new psychotropic drugs, especially antipsychotics, during this time. The role of drugs in the history of psychiatric deinstitutionalisation has long been debated, with a common argument being that drugs did not lead to deinstitutionalisation, but helped to accelerate it (e.g. Gronfein 1985). Another argument is that psychotropics developed since the 1950s triggered the "deinstitutionalization of psychiatry and psychiatrists rather than patients" (Healy 2008, 428), in the sense that drugs allowed doctors to leave the asylums and work privately instead. Another trigger for deinstitutionalisation was the attempt to save money: asylums were seen as too expensive to be continued at a large scale.

MGMH advocates claim deinstitutionalisation in the Global North as one of its roots (Patel et al. 2018, 5). While arguing for better government mental health services, MGMH tends to be critical of brick-and-mortar mental institutions, as places of poor treatments and human rights abuses. MGMH strategies favour "care in the community" and providers from outside of institutions. The notion of community care has gathered pace since the 1960s, and eventually became the dominant discourse in the 1980s. In India, for example, the first Mental Health Programme (NMHP), launched in 1983, called for the deinstitutionalisation of psychiatry and for a move towards community care (Jain and Jadhav 2008). The "community care" and "human rights" pillars of MGMH both stem from this turn against asylum-based care. If there had been as many asylums in the Global South as in the Global North, MGMH would have taken a different turn. But the mental asylums in European colonies during the nineteenth century were thin on the ground and almost exclusively catered to Europeans and not to the "natives". There were not many institutions in the South that could ever be deinstitutionalised.

The landmark World Health Report of 2001 (whose principal author was the NIMHANS psychiatrist R.S. Murthy) embraced all the assumptions of the DALY era: mental illnesses are widespread and highly burdensome; effective drugs exist but are neither widely available nor affordable; and closing the treatment gaps should be a top priority of global health interventions. The Report warned about an "increasing" burden of mental disorders and a "widening" treatment gap: "Today, some 450 million people suffer from a mental or behavioural disorder, yet only a small minority of them receive even the most basic treatment" (WHO 2001, 3). It went further by pointing out that "the poor and the deprived have a higher prevalence of disorders, including substance abuse" (ibid., xiv). The treatment gap is deeper not just because services are not offered to the poor but because the poor are suffering more. The 2001 Report moved depression to the top of the intervention agenda by arguing that this disease would become the world's second-leading health problem by 2020.

In the 2001 Report, psychotropics hold the promise of better treatment for all, and "new" hope comes particularly with "new" drugs. Drugs "provide the first-line treatment" (ibid., xi). Psychotherapy, counselling, and other nonpharmaceutical interventions are favourably discussed. But the Report questions if they could be cost effective, and if the lack of skilled personnel does not rule them out as a viable option for poorer countries (ibid., 62). The problem that needed a policy solution is to make psychotropics accessible to everyone, especially to poorer people. "Make psychotropic drugs available" is the second out of ten points for future policies (ibid., xi). "Essential" drugs should be on every country's essential drugs list, and "the best drugs" should be available "whenever possible" (ibid.). In the antidepressant segment, drugs are said to be effective "across the full range of severity" (ibid., 65) including mild depressive symptoms. The "new" drugs – presumably SSRIs, though this is never explicitly stated – are seen as highly effective for all forms of depression, including severe depression. There are no doubts about the efficacy of antidepressant drugs, and no doubts about using them across the world as a first-line treatments. The new antidepressants are costlier than the older ones, but their better side effect profile means a "reduced need for other care and treatment", so that even expensive drugs are ultimately more cost effective (2001, 61). No one in the world should be "deprived, on economic grounds only, of the benefits of advances in psychopharmacology" (2001, 61).

The confidence in "new" drugs as best first-line treatment peaked in the 2000s. Later publications by the WHO maintained the severity and depth of the global treatment gap but became more reluctant to tout drugs as the best first-line treatment. For example, the WHO-sponsored Mental Health Gap Action Programme (mhGAP) Report of 2008 calculated that there were vast gaps between what national governments were investing into mental health and what was needed. The Report held that the treatment gap was "more than 75%" worldwide, that is, only 25 per cent of people who need treatment received it. Divided by different types of mental disorders, the treatment gap was found to range from 32 per cent for schizophrenia to 78 per cent for alcohol use disorders. Depression treatments showed a gap of 56 per cent. The same report also listed "treatment with antidepressant medicines" as the first of two "evidence-based interventions", the second being "psychosocial interventions" (2008, 11).

In the 2010s, WHO started to shy away from an all-out embrace of psychotropics, with all major mental disorders. Depression treatments became less pharmaceuticalised. The mhGAP Intervention Guide, first published in 2010 with a second edition in 2016, split "mild" depression from moderate and severe depression and moved it into a separate section for "other significant emotional or medically unexplained complaints" (2010, 80). (Why "mild depression" should not count as "depression" is not explained.) Moderate and severe depression, meanwhile, are said to be best treated by nonpharmacological interventions, such as addressing psychosocial stressors or reactivating social networks (ibid., 10). The demotion of antidepressants from first-line treatment to an intervention to be merely "considered" can only be read between the lines.

The WHO Mental Health Action Plan 2013-2020, published in 2013, only mentions the treatment gap once, and only in an annexe (2013, 35). Whenever the treatment gap gets less attention, psychotropic treatments also get less attention. The *Action Plan* does not make any statements about psychotropics. In this document the word "drug" only refers to illegal and addictive substances, not to psychotropics. At one point, the availability of "basic medicines for mental disorders in primary healthcare" is said to be low, but so was the availability of "nonpharmacological approaches" (ibid., 9). The action plan insists that "mental health strategies and interventions for treatment, prevention and promotion need to be based on scientific evidence and/or best practice, taking cultural considerations into account" (ibid., 10). Is not spelled out what the best evidence is for psychotropics, but statements like these can be taken as a nod to the growing doubts about the efficacy of medications.

When MGMH calculates treatment gaps for countries of the global South, private-sector services are entirely excluded. The exclusive focus on what happens in the public sector produces a skewed picture of treatment gaps in countries of the South. Not only are private-sector pharmaceutical prescriptions ignored by MGMH, but private practitioners providing mental health care are also ignored. When MGMH say that there are, for example, only "0.31 mental health professional per 100,000 population in India" (WHO 2008), then this captures only specialised personnel in public sector facilities. The fact that at least 90 per cent of all mental health treatments are given by non-specialists and in the private sector is never even considered as a possibility. Nor is the possibility ever entertained that psychotropics are used by unlicensed people as well. In India, people who work in medicine shops and unlicensed "quack" doctors are often the first point of call (Ecks and Basu 2009). MGMH calculation of mental health treatment gaps is faulty because it ignores everything happening outside the public biomedical sector.

MGMH's key idea for closing the treatment gap is "task sharing" (formerly known as "task shifting"). Given that it was impossible to train enough specialised psychiatrists in poorer countries, the only solution was to tone down the training requirements and to employ low-skilled health workers. This is not a shift in tasks, but a shift in who is performing tasks: "specific tasks are moved, where appropriate, from highly qualified health workers to health workers with shorter training and fewer qualifications" (Patel, Koschorke and Prince 2011, 11). With basic supervision by a psychiatrist or similar specialist, these low skilled health workers were just as good at diagnosing problems, dispensing drugs, and offering behavioural therapy. The "mobilization and recognition of nonformal resources in the community – including community members without formal professional training", was the essential element in delivering services for all (ibid.).

One of the many problems of task sharing is that it embraces a kind of strategic ignorance about therapeutic spaces and healers that are deemed unqualified or irrelevant (Ecks and Basu 2014). The wide variety of treatment options for mental health problems, especially in countries of the Global South (cf. chapters x, y, z), gets pushed aside (Fernando 2014). The way that MGMH operationalises the treatment gap is based on a biomedicalised concept of healing (Ingleby 2014). Scaling up biomedical services through task sharing treats forms of healing that do not fit into the MGMH agenda as quackery, or ignores them altogether. Many countries have informal biomedical providers, who can easily outnumber trained formal providers. The presence of these informal providers gets entirely ignored. In other fields, such as tuberculosis control, the presence of these informal practitioners is not only recognised but also utilised for the extension of treatment protocols in areas where no formal provider would be present, but not (yet) in MGMH (Ecks and Basu 2014). It is also well-established that many forms of distress are helped by religious and ritual practices (Sax 2014; Heim and Schaal 2014).

Global Mental Illness, Local Mental Health

During fieldwork on the uses of psychotropics in India, I explored how Rural Medical Practitioners (RMPs) in West Bengal make sense of depression (e.g. Ecks and Basu 2009, 2014). RMPs have no formal training in biomedicine and are viewed as illegal quacks by the government. But in rural areas, they outnumber trained biomedical practitioners by a large margin. As a first point of call for people with health problems, the police tolerates their presence. RMPs are not meant to know anything about how depression is diagnosed, how it is treated, and what its causes are. Yet all of them spoke about how many patients nowadays come with depression symptoms and how they treat them routinely with drugs. The drugs are supposed to be "by prescription from licensed practitioner only", but RMPs have no trouble sourcing antidepressants from drugs wholesalers.

The RMPs said that depression was increasing by leaps and bounds among the rural poor: "A recent addition to the list of diseases has been depression. It has reached frightening proportions" (RMP Malla). The present era was clearly more stressful and unhappy than previous times. The cause of rising rates of depression was rampant socioeconomic change, which in turn was caused by globalisation and market capitalism: "Anxiety, depression is increasing. It is mainly because of the economic situation. This is our analysis and we are sure of this conclusion. In my fifteen years' experience, I have seen the number of patients coming with such problems has increased" (RMP Sasumal). People used to be more content with their situation in previous times. But now TV shows them affluent lifestyles of the big city folks, while their own economic status seemed to become ever more precarious. If the root cause of depression was socioeconomic, the psychotropic drugs could only tinker with symptoms: "I don't think this problem can be solved with medicines. The cause is socioeconomic. But we use medicines to take care of the symptoms" (RMP Ghosh). Echoing popular ideas about how to deal with low moods and the mind "feeling bad" (Ecks 2013), the RMPs also used nonpharmacological treatments: counselling ("don't think too much"), practical advice on life problems, and spiritual encouragement ("try praying").

Even small insights into local practices trouble key assumptions of Global Mental Health. MGMH says that there is a huge gap between rich and poor countries both in the awareness of mental disorders and in the effective treatments provided. MGMH holds that rising levels of material wealth around the world lowers the risks of suffering from mental illnesses. The treatment gap in poor countries is so severe that only the drafting of lay people into psychiatric task-sharing schemes can begin to close it. However, the example of rural medical practitioners in West Bengal shows that, on the contrary, there are many more mental care providers in the real world than is acknowledged in MGMH policies; that treatment deemed to be effective by MGMH circulates much deeper and further than is apparent; that mental illnesses are not nearly as unknown or stigmatised as MGMH assumes; and that rising levels of wealth are not necessarily good for mental health.

One point that MGMH representatives and RMPs agree on is that mental suffering continues to be on the rise. Both MGMH advocates and RMPs hold that the available treatments can have a limited positive effect on some individual patients, but none of the treatments seem to get a grip on the actual underlying problems. Even The Lancet Commission admits that "pharmacological and other clinical interventions for mental disorders [...] could have limited effects on the population-level burden of mental disorders" (Patel et al. 2018, 8). In rich countries, the prevalence of mental health problems "has not decreased, despite substantial increases in the provision of treatment (particularly antidepressants) and no increase in risk factors" (ibid., 8). That mental ill health increases during the same era when more money is put into improving mental health is one of the fundamental paradoxes that MGMH needs to face. Only an approach that looks at mental health *beyond* the brain can provide an answer. There can be no global mental health without understanding *social* mental health.

References

Bhugra, Dinesh, and Anastasia Mastrogianni. 2004. "Globalisation and Mental Disorders: Overview With Relation to Depression." *British Journal of Psychiatry* 184 (1): 10-20.

Brhlikova, Petra, Allyson M. Pollock, and Rachel Manners 2011. "Global Burden of Disease Estimates of Depression: How Reliable Is the Epidemiological Evidence?" *Journal of the Royal Society of Medicine* 104 (1): 25-34.

BlueCross BlueShield. 2018. "Major Depression: The Impact on Overall Health." Published 10 May 2018. Accessed 8 July 2020. https://www.bcbs.com/the-health-of-america/reports/major-depression-the-impact-overall-health#five.

Bromet, Evelyn J., and Ezra Susser. 2006. "The Burden of Mental Illness." In *Psychiatric Epidemiology: Searching for the Causes of Mental Disorders*, edited by Ezra Susser, Sharon Schwartz, Alfredo Morabia, and Evelyn J. Bromet, 5-14. Oxford: Oxford University Press.

Bromet, Evelyn J., Laura H. Andrade, Irving Hwang, Nacy A. Sampson, Jordi Alonso, Giovanni de Girolamo, Ron de Graaf, et al. 2011. "Cross-National Epidemiology of DSM-IV Major Depressive Episode." *BMC Medicine* 9 (1): 90.

Chisholm, Dan, Kim Sweeny, Peter Sheehan, Bruce Rasmussen, Filip Smit, Pim Cuijpers, and Shekhar Saxena. 2016. "Scaling-Up Treatment of Depression and Anxiety: A Global Return on Investment Analysis." *The Lancet Psychiatry* 3 (5): 415-24.

Cohen, Alex, Vikram Patel, and Harry Minas. 2014. "A Brief History of Global Mental Health." In *Global Mental Health: Principles and Practice*, edited by Vikram Patel, Harry Minas, Alex Cohen, and Martin J. Prince, 3-26. New York: Oxford University Press.

Collins, Pamela Y., Vikram Patel, Sarah S. Joestl, Dana March, Thomas R. Insel, Abdallah S. Daar, Isabel A. Bordin, et al. 2011. "Grand Challenges in Global Mental Health." *Nature* 475 (7354): 27-30.

Cuthbert, Bruce N. 2014. "The RDoC Framework: Facilitating Transition from ICD/DSM to Dimensional Approaches That Integrate Neuroscience and Psychopathology." *World Psychiatry* 13 (1): 28-35.

Desjarlais, Robert, Leon Eisenberg, Bryon J. Good, and Arthur Kleinman. 1995. *World Mental Health: Priorities, Problems and Responses in Low-income Countries.* New York: Oxford University Press.

Durkheim, Emil. 1951 [1897]. *Suicide: A Study in Sociology.* Glencoe: Free Press.

Ecks, Stefan. 2013. *Eating Drugs: Psychopharmaceutical Pluralism in India.* New York: New York University Press.

—. 2018. "Biocommensurations." *Anthropology News* 59 (4): 162-65.

Ecks, Stefan, and Soumita Basu. 2009. "The Unlicensed Lives of Antidepressants in India: Generic Drugs, Unqualified Practitioners, and Floating Prescriptions." *Transcultural Psychiatry* 46 (1): 86-106.

—. 2014. "'We Always Live in Fear': Antidepressant Prescriptions by Unlicensed Doctors in India." *Culture, Medicine, and Psychiatry* 38 (2): 197-216.

Ecks, Stefan, and William S. Sax. 2005. "Introduction: Special Issue: The Ills of Marginality: New Perspectives on Subaltern Health in South Asia." *Anthropology & Medicine* 12 (3): 199-210.

Eisenberg, Leon, and Laurence B. Guttmacher. 2010. "Were We All Asleep at the Switch? A Personal Reminiscence of Psychiatry from 1940 to 2010." *Acta Psychiatrica Scandinavica* 122 (2): 89-102.

Faris, Robert E. L., and Henry W. Dunham. 1939. *Mental Disorders in Urban Areas: An Ecological Study of Schizophrenia and Other Psychoses.* New York: Hafner.

Fernando, Suman. 2014. *Mental Health Worldwide: Culture, Globalization and Development.* New York: Palgrave Macmillan.

Friedli, Lynne, and World Health Organization. 2009. *Mental Health, Resilience and Inequalities.* Copenhagen: WHO Regional Office for Europe.

Fu, Cynthia H., and Sergi G. Costafreda. 2013. "Neuroimaging-Based Biomarkers in Psychiatry: Clinical Opportunities of a Paradigm Shift." *The Canadian Journal of Psychiatry* 58 (9): 499-508.

Geppert, Cynthia. 2017. "Introduction: More Dives and Intellectual Jujitsu." *Psychiatric Times*, 31 May 2017. Accessed 8 July 2020. http://www.psychiatrictimes.com/special-reports/introduction-more-dives-and-intellectual-jujitsu.

Gronfein, William. 1985. "Psychotropic Drugs and the Origins of Deinstitutionalization." *Social Problems* 32 (5): 437-54.

Hacking, Ian. 2013. "Lost in the Forest." Review of *DSM-5: Diagnostic and Statistical Manual of Mental Disorders, Fifth Edition*, by the American Psychiatric Association. *London Review of Books* 35 (15): 7-8.

Healy, David. 2008. "The Intersection of Psychopharmacology and Psychiatry in the

Second Half of the Twentieth Century." In *History of Psychiatry and Medical Psychology*, edited by Edwin R. Wallace, and John Gach, 419-42. New York: Springer.

Heaton, Matthew M. 2013. *Black Skin, White Coats: Nigerian Psychiatrists, Decolonization, and the Globalization of Psychiatry*. Athens, OH: Ohio University Press.

Heim, Lale, and Susanne Schaal. 2014. "Rates and Predictors of Mental Stress in Rwanda: Investigating the Impact of Gender, Persecution, Readiness to Reconcile and Religiosity via a Structural Equation Model." *International Journal of Mental Health Systems* 8 (1): 37.

Hidaka, Brandon H. 2012. "Depression as a Disease of Modernity: Explanations for Increasing Prevalence." *Journal of Affective Disorders* 140 (3): 205-14.

Horwitz, Allan V., and Gerald N. Grob. 2011. "The Checkered History of American Psychiatric Epidemiology." *Milbank Quarterly* 89 (4): 628-57.

Horwitz, Allan V., and Jerome C. Wakefield. 2007. *The Loss of Sadness: How Psychiatry Transformed Normal Sorrow Into Depressive Disorder*. Oxford: Oxford University Press.

Ingleby, David. 2014. "How 'Evidence-Based' is the Movement for Global Mental Health?" *Disability and the Global South* 1 (2): 203-26.

Insel, Thomas R. 2008. "Assessing the Economic Costs of Serious Mental Illness." *The American Journal of Psychiatry* 165 (6): 663-65.

—. 2013. "Transforming Diagnosis." NIMH Director's Blog, 29 April 2013. Accessed 8 July 2020, https://www.nimh.nih.gov/about/directors/thomas-insel/blog/2013/transforming-diagnosis.shtml.

—. 2014. "Mental Health in Davos." NIMH Director's Blog, 27 January 2014. Accessed 8 July 2020. https://www.nimh.nih.gov/about/directors/thomas-insel/blog/2014/mental-health-in-davos.shtml.

Insel, Thomas R., and Jeffrey A. Lieberman. 2013. "DSM-5 and RDoC: Shared Interests." NIMH Press Release, 13 May 2013. http://www.nimh.nih.gov/news/science-news/2013/dsm-5-and-rdoc-shared-interests.shtml.

Jain, Sumeet, and Sushrut Jadhav. 2009. "Pills That Swallow Policy: Clinical Ethnography of a Community Mental Health Program in Northern India." *Transcultural Psychiatry* 46 (1): 60-85.

Kupfer, David J., Michael B. First, and Darrel A. Regier. 2002. *A Research Agenda for DSM-V*. Washington, D.C.: American Psychiatric Association.

Lock, Margaret. 2001. "The Tempering of Medical Anthropology: Troubling Natural Categories." *Medical Anthropology Quarterly* 15 (4): 478-92.

Lorant, Vincent, Christophe Croux, Scott Weich, Denise Deliège, Johan Mackenbach, and Marc Asseau. 2007. "Depression and Socio-Economic Risk Factors: 7-year Longitudinal Population Study." *The British Journal of Psychiatry* 190 (4): 293-98.

Lovell, Anne M. 2014. "The World Health Organization and the Contested Beginnings of Psychiatric Epidemiology as an International Discipline: One Rope, Many Strands." *International Journal of Epidemiology* 43 (suppl. 1): i6-i18.

Lund, Crick, Mary De Silva, Sophie Plagerson, Sara Cooper, Dan Chisholm, Jishnu Das, Martin Knapp, and Vikram Patel. 2011. "Poverty and Mental Disorders: Breaking the Cycle in Low-Income and Middle-Income Countries." *The Lancet* 378 (9801): 1502-14.

Lupien, L. J., M. Sasseville, N. François, C. E. Giguère, J. Boissonneault, P. Plusquellec, R. Godbout, et al. 2017. "The DSM5/RDoc Debate on the Future of Mental Health Research: Implication for Studies on Human Stress and Presentation of the Signature Bank." *Stress* 20 (1): 2-18.

Marmot, Michael. 2005. "Social Determinants of Health Inequalities." *The Lancet* 365 (9464): 1099-104.

Patel, Vikram. 2014. "Rethinking Mental Health Care: Bridging the Credibility Gap." *Intervention* 12 (1): 15-20.

Patel, Vikram, Shekhar Saxena, Crick Lund, Graham Thornicroft, Florence Baingana, Paul Bolton, Dan Chisholm, et al. 2018. "The Lancet Commission on Global Mental Health and Sustainable Development." *The Lancet* 392 (10157): 1553-98.

Patel, Vikram, and Arthur Kleinman. 2003. "Poverty and Common Mental Disorders in Developing Countries." *Bulletin of the World Health Organization* 81: 609-15.

Patel, Vikram, Mirja Koschorke, and Martin Prince. 2011. "Closing the Treatment Gap." In *Mental Health in Public Health: The Next 100 Years,* edited by Linda B. Cottler, 3-22. Oxford: Oxford University Press.

Prince, Martin, Vikram Patel, Shekhar Saxena, Mario Maj, Joana Maselko, Michael R. Phillips, and Atif Rahman. 2007. "No Health Without Mental Health." *The Lancet* 370 (9590): 859-77.

Romelli, Katia, Alessandra Frigerio, and Monica Colombo. 2016. "DSM Over Time: From Legitimisation of Authority to Hegemony." *BioSocieties* 11 (1): 1-21.

Sax, William S. 2014. "Ritual Healing and Mental Health in India." *Transcultural Psychiatry* 51 (6): 829-49.

Shorter, Edward. 2013. *How Everyone Became Depressed: The Rise and Fall of the Nervous Breakdown.* Oxford: Oxford University Press.

Solomon, Harry C. 1958. "The American Psychiatric Association in Relation to American Psychiatry." *American Journal of Psychiatry* 115 (1): 1-9.

Stein, Dan J., Crick Lund, and Randolph M. Nesse. 2013. "Classification Systems in Psychiatry: Diagnosis and Global Mental Health in the Era of DSM-5 and ICD-11." *Current Opinion in Psychiatry* 26 (5): 493.

Wilkinson, Richard G. 2002. *Unhealthy Societies: The Afflictions of Inequality.* London: Routledge.

Wilkinson, Richard G., and Kate Pickett. 2010. *The Spirit Level: Why Equality is Better for Everyone*. London: Penguin.

World Bank. 1993. *World Development Report 1993: Investing in Health*. New York: Oxford University Press.

World Health Organization. 2001. *Mental Health: New Understanding, New Hope: The World Health Report 2001*. Geneva: World Health Organization.

—. 2008. *mhGAP: Mental Health Gap Action Programme: Scaling up Care for Mental, Neurological, and Substance Use Disorders*. Geneva: World Health Organization.

—. 2013. *Mental Health Action Plan 2013-2020*. Geneva: World Health Organization.

About the Author

STEFAN ECKS co-founded Edinburgh University's Medical Anthropology programme. He teaches social anthropology and directs postgraduate teaching in the School of Social and Political Sciences. He has conducted ethnographic fieldwork in India, Nepal, and the UK. Recent work explores value in global pharmaceutical markets, changing ideas of mental health in South Asia, poverty and access to health care, as well as multimorbidity. His publications *include Eating Drugs: Psychopharmaceutical Pluralism in India* (New York, 2013) and *Living Worth: Value and Values in Global Pharmaceutical Markets* (forthcoming), as well as numerous journal articles on the intersections between health and economics.

3   Schizoid Balinese?

Anthropology's Double Bind: Radical Alterity and Its
Consequences for Schizophrenia

Annette Hornbacher

Abstract

This contribution explores "schizophrenia" as a contested Western discourse fluctuating between biomedical naturalism and anti-psychiatric
cultural relativism. Although the latter was seen as an epistemic coun-
terweight to, and critique of, a modern Western paradigm of normality,
I argue that this alternative is couched in a Eurocentric ideology about
radical alterity that ignores local interpretations along with practices of
social reintegration. I will elucidate this in view of Mead's and Bateson's
interpretation of the allegedly "schizoid" Balinese and its entanglement
with the anti-psychiatric movement, which I will contrast with my
fieldwork in Bali that illustrates how deviant behaviour and dissociation
are integrated in social life via local interpretations and ritual practices.

Keywords: history of psychiatry, schizophrenia, Bali, anthropology, radical
alterity

This contribution analyses "schizophrenia" as a contested Western discourse
fluctuating between a modern, naturalist or biomedical position, on the one
hand, and psychosocial, anti-psychiatric and culturally relativist interpretations on the other. But while the latter were seen as epistemic alternatives
to modern Western paradigms of normality and politics, I argue that this
very "alternative" is part of a Eurocentric discourse opposing biomedical to
psychosocial explanations of radical alterity. In either case, other interpretations of alterity and dissociation, along with practices of social reintegration,
are ignored. I will elucidate this argument by a close reading of Mead's and
Bateson's ethnographic research and interpretation of the exotic – and

---

Sax, William, and Claudia Lang (eds), *The Movement for Global Mental Health: Critical Views
from South and Southeast Asia.* Taylor & Francis Group, 2021
DOI: 10.5117/9789463721622_CH03

allegedly "schizoid" – Balinese and its ambiguous entanglements with both early schizophrenia research and anti-psychiatric theories. In contrast, I conclude with an ethnographic case study from Bali illustrating how deviant behaviour and dissociation can be integrated into social life via local interpretations and ritual practices.

Preliminary Thoughts on Schizophrenia and *the Movement for Global Mental Health*

A diagnosis of schizophrenia refers to a severe mental and behavioural disorder regarded by modern psychiatry as a universal disease affecting people in societies all around the world and therefore assumed to be a natural kind with physiological and genetic causes even though its exact aetiology remains unclear (Walker et al. 2004). This epistemic assumption also informs the medical treatment of schizophrenia with antipsychotic drugs, which are regarded, not as a cure but as an efficient treatment and prevention of psychotic episodes that helps some (but not all) patients to lead a normal life (de Mari et al. 2009). Statistics suggest that 10 per cent of the patients diagnosed with schizophrenia die within a 10-year period, mostly from suicide or the side effects of their medication (e.g. diabetes). Only 25 per cent recover completely.[1]

Despite remaining uncertainties regarding aetiology and the general consensus that schizophrenia is ultimately a complex and multicausal illness with both hereditary and socio-psychological factors, it seems that psychiatry in general and the movement for global mental health (MGMH) in particular favour a biomedical treatment and regard social, political, and cultural circumstances both of schizophrenia and psychiatry itself at most as factors of secondary importance.[2] This assumption has important political, scientific and therapeutic consequences: it suggests above all that the diagnosis of and antipsychotic medication for schizophrenia can and arguably must be applied transculturally because it responds to a universal human nature thus providing the most effective treatment.

1   See the homepage of the World Fellowship of Schizophrenia and Allied Disorders, a grassroots organisation linked to the agenda of the Movement for Global Mental Health. http://world-schizophrenia.org/disorders/schizophrenia.html (Accessed 06 August 2019)

2   Therefore the earliest possible medication with antipsychotic drugs is recommended because it reduces the severity of symptoms. This motivates also attempts to identify – and eventually to medicalise – conditions diagnosed as subthreshold schizophrenia in order to prevent the manifestation of schizophrenia (de Mari et al. 2009).

This conviction – and its ontological implications regarding the nature of the human mind and mental health – also informs the policy of the MGMH, which is based on the claim that low-income countries of the Global South suffer from a psychiatric "treatment gap" especially regarding serious mental disorders like schizophrenia, which involves a lack of proper diagnosis, no access to medical treatment, and the stigmatisation and social exclusion of patients with psychotic or eccentric behaviour. To bridge this gap, MGMH promotes several measures: the adoption of a secular, Western disease model as a universal explanatory framework for mental health, the formation of "community based rehabilitation" (CBR) groups consisting of local social workers and family members, and effective treatment based on antipsychotic drugs (Chatterjee et al. 2003, 58).

In what follows, I will critically examine such ontological implications regarding radical alterity from an anthropological perspective and by analyzing the psychiatric category of "schizophrenia" not as a universal fact but as an evolving and contradictory Western discourse that was shaped, on the one hand, by a physiological disease model, and on the other hand, by early anthropological attempts to explain the radical alterity of Balinese culture.

To reflect upon "schizophrenia" from an anthropological and cultural historical perspective and thus as an emerging discourse rather than a fact is particularly important in view of the universalist and yet reductionist assumptions of the MGMH: the biomedical disease and treatment model of schizophrenia acknowledges mainly the hereditary and neurobiological causation of mental illness but pays scant attention to socio-psychological factors and political or social inequality, which are possibly of much greater significance for recovery and wellbeing, as Tanya Luhrmann has argued. Her research suggests that in the USA, vulnerability to and recovery from schizophrenia is directly correlated to class, race and wealth but not necessarily to drugs.[3]

Moreover, the diagnosis of schizophrenia implies certain assumptions about reality in general and about the human mind in particular, which are not necessarily universal: What counts as a hallucination in a modern Western setting may be regarded as a mystical vision in another cultural or historical context. To impose a universal paradigm for mental health and normality potentially entails epistemic and ontological violence and the exclusion of alterity on different levels.

---

3   She describes a schizophrenic patient who is able to cope with her paranoid delusions after obtaining her own apartment, but without medication: "That apartment was the most effective antipsychotic she had ever taken" (2012, 28).

It is not only anthropologists who have expressed their concerns but also philosophers. Whereas Luhrmann emphasises the importance of social and economic factors rather than purely biological explanations of schizophrenia, philosophers like Foucault, Hacking, and Deleuze and Guattari have criticised modern Western categories of mental illness – especially schizophrenia – for more theoretical and epistemological reasons, arguing that the diagnosis is part of a political attempt to "normalize" radical alterity by treating it as a pathological individual deviance that must be corrected by the modern disciplinary society (Foucault 1975, Szasz 1976), or of a sociopolitical "looping" process, in which diagnostic categories cum practices do not represent but rather interactively create the human kinds and disease entities they presume (Hacking 1995).

A similar political and epistemological critique informed the anti-psychiatry movement of the 1960s and 70s. Interestingly, such criticism seems to have almost disappeared since the 1980s, under the powerful influence of "the factual", in this case, the development of new antipsychotic drugs influencing the function of neurotransmitters, and making it possible to interrupt psychotic episodes rather than merely sedating patients with tranquilisers (Harrington 2019,116). But the fact that strong neuroleptics are able to influence some of the symptoms of some patients efficiently – albeit at the cost of severe side effects – tells us nothing about its causation, and certainly does not prove that schizophrenia is a natural kind. Such unresolved epistemic problems have led to a fundamental critique of the nosological concept of schizophrenia and to the suggestion that it should be replaced with the concept of "psychotic spectrum disorder" (van Os 2016; Guloksuz and van Os 2017). Although this may be a suitable response to the epistemic problems of schizophrenia as a nosological category, it is unlikely to change the medicalisation of symptoms formerly classified as "schizophrenia".

In my discussion below, I do not defend social versus biological aetiologies or nosological categories, rather I take a strictly anthropological view by looking at "schizophrenia" as the centre of a contested multidisciplinary Western discourse, in which the boundaries between acceptable and non-acceptable deviance – or the radical alterity of human mind and behaviour – are defined, maintained and established on local and increasingly international scales, for example by the MGMH.

I will begin my analysis by elucidating the ontological and epistemological implications and therapeutic consequences of these two rival interpretations by summarising a discourse that emerges from the opposition of a psychiatric disease model of schizophrenia and its psycho-social critique. Whereas the nosological category of schizophrenia seems to represent – and to globally impose – an exclusively Western system of psychiatric thought (Guloksuz and van Os 2017, 238) I argue that it emerges from a discourse that has been strongly influenced by the anthropological encounter with cultural alterity. This applies particularly to the critique of the psychiatric disease model inspired by Gregory Bateson's "double bind theory" that was immensely influential for anti-psychiatry in the 60s and 70s, and still receives attention. But closer examination shows that this first socio-psychological aetiology for schizophrenia is actually based on the ethnographic work of Bateson's ex-wife Margret Mead's wo developed her theory of the "schizoid" "Balinese Character" more than ten years earlier.

> In the historical context of anti-psychiatry – and as part of a new and critical discourse about psychiatric normalisation and alterity – Michel Foucault developed his theory that the humanities contribute to the normalisation and medicalisation of deviance and madness because they presume a universal and identical human subject, whereas anthropology offers the unique opportunity to think radical alterity in the other's terms and is therefore a "contre-science' (Foucault 1966, 392).

But what would that mean, and does it apply to Mead's and Bateson's ethnographic theory about 'the' Balinese? How did anthropology contribute to the discourse about schizophrenia, and how could it open new horizons regarding the social response to radical alterity?

In my close reading of their work on Bali, I will argue that although Mead and Bateson introduced a socio-psychological aetiology of schizophrenia as a critique of the physiological disease model, their interpretation is also couched in a Eurocentric ontology and anthropology without taking Balinese thoughts about dissociation, mental health and the human mind into serious consideration. In this sense, Bateson and Mead missed a genuinely anthropological chance to develop the "contre-science" envisioned by Foucault, which in this case would have opened a more diverse, transcultural – and in that sense global – perspective on radical alterity, mental health, madness and healing, as I will show in view of an example from my own fieldwork in Bali.

Mental Health Between Clairvoyance, Disease and Social Resistance – the Emergence of 'Schizophrenia' in European History

The introduction of the new nosological category "schizophrenia" was a pathbreaking step in the history of early psychiatry. The Swiss psychiatrist

Eugen Bleuler coined the term in 1908, and slowly it came to replace Emil
Kraepelin's earlier concept of "dementia praecox" (Bleuler 1911; Aderibigbe
et al. 1999, 339 f.). Both concepts refer to a syndrome consisting of severe
cognitive, affective and behavioural disorders, and both were used interchangeably for some time – as Margret Mead's work shows – even though the
assemblages of symptoms as well as the prognosis described by Kraepelin
and Bleuler differ significantly. Kraepelin regarded dementia praecox as
the final and irreversible stage of a disease that – in his understanding – affected the human brain, and led to a range of different symptoms including
complete withdrawal from reality, flattening of emotions, catatonia, and
hallucinations. Bleuler on his part differentiated various forms of schizophrenia, distinguished primary from secondary symptoms, and regarded
hallucinations only as secondary symptoms that may or may not occur
(Aderibigbe et al.1999, 340). Moreover, he was more optimistic regarding a
possible recovery from schizophrenia than Kraepelin was with regard to
dementia praecox.

In any case, both terms combine sets of very different symptoms into a
single category, defined as a natural disease entity which has one significant
common denominator: All of these various symptoms contradict enlightenment ideals of universal human reason, individual freedom, and subjective
identity. Persons diagnosed with "dementia praecox" or "schizophrenia"
seem to lose – at some point of their biography – the genuinely human
ability of reasonable thought, adequate communication, and a consistent
sense of self along with the capacity for emotional self-regulation. Moreover,
they seem unable to distinguish objective reality from internal fantasy,
and they withdraw from a shared sociocultural reality into idiosyncratic
dissociative states and/or paranoid ideas. The creation of this new disease
entity can thus be regarded as a specifically modern attempt to deal with
radical alterity in a rational secular society – by pathologising it.

But although the assertion that these heterogenous symptoms were
indicators of a single disease was new, some of them had formerly been
described in religious and moralistic terms. This led – as Foucault and
others have shown – to disciplinary measures and behavioural control in
different types of asylums or "discipline-, work- and madhouses" that were
fundamental for the treatment of deviant people during the eighteenth and
nineteenth century (Foucault 1961, 1975; Schott and Tölle 2006, 437). But
there were even older – religious – interpretations that, until the nineteenth
century, coexisted with the moralistic and rational enlightenment paradigm
of discipline and self-control. A famous example is the German physician
Justinus Kerner, a widely respected scientist in his day, who was open to

the self-understanding of his patient Friederike Hauffe as a clairvoyant communicating with the "spiritual world" (Kerner 1829). However, soon after Kerner's death such ideas were dismissed by psychologists and psychiatrists who re-interpreted his detailed case study as a result of self-deception, as a "widely accepted" belief in Germany or as a side effect of his patient's malnutrition, thereby supporting the physiological disease model of modern psychiatry (Podmore 1909, 2005 ff.; Falzeder 2018).

At about the same time, the German psychiatrist Kraepelin in Heidelberg was promoting the idea that mental diseases were universal, physiological "disease entities" with as yet unidentified neurological causes. He developed this hypothesis both on the basis of intercultural comparison with Java, which he had visited (Leitner 2014), and in analogy with the physiological brain damage caused by syphilitic paresis (*dementia paralytica*), which had been discovered in 1822 and became in many ways the paradigm for mental disorders in early psychiatry: As Szasz (1976) reminds us, before the advent of penicillin, 20 to 30 per cent of patients in mental hospitals suffered from neurosyphilis, and Kraepelin was looking for similar relations between physiological brain degeneration and cognitive or behavioural disorders. He was passionately against psychoanalysis and in favour of a universalist physiological disease model of dementia praecox because he believed that the identification of the physiological causes was only a matter of time (Read 2013, 21). But since the aetiology of the disease that he believed to have found remained unclear, it was hardly possible to develop an effective therapy. This was perhaps not a major problem for Kraepelin, for whom dementia praecox was an irreversible and final state of physiological degeneration. In fact, when certain cases diagnosed as "dementia praecox" later showed improvement, Kraepelin simply pronounced the diagnosis false (Read 2013, 22).

Kraepelin's Swiss colleague Bleuler was initially more open with regard to psychoanalysis and certainly more optimistic regarding the prognosis and treatment of schizophrenia, but still his therapies were little more than attempts to make patients docile and obedient. This meant in the first place that patients had to adopt the disease model and to accept that they were ill rather than insisting on their delusions or defending their eccentric behaviour as a normal reaction to "stimuli and irritations of their environment", which seems to have happened so often that Bleuler mentions the rejection of the disease model as a symptom of the disease that he believed he had discovered (1950, 257; cf. Read 2013, 31). In other words, it seems that for the restoration of mental health the adoption of the psychiatric disease model was a necessary and the restoration of normal behaviour a sufficient condition.

This epistemic and behavioural normalisation was enforced with dubious methods like incarceration, prolonged baths, enforced bed rest, and, if patients showed no compliance, sedative drugs like veronal, or drugs that artificially induced vomiting. Bleuler did not claim that this was a form of healing, but rather understood his treatment as a disciplinary intervention that made "negativistic patients appear more docile and obey medical rules" (ibid., 31-32).

Such iatrogenic cruelty and the gap between the weakness of psychiatric theory and aetiology on the one hand, and the violence of its therapy on the other, provoked political and ethical criticism, especially from the 1960s onward, where schizophrenia became a transdisciplinary topic for critical psychiatrists, anthropologists and philosophers. Psychiatrists who were directly confronted with the therapeutic shortcomings of sedation and enforced hospitalisation began to re-examine the epistemic basis of Kraepelin's and Bleuler's model of schizophrenia and tried to relocate the biomedical diagnosis and nosology in a sociopolitical context.

The fundamental epistemological critique of the naturalised disease model emerges from the argument that it is impossible to identify schizophrenia, or for that matter any disease, on the basis of a collection of random symptoms, none of which indicates mental health or illness per se: The perception of immaterial agents for instance can either be understood as a religious belief, a mystical experience, or simply a delusion and hallucination of the patient, the difference depending solely on the dominant ontological assumptions of a given social context. And since the relation between symptoms and causation remains unclear, and biological markers turn out to be unreliable, the term schizophrenia remains contested within psychiatry until today, where some believe to have found genetic or biomarkers while others – like Szasz (1976, 311) and most recently van Os – are convinced that "schizophrenia" does not even exist (Guloksuz and Van Os 2018).

Such nosological uncertainties have diagnostic consequences, as is shown by a study where, confronted with a detailed symptom description of a patient, 69 per cent of a group of American psychiatrists diagnosed "schizophrenic" whereas only 2 per cent of a British group of psychiatrists did so (Read 2013, 48).[4]

And yet, the MGMH presumes that an early and reliable diagnosis is possible and has to be made available for everyone.

---

4   Another meta-analysis shows, moreover, a significant interrelation between groups of migrants and the incidence of schizophrenia, which suggests that migration itself affects rates of schizophrenia and is thus directly opposed to the genetic disease model (Pérez-Alvarez et al. 2016, 9).

In the 1960s, such inconsistencies were related to a discursive paradigm shift concerning schizophrenia. Foucault (1961, 1975) investigated the historical and cultural relativity of normality and madness, reason and un-reason as an epiphenomenon of social, political and epistemic power relations aiming at the exclusion or normalisation of the "other". At that point schizophrenia became a matter of political concern and a topic of interdisciplinary discussion among philosophers and critical psychiatrists from the anti-psychiatry movement. Its central figures like the psychiatrists Szasz, Cooper, and Laing argued against the idea of a natural disease entity, claiming that "schizophrenia" had become the "panchreston" – that is, a catchall explanation – of madness but was in fact a "myth" (Szasz 1960). The Marxist psychiatrist David Cooper argued that the very category of schizophrenia as a natural disease entity was untenable and suggested a reinterpretation in the context of its social environment as a "micro-social" crisis situation in which an individual is denied his or her perceptions and at some point declared as insane by the group (1967, 14). In his opinion, it was not the incarcerated patient but rather his social environment that was the problem.

Thus, during the 1960s and 1970s the discourse of schizophrenia had shifted from pathologisation and medicalisation to a discussion of epistemic and sociopolitical problems and an analysis of the obscure connections between nosology and power. Philosophers as well as anti-psychiatrists emphasised the political aspect, not only in the diagnosis of schizophrenia but also in its therapy, since they saw the psychiatrist as the state's incarcerating agent.

This was particularly obvious regarding the instrumentalisation of the psychiatric disease model in totalitarian systems like Nazi Germany and the Soviet Union, but eugenic programmes and compulsory sterilisation for the "feeble-minded" and mentally degenerated were not an invention of totalitarian states but originated as a scientific conviction in American democracy (Harrington 2019, 49-51). Eugenic programmes were launched by some US states around 1907, and similar laws were passed in Norway, Denmark and Sweden during the 1930s before they reached their horrendous apex in the National socialist laws for *Rassenhygiene* or "racial health", which included the euthanasia of people with hereditary diseases (Masson 2013, 35f.).

Ethical problems emerge thus as a structural side effect of the biological disease model of schizophrenia and are by no means only restricted to psychiatry in totalitarian regimes:[5] It seems that the axiomatic assumption

5   To avoid such detrimental effects from the biological diagnosis, health ministries in some East Asian countries like Japan and Hong Kong have therefore replaced the term "schizophrenia"

of schizophrenia as a hereditary and physiological disease entity distorts human perception in democracies as well, as the Rosenhahn experiment during the 1970s suggests (Rosenhahn 1973). Completely sane people who falsely claimed to experience hallucinations were hospitalised and then systematically depersonalised, ignored, and repressed in American mental hospitals because the staff was unable to distinguish them from "truly disturbed" patients and to judge their sanity or insanity on the grounds of their actual behaviour. The axiomatic assumption that they suffered from an incurable disease led to their extended hospitalisation even though, after hospitalisation, they had stopped pretending to hallucinate, and did not show any deviant behaviour. Moreover, even when the staff was informed that some of their patients were actually sane they were unable to identify which ones they were, and when the pseudo-patients were discharged they were never diagnosed as "healed" but only as "symptom free" because schizophrenia had been defined since the time of Kraepelin as an incurable disease. A similar circular or totalitarian logic – with more serious consequences – had already informed Bleuler's consideration that it might be better to inject emetics to stop agitated patients because it was better to make them suffer than to annoy an entire roomful of other patients (in Read 2013, 32). Beyond that, Bleuler defended eugenic programmes and considered euthanasia an ethical option for certain schizophrenic patients because it would, as he saw it, reduce their incurable suffering.

This short summary may suffice to illustrate that the universal biological disease model of schizophrenia is not only based on problematic epistemological assumptions, but also associated with questionable therapeutic consequences, which provoked the critiques of anti-psychiatrists and philosophers who analysed the political and social power relations behind – and below – the disease model of schizophrenia and suggested its reinterpretation in social, economic and political terms.

The philosopher-psychiatrist team Deleuze and Guattari was quite explicit in this regard when they theorised "the Schizo" as no longer a deviant individual but as the paradigmatic rebel against the capitalist system and its control of human desire. Similar ideas inspired the perhaps most radical therapeutic experiment in this regard: the formation of a revolutionary "socialist patient's collective" in 1970 by the psychiatrist Wolfgang Huber at the same psychiatric university hospital in Heidelberg where Kraepelin had

---

with "psychotic syndrome" because in cultures informed by shame, the diagnosis of a hereditary mental disease is connected to stigmatisation and interpreted as a tacit recommendation for suicide. (See van Os: https://www.spektrum.de/news/schizophrenie-gibt-es-nicht/1682902)

developed his disease model of dementia praecox eighty years previously. In sharp contrast to his naturalistic predecessor, Huber and his patients understood schizophrenia as "weapon" in a collective fight against the capitalist class society that was identified as the cause of mental suffering. Yet the experiment failed, even though the University appointed a committee of three experts, who recommended giving the programme qualified support. Evidently this was not what was wanted – perhaps because the group was falsely associated with the Baader-Meinhof Gang – and the medical faculty presented its own set of negative evaluations, which provided the hoped-for results. After heated discussions the patient's collective was dissolved by the police and Huber arrested for illegal possession of weapons (Böhlich 1972; Spandler 1995).

This political appropriation of mental suffering was certainly a rare exception which has to be seen in the wider context of a critical political discourse that affected many Western societies during the cold war and involved a radical change in former paradigms of legitimate power, authority and authoritarian education.

Yet it would seem that the discursive shift from investigating "schizophrenia" as an individual disease to a politically engaged analysis of its social context was only a temporary intermezzo that did not lead to a paradigm shift in psychiatric research, but was later dismissed as a form of "social romanticism" (Arenz 2008, 11) and ignored in favour of a new neurobiological approach to schizophrenia (Luhrmann 2007). This may be related – as some US scholars have argued – to the disillusion or even to the collective embarrassment of American psychiatry following awareness of the immense damage that had been done in the name of one of its most prominent tropes: the "schizophrenogenic mother" (Fromm-Reichmann 1948),[6] which was related to the psychoanalytical influence on US psychiatry and dominated the field during the 1950s and 1960s until a critical restudy in 1982 (Johnston 2013, 802). But as Johnston emphasises, the critique of this simplistic psychoanalytical model does not mean that social relations and parenting play no role for the mental health of the children and adults but rather that entire family systems need help and not just the symptom bearing child. Yet she observes that psychotherapeutic treatment has consistently declined while a purely pharmaceutical-based therapy has become more

---

6   It is worth noticing that Frieda Fromm-Reichmann for her part came to the USA as a German refugee who had previously worked at the Frankfurt psychoanalytical institute as a colleague of the sociologist Horkheimer, and that both saw mental illness as aspect of larger sociopolitical dynamics (Hartwell 1996, 277).

prominent, as statistical data from the USA between 1998 and 2007 suggest (Johnston 2013, 803).

A decisive aspect in this process of depoliticisation was the development and marketing of new antipsychotic medications that were made available during the 1970s and responded to one of the major challenges of anti-psychiatry: After decades of mere sedation, these new drugs were able to influence key symptoms of psychosis thus making it possible to release patients from enforced hospitalisation.[7] This development and, more recently, new possibilities for brain imaging and attempts to identify sub-threshold schizophrenia via hereditary factors and bio markers indicate, on the one hand, a new shift toward a neurobiological disease paradigm and increasing medicalisation, and on the other hand the decrease of psychoanalytical or psychological therapies that Johnson observes and that goes together with the marginalisation of a politically sensitised and culture critical examination of mental health in modern Western societies – as opposed to alternatives.

This corresponds to a de-politicised disease model that provides treatment for individuals who are expected to adjust to a given society rather than changing it, and it is this paradigm of medicalisation cum social integration that informs also the global mental health politics and its attempt to bridge the "treatment gap" in low income countries of the global South.

Pasung and the Movement for Global Mental Health from a Balinese Perspective

To understand why clinicians and patients not only in the Global North, but in the Global South as well, are in favour of this disease model, thus embracing (at least implicitly) the theory and policy of the MGMH, it is helpful to take a look at the Indonesian island of Bali.

Paradigmatic for the implementation of global mental health politics is the current campaign of the renowned Balinese psychiatrist Prof. Dr. Luh Ketut Suryani for the institutionalisation of psychiatric treatment and particularly for the treatment of Indonesians diagnosed with schizophrenia. Suryani complains that the Indonesian medical system does not support patients with mental illness, especially those with schizophrenia. Their

---

7   It is important to note that the influence of drugs like Haloperidol is limited to the psychotic symptoms of schizophrenia, but does not alleviate other symptoms such as lack of motivation or interpersonal problems, which might cause much more personal suffering (Harrington 2019, 116).

suffering is simply ignored even though the latest data of the Indonesian Basic Health Research suggest that Bali is the Indonesian province with the highest incidence of schizophrenia, and similar observations have been made regarding a high incidence of suicides.[8] Suryani complains that patients who are unable to adjust to social rules are stigmatised and left in the custody of overburdened and psychologically untrained family members and local healers because there is only a handful of psychiatrists for four million of Balinese. As a consequence, families rely often on the method of *pasung*: They chain their deviant family members in the house or lock them in cages for years and neglect them, often in miserable and inhuman conditions, sometimes until they die. I was told that similar practices are also reported in Java and other islands.[9] Suryani and her *Institute for Global Mental Health* discovered such cases while she was doing a first epidemiological survey on the number of mentally ill people in Bali. Since then she has regularly sought to intervene by freeing patients from chains so as to avoid extended periods of hospitalisation, and reintegrating them into social life by providing antipsychotic medication. According to her estimation, there are dozens if not hundreds of Balinese chained by their families, and hundreds or perhaps thousands of mentally ill people who are left without support from the official medical system, a number that may be growing, as the increasing suicide rate on the island suggests.[10] To change this situation, Suryani tries to convince families practicing *pasung* to accept antipsychotic medication, which she offers free of cost, mainly with the help of funding from Europe. She regards this medicalisation as the mainstay of biological treatment of schizophrenia but combines it with social and cultural reintegration, and local ideas of harmony and spirituality or meditation. To realise a local version of global mental health, Suryani trains social workers and physicians, establishes community-based intervention, offers a combination of medicalisation spiritual and social treatment and, last but not least, tries to raise political and global awareness by cooperating with groups of international scholars and national and international media, launching documentaries and photo exhibitions in Bali and Europe about the inhuman practice of *pasung*.[11]

8   https://www.facebook.com/pg/suryaniinstitute/posts/?ref=page_internal. Accessed 10 August 2019.

9   Personal communication, Dr. Agus Mahar, Javanese psychiatrist. August 2019.

10   For more information see: Hornbacher 2013.

11   http://www.suryani-institute.com/our-programs/ Accessed 10 August 2019.
http://www.suryani-institute.com/in-the-media/ Accessed 10 August 2019.

Obviously, Suryani's *Institute for Mental Health* embraces some of the core ideas and treatment schemes of the MGMH regarding schizophrenia, which she too regards as a universal disease that in many cases requires long-term treatment with antipsychotic drugs. This connection between schizophrenic patients and injections of antipsychotics is also propagated with several photos on the *Facebook* account of her Institute for Mental Health. But her ultimate goal is the integration of medication, Balinese culture, and spiritual techniques, for example by combining local purification rituals with antipsychotic medication.

But despite her efforts to reconcile local and global ideas and therapies in a "biopsychospiritsociocultural approach" as a Facebook post from 9 February 2018 calls it, Suryani leaves no doubt that in her understanding, the key element for a successful therapy for schizophrenia is neither rituals nor meditation but antipsychotics as a precondition for socially reintegrating of people who would be chained up without them. The rituals which are of crucial importance for her patients and families seem to represent the symbolic framework of Balinese culture in contrast to the actually effective drugs.[12] Accordingly, she insists that even though her Balinese patients tend to treat her as a healer or priest, she regards herself as a psychiatrist in the modern sense.[13] Thus, for her, the combination of rituals and drugs does not represent a symmetrical but rather a hierarchical relation between incommensurable ontologies and epistemic fields, because it distinguishes a symbolic set of ritual actions and cultural values and traditions from universally effective pharmaceutical treatment.

The beneficial effects of Suryani's work and her sociopolitical campaigning are obvious, especially for patients who have been living under terrible conditions when families could not cope with their disobedient members. In this regard, her campaign is paradigmatic of the benefits of a culture-sensitive psychiatry. And yet, it leaves important questions unanswered. For example, a documentary showing her efforts to release patients from their chains does not ask whether the practice of *pasung* is always a response to schizophrenia or perhaps sometimes to other forms of social disobedience as well. Nor does it explain whose diagnosis led to the incarceration. Could it be that rebellious family members were also chained? Would that explain why some families reject free medical treatment for those whom they have chained? Moreover, antipsychotic medication is not always linked to success stories, as I learned during my conversation with Prof. Suryani

12   https://www.facebook.com/suryaniinstitute/ Accessed 10 August 2019.
13   Personal communication, September 2016.

in 2016. Some of the patients whom she had freed from their chains refused to continue with the medication after a while because they felt alienated from themselves or suffered from its side effects, and this is reminiscent of what some Western patients report.

It is well known that antipsychotics have serious neurological and emotional side effects that involve further suffering and may lead to secondary diseases, as the statistically significant compensatory alcohol abuse of medicalised patients with schizophrenia shows (Walker et al. 2004; Seemann 2006, 368; see also Harrington 2019, 117). The existence of such side effects makes it difficult to see antipsychotics as an optimal form of therapy, and in any case few people would claim that such drugs "heal" mental disorders. In other words, it is important not to confuse the effect of these drugs on psychotic episodes with healing, or to regard them as an answer to the still open question of aetiology. If Bali does indeed have higher rates of suicide and schizophrenia than other Indonesian islands, as Suryani and others have found, this suggests reconsidering the role of local social factors rather than imposing a universalist biomedical paradigm of mental disease and therapy.

It is worth remembering at this point that the MGMH involves not only a set of new therapeutic options but also and primarily a universalist epistemic regime which involves reality assumptions and creates power relations and hierarchies even as it denies their existence, just as Foucault reminded us, by marginalising alternative interpretations of the human soul and subordinating other paradigms of healing. Such ontological and epistemic power hierarchies are a constitutive aspect of the neurobiological disease model with its claims to universality, a model that is not easily overcome, even for Suryani who is trying to combine Balinese traditions with biomedical treatment schemes. But whereas the idea of combining the different traditions sounds convincing in theory, in practice it involves the subordination not only of rituals but also of the ontological assumptions that make them convincing (Sax 2014): for example the assumption that there are non-human agents who cause what psychiatrists call the "florid" behaviour of humans.

Such differences cannot always be reconciled, and this leads in practice rather to subordination than to a symmetrical integration of different ontologies and healers, as I understood during my fieldwork in East Bali. I have worked for years with a healer-priest, a Jero Balian, who told me that he had been invited to Suryani's *Institute for Global Mental Health* but refused, after a long discussion with her assistants, to cooperate, because he felt that his perspective on mental healing – which involved witchcraft and spirits – was not sufficiently respected. This seemed evident to him for two reasons: First of all, he thought that although one of Suryani's assistants was afflicted by witchcraft – according to his diagnosis – he did not receive adequate help from the Institute. Second, Suryani had not come to invite him personally, which indicated that she did not take his diagnostic system seriously. Thus, even though he regularly performs purification rituals and exorcisms for mentally and physically afflicted people who are disturbed by black magic and spirits, this healer was hesitant to go to Denpasar just in order to subordinate his expertise to the programme of the *Institute for Global Mental Health*.

Anthropology in the Psycho-Social Interpretation of "Schizophrenia"

These glimpses of a shifting debate about causes and therapies suggest that schizophrenia was, from the outset, much more than a psychiatric condition or a natural disease. It reveals a contested transdisciplinary – and transcultural – discourse in which a modern secular society defines the limits of and rules for normal subjectivity and acceptable alterity against the backdrop of religious, mystical and moralistic ideas about human beings which are potentially open to manifestations of non-human agents.

What is at stake in this discourse is therefore not only therapies for a universal disease but also the defence of a secular modern anthropology and ontology that allows for only two interpretations of radical alterity: a physiological disease model based on brain damage, genetics and neurobiological factors, or a social explanation of psychological deviance. Spiritual or religious interpretations simply cannot be thought within the limits of this secular discourse about schizophrenia, they are no longer "dans le vrai" as Canguilhem (1988, 46) put it. Within the "truth" of this modern discourse are social interpretations of schizophrenia that have assumed a critical stance against the universalistic biomedical disease model because they reflect the social and political power relations that inform the diagnosis and treatment.

But what about radically different concepts of the human being which include different ideas about madness and mental health and may be irreconcilable with the powerful modern paradigm of mental health – as the example of the Balinese healer suggests? This brings me back to the initial question of anthropology and its specific role within the discursive field of schizophrenia. I have argued that psychiatry and anthropology are comparable insofar as both deal with the radical alterity of human thought and behaviour albeit in different and even contradictory ways. Whereas psychiatry tries to normalise a behavioural, cognitive, and emotional alterity regarded as individual disease, anthropology tries to understand the alterity of sociocultural realities in its own terms and by analysing the internal logic of radically different lifeworlds. But sometimes boundaries and roles are blurred as early anthropological attempts show that describe shamanism as "Arctic Hysteria", "psychosis", or schizophrenia on the basis of Western disease models and psychology (Bogoras 1909; Silverman 1967, Mitrani 1992). On the other hand, proponents of sociopolitical and socio-psychological explanations draw on ethnographic examples to emphasise the cultural relativity of normality standards and for that matter of symptoms. This applies also to the critical discourse of schizophrenia.

It is a little known but significant fact that David Cooper's anti-psychiatric critique of the disease model and his reinterpretation of schizophrenia as a "microsocial crisis" was directly influenced by anthropological research via the "double bind" theory, which the anthropologist Gregory Bateson, together with Jackson, Healy, and Weakland published as an alternative theory of schizophrenia in an influential article in 1956. Bateson offered a socio-psychological interpretation of the nature and aetiology of schizo-phrenia, hypothesising that schizophrenia is not an individual disease with internal or neurological causes, but the expression of an unresolvable cognitive and emotional conflict emerging from ambivalent communica-tion patterns in intense and dependent social relationships (Bateson et al. 1956, 251). This applies paradigmatically to the relation between mother and child, but it can also include entire family systems "victimizing" one member. The double bind theory draws on psychoanalytical explanations of repressed motives of communication, but it argues against a strictly Freudian approach by claiming that schizoid behaviour is not caused by one traumatic childhood event but is the manifestation of a repetitive pattern of distorted communication in intense relationships. The distortion happens when contradictory messages and orders are simultaneously delivered on different scales of communication, confronting a person with an aporetic situation because explicit verbal messages are contradicted by metalin-guistic messages including gestures and tones of voice, which are crucial for understanding utterances. Moreover, in double-bind relationships, the victim is punished if he or she dares to address the contradiction explicitly, which leads to an irresolvable cognitive and emotional dissonance. A victim in a double bind relationship can either defend his or her percep-tions and feelings, or s/he can defend the relationship by giving up his/ her own feelings. Such communicative dilemmas lead to disorientation, confusion, anger, and panic, and the more often they occur the greater are these negative emotions so that, according to Bateson, they may even lead to psychotic breakdowns or other symptoms of schizophrenia, such as hallucinations and complete emotional withdrawal or dissociation from one's own authentic perceptions and feelings in an attempt to preserve the relationship. From the perspective of this theory, it is not the psychotic individual who is schizoid but the relationship itself, the communicative network, in which s/he is trapped.

It is not surprising that Cooper refers repeatedly to the double bind theory to explain why, in his understanding as well, patients with schizophrenia are not suffering from an individual illness but from a distorted pattern of social interaction, usually within the family (1970, 57). Moreover, this interpretation of schizophrenia as the effect of a micro-social environment is based on an ultimately anthropological method that Cooper adopts from Bateson: Rather than observing the weird behaviour or describing the symptoms of the schizophrenic, he recommends the detailed "participant observation" of entire family interactions and especially the analysis of metalinguistic messages. In other words, he replaces the distant and controlling psychiatric gaze at a mad individual with the classical anthropological participation of a social situation observed from "the inside", and shows how the psychotic patient is confronted with and reacts to a communicative dilemma (ibid., 63). But shifting from an observation of the patient to "participant observation" within the family situation is only one aspect of the influence of anthropology on the anti-psychiatric reframing of schizophrenia. Closer inspection reveals that Bateson's new aetiology is the direct result and application of a groundbreaking ethnographic research in Bali in which he was involved.

Schizoid Balinese? An Anthropological Double Bind Theorised

Even though Bateson does not mention the ethnographic sources for his new theory of schizophrenia, there is no doubt that it is directly related to former fieldwork on Bali. His hypothesis that ambivalent social communication triggers anger, panic, and eventually emotional withdrawal is obviously an extension of an earlier work to which he contributed: The seminal ethnography *Balinese Character*, co-authored by Bateson and his then wife, the anthropologist Margret Mead, and published in 1942. The couple conducted more than a year of fieldwork at various periods between 1936 and 1938 on the island of Bali, and although Bateson did not write the ethnography, he contributed substantially to it with dozens of photographs providing evidence for Mead's theoretical claims. The monograph is remarkable in several respects: It is the first ethnography of Bali, and it links basic aspects of family life, spatial orientation, embodied learning, ritual drama, and dissociation with mother-child interactions. Beyond that, it introduces a new form of presentation. Dissatisfied with the translation of local concepts in Western terms and critical of the description of "culture" as a set of norms and rules, Mead was trying to grasp the process of acculturation or embodiment, for example in childrearing practices, and she decided that photographs were able to show the interaction of people more clearly than statements. She and Bateson used series of photographs to depict the spoken and tacit information conveyed by social interaction, an approach that can also be understood as the first example of visual anthropology (Jacknis 1988). The book combines a relatively short text in which Mead explains basic features of Balinese society and socialisation with Bateson's photograph series illustrating Mead's psychoanalytical thesis that Balinese mother-child interactions lead to a culture-specific Balinese character.

Both anthropologists contributed with this work to seminal theories of their time: Bateson's double bind theory inspired family therapy and anti-psychiatry, Mead's ethnography was a major contribution to the "Culture and Personality School" that she developed with Ruth Benedict, combining psychoanalysis and participant observation which befitted Mead's academic training in psychology. The Culture and Personality School was prominent in the US anthropology between the two world wars and investigated the interrelation of cultural values and ideas on the one hand, and individual psychological patterns, on the other claiming that cultures develop characteristic personality traits. Other influential proponents were former students of the cultural relativist Franz Boas such as Mead's friend Ruth Benedict who analysed the character patterns of selected tribal cultures such as the Zuni and the Kwakiutl in Nietzsche's terms as "apollonian" and "dyonisian". Her book *Patterns of Culture*, which was released shortly before Mead started her fieldwork in Bali, was inspirational for Mead, but Benedict's later work shows also the limits and dangers of this theoretical framework: She wrote her last work on the Japanese character during the Second World War and at the invitation of the American Office of War Information in order to make the "enemy" more predictable for the government. But whereas, owing to the circumstances of war, Benedict had to rely on media, historical sources and interviews with Japanese Americans or war prisoners, Mead was lucky enough to conduct fieldwork in pre-war Bali. She was convinced that Balinese culture and personality differed from Western society more radically than any other, and she ascribed this alterity to the culture-specific "schizoid" personality of the Balinese in general (Bateson and Mead 1942, xvi). From an anthropological perspective, this diagnosis seems contradictory and disturbing because it attributes symptoms of a severe mental disorder to a well-functioning and resilient society that was described by other travellers of that time as one of the happiest they had seen: Why would an anthropologist trained in cultural relativism interpret an entire society in terms of a Western illness category in the first place?

An examination of Mead's research plans during the mid-1930s suggests rather profane reasons: After her fieldwork in Samoa and Papua New Guinea Mead was seeking funds for a research project in yet-unspecified field sites about the development of character and became aware of Bali after she learned about the exotic phenomena of trance possession for which Balinese rituals were notorious (Sullivan 1989, 67). But a second coincidence was perhaps even more decisive for her decision to do her research in Bali. In the same year (1935), she was approached by the American "Committee for Research in Dementia Praecox", a newly founded branch of the institute for mental hygiene that was formed to explore the unknown aetiology of the final stage of "Schizophrenia" (Sullivan 1998, 72f.). More research regarding the causes of this disease was thought to be urgently necessary because the USA faced a dramatically growing number of schizophrenia diagnoses during the 1920s and 1930s. The new mental disease was regarded as incurable, which involved the threat of expensive and time consuming care for which the US health system was not prepared. Statistics show that during those years 50 per cent of the beds in mental hospitals were occupied with patients diagnosed with dementia praecox, which became a major economic threat for the public health system (Sullivan 1989, 75). The identification of possible social or socio-psychological factors other than a merely hereditary or biological aetiology was thus promising for both therapeutic and economic reasons: it would have offered new possibilities for treatment, and these might well be cheaper. At any rate, it would be much less expensive to send patients home than to keep them in hospitals for the rest of their lives.

For her part, Margaret Mead was not only seeking to obtain funding for a new research project, she was also eager to prove the practical use and scientific value of anthropological research, and during a conversation with Nolan Lewis, the research coordinator of the "Committee of Research in Dementia Praecox", she convinced him that she would be able to make an important contribution for the solution of this problem (Lewis 1936; 99). He was obviously thrilled by the prospect of evaluating the hereditary, cultural, and individual aspects of "mental disorder" (Sullivan 1989, 73). In her introduction to *Balinese Character* Mead emphasises this pragmatic dimension of her ethnographic fieldwork and the radical alterity of Bali quite frankly:

> Balinese culture is in many ways less like our own than any other which has yet been reported. It is also a culture in which the ordinary adjustment of the individual approximates in form the sort of maladjustment which, in our own cultural setting, we call schizoid. As the toll of dementia praecox in our own population continues to rise, it becomes increasingly important to us to know the bases in childhood experience which predispose to this condition[.] (Mead and Bateson 1942, xvi)

Lewis encouraged Mead and Benedict to submit proposals for an anthropological study pertinent to the development of schizophrenia. Most likely, the suggestion that there were lavish funds available convinced her to abandon her former research plans and to shift her interest to Bali as the ideal place to investigate the cultural preconditions of schizophrenia, and that is what she did (ibid., 72). It turned out however, that the "Committee of Research in Dementia Praecox" was not as convinced of the benefits of anthropological research as Lewis, and the money granted to Mead and her husband Bateson was ultimately much less than she had expected, but still enough for a small team of scholars and advanced students.

Since both of them were anxious to contribute to a socio-psychological explanation of schizophrenia, the research goal and analytical terminology was from the outset based on Western psychiatric categories and informed by a modern Western paradigm of mental health, which none of them ever questioned or reflected. In other words, their "knowledge interest" aimed at the production of useful results for the national mental health policy of the USA, but its analytical terms did not reflect the Balinese tradition which includes quite complex ideas about the soul, trance-possession, and mental disease. Following the analytical distinction of Adorno's and Horkheimer's "Kritische Theorie", we could say that the entire research plan was based on "instrumental" rather than "critical" or emancipatory reason: It provided explanations for a purpose imposed by a donor organisation rather than analysing the power relations and axiomatic presumptions of their psychiatric terminology in relation to Balinese thought and practice. The result was indeed a kind of non- or even anti-anthropology, because it led to ethnographic and epistemic distortions and ultimately to a kind of "double bind" – a deep

ambivalence – in this case between Bateson and Mead's anthropological
goal of understanding the exotic Balinese, and their personal interest in
producing pragmatic knowledge based on psychoanalytical theories for
their funding organisation.

This ambivalence and epistemic distortion is obvious in several respects.
First of all, and from the outset, the project involved a certain pathologisation
of the Balinese: Mead looked for a Balinese field site that was "pathological".
She decided to go to the remote mountain village of Bayung Gede, because
she saw it as a simpler version of the more complex Balinese culture in the
royal centres of South Bali. She argued that life and cognitive processes in
the mountains were much slower – and thus easier to observe – because
people in this region were suffering from a "thyroid condition", by which
she probably meant thyroid hypofunction (Bateson and Mead 1942, xiii).
Whereas there may indeed have been a high incidence of goitre, Mead's
conclusions and ethnographic assumptions concerning the culture of the
mountain villages are simply wrong: Mountain people are neither mentally
slower nor retarded, nor is Bayung Gede a culturally simpler version of the
royal centres, but simply different. It preserves until today a unique old
Balinese tradition that differs significantly from the feudal caste and ritual
system of South and central Bali (Reuter 2002). This is obvious not only from
the cosmological and social village structure but also from several unique
traditions that escaped Mead's attention. Significant, for example, is the
lack of cremation, which is the most emblematic life cycle ritual in South
Bali, as well as the existence of a cemetery that can be found only in this
region: for placentas, which are stored in coconut shells and hung in trees.

The second epistemic distortion is even worse: In her attempt to provide
empirical evidence for her theory about "the" schizoid Balinese character,
Mead ignores almost completely Balinese ideas and interpretations regarding
the nature of the person, mother-child interactions, ritual drama, and trance
possession, and relies instead on the analytical framework of psychoanalysis
and psychiatry. She thus does not even try to understand the local society
in its own terms, as these might challenge the theoretical assumptions of
the anthropologist. Instead, she presents an analysis of Balinese society that
is based on Freudian aetiology and uses the nosology of psychiatry. Unlike
Kraepelin, Mead describes the schizoid Balinese character therefore not as
the result of a biological disease but of a culture-specific socialisation based
on permanently frustrating childhood experiences, with ambivalent mothers
forcing their infants to gradually dissociate from their real emotions and
from their sense of a coherent self until they develop the culture specific-
character traits of schizophrenia or dementia praecox: mainly emotional

withdrawal and dissociation.[14] Mead suggests that the investigation of the cultural mechanisms that trigger this schizoid dissociation helps to understand how the "predisposition" of schizophrenia can be culturally handled "so that it does not become maladjustment", which implies that although the normal Balinese socialisation processes force infants to develop a schizoid character, this does not lead to schizophrenia because of culture-specific compensation mechanisms.

But what is so traumatising about Balinese socialisation processes, and how do Balinese cope with them? Following Mead, Balinese mothers treat their infants in a highly ambivalent, indeed a covertly sadistic way: They provoke strong emotional reactions in their babies, which they proceed to ignore. Mothers threaten their infants by shouting that a tiger (policeman, white person, etc.) will come and take them away, or by claiming that they will abandon them and take another baby until their own baby starts to cry, which they invariably ignore. They also tease their babies in an exaggerated and theatrical way to evoke desire and positive responses in their child. They flirt, offer their breast, stroke the child's genitals, and so forth. However, following Mead, all of this threatening, teasing and over-excited flirting has only one aim: to ignore the child completely as soon as it shows the expected strong emotional response, and starts crying, suckling, laughing and so forth. In this very moment, the mother withdraws disinterestedly from her emotionally responsive child. She withdraws with an empty gaze that avoids eye contact, turns her head or starts discussing banalities with her neighbour – while keeping physical contact and granting her breasts to the baby.

Thus, Balinese infants are caught in what Bateson later called a "double bind". They must come to terms with an irritating and confusing contradiction between the teasing and evoking of emotions on the one hand, and the frustrating emotional withdrawal of their mothers on the other, mothers who are physically present and who grant their breasts while verbally threatening to leave the infant. This deeply ambivalent mode of communication culminates – following Mead – when the next baby is born and the first child, who until then was at least carried around and suckled by his mother, has to accept abrupt weaning. This situation, claims

14 Not only is Mead's interest in mother-child interactions an extension of her former fieldwork in Samoa and Papua New Guinea: All of her work is informed by a theoretical framework based on psychology and namely Freudian theories. These mirror her first majoring subject at Barnard – psychology – and her cooperation with psychiatrists and psychoanalysts like Kardiner and Linton. majoring subject at Barnard: psychology, and her cooperation with psychiatrists and psychoanalysts like Kardiner and Linton.

Mead, leads to a serious emotional crisis starting with violent tempers on the side of children, who gradually come to accept the situation by way of resignation: At that point, small children begin to withdraw fully from their own feelings, become emotionally numb and enter permanently the trancelike state of "awayness" or dissociation both from their feelings and from their environment developing what Mead described as the "schizoid" Balinese character.

The similarities between Mead's description of Balinese mother-child interactions and Bateson's explanation of the double bind theory are obvious even though Bateson does not mention his source of inspiration: Both describe an intense but highly ambivalent relationship, usually between mother and child, and a crisis that emerges from a permanent contradiction between different scales of implicit and explicit communication. Both analyse reactions of fear, anger and panic as the result of ambivalent relationships causing emotional withdrawal, dissociation, a lack of responsiveness, or in other words: a "schizoid" or catatonic behaviour. And both contribute thereby to the influential psychoanalytical paradigm of US psychiatry: the schizophrenogenic mother (Seemann 2006).   But there are significant differences, as well. Mead describes the emotional "awayness" and trancelike dissociation of the Balinese as their normal state of mind because it is her goal to describe cultural coping strategies that prevent from schizophrenia and can thus be applied to the USA as well. Bateson on the other hand, uses her analysis of Balinese mother-child interactions to develop a universal socio-psychological aetiology for schizophrenia, which suggests that in his understanding there is no cultural compensation for such distorted forms of communication within the family. Finally, whereas Mead does not ask why Balinese mothers treat their infants in such a cruel way, Bateson hypothesises that the victimiser in double bind situations is unaware of his or her own contradictions and projects them on a dependent family member. His aim is the explanation of schizophrenia on the grounds of distorted family systems, while Mead's interest is a consistent anthropological theory that explains why habitualised schizoid patterns do not always result in manifest illness.

Mead finds her solution to the problem by linking the axiomatic "awayness" of the Balinese to a second claim: Balinese avoid focused intellectual concentration, performative climaxes, and the expression of authentic emotions or strong emotional connections, for example between spouses. She states that Balinese men discover – to their disappointment – that their wives are reproducing the emotionally ambivalent behaviour of their mothers, but interestingly, she assumes that men do not reproduce the same ambivalent relationships. She depicts fathers as the warm, emotionally connected, and reliable counterpart to the pain- and fear-evoking ambivalent mothers and claims that even their teasing of children is different.

One is tempted to speculate about Mead's own unresolved ambiguities, which might have inspired such firm statements about Balinese and their feelings, but what matters here is her theory about the culture-specific compensatory mechanism that prevents Balinese from a pathological form of schizophrenia. Even though she is not too explicit in this regard, she suggests a correlation between the schizoid and emotionally withdrawn Balinese character, ritual trance-possession, and the theatrical expression of exaggerated feelings. All of these features are connected in the ritual drama *Calonarang*, where an evil witch transforms into the demonic but sacred mask-being *Rangda*, the goddess of the graveyards and of witchcraft who threatens to destroy the world until she is conquered by a benevolent male dragon, the mask-being *Barong*. This ritual drama involves spontaneous trance-possessions both of dancers and audience trying to kill *Rangda*, which Mead interprets as a cathartic re-enactment of the ambiguous interaction between mothers and infants. In her interpretation, *Rangda* embodies the Balinese mother, *Barong* the father, and the entire ritual drama is not only a re-enactment of the primordial childhood trauma, but also a compensatory mechanism for dissociated feelings of fear and anger.

Anthropology and Schizophrenia – Concluding Remarks

It is perhaps unnecessary to add that Mead's psychoanalytical interpretation of Balinese mother-child interactions and ritual trance-possession hardly corresponds to anything Balinese would say about themselves, as I can confirm after two decades of fieldwork. Quite the contrary, her interpretation of "Balinese Character" has provoked strong criticism from the Balinese psychiatrist Suryani, mentioned above, who wrote an entire book about "the people of Bali" as a critical reassessment of Mead's description, and namely of her attempt to use a Western category for mental illness to describe completely sane people and their intimate relationships and feelings (Suryani and Jensen 1992).

Similarly trance-possession – and for that matter dissociation – is a complex feature of many Balinese rituals and it has different social and political functions ranging from the manifestation of divine presence and power to the public revelations of oracular speech. In other words, possession cannot be limited to the compensatory function of the individual psyche nor to the witchcraft drama *Calonarang* on which Mead is focusing due to her theoretical interests. And even in this regard, she ignores local interpretations that would have shown that *Calonarang* performances have little to do with mother-child relations but a lot with Balinese ideas about the socially repressed emotional background of witchcraft: mainly feelings of envy or jealousy within extended families or between neighbours.

It is worth noticing at that point that the Dutch psychiatrist van Wulfften Palthe, who examined Balinese trancers at the request of Mead's student Jane Belo (who investigated Trance-possession in Bali), could not find any abnormal or pathological personality features (Belo 1960, 5). On her part, Belo refers to Mead's hypothesis rather reluctantly, and emphasises that trancers are psychologically indistinguishable from people who go never in trance in their normal life, which was confirmed by psychological "sorting tests" used in US psychiatry to distinguish schizophrenics (ibid., 10). Thus from the perspective of psychiatry, Balinese trancers were mentally and emotionally perfectly normal and healthy in their daily lives, they showed no deviance, their trance-possession was limited to the context of rituals, and they showed no symptoms of mental disturbance if they did not participate in the ritual.

This supports what I learned from several Balinese who were regularly possessed during rituals but who knew that they could avoid such physically exhausting transformations if they stayed away from the temple rituals because in their understanding, possession was their ritual service for the temple community (*ngayah*) and not an expression of or relief from their repressed personal feelings. People going in trance-possession are therefore regarded in Balinese terms as *kulit* ("skin"), *pelinggihan* ("shrines"), or *tapakan*, the "sitting place" of a deity who manifests to demonstrate his or her presence and power or to communicate their concerns and wishes to the temple community. In other words: according to Balinese ideas trance-possession is neither a dissociation of the human mind nor a form of mental disease, but the arrival (*kerauhan*) of a divine being, which can only manifest if the personal soul temporarily withdraws (Hornbacher 2011).

To leave one's body and become literally selfless, so that these powerful agents from the invisible dimension (*niskala*) of the material and visible (*sekala*) world can manifest, is crucial for the understanding of Balinese trance-possession, which is regarded as an individual service for the gods and the temple community but irreconcilable with a psychological interpretation that regards dissociation as an individual psychological deviation. Unfortunately, such conceptual differences are ignored by Mead and Bateson, who present "the Balinese" as paradigm of Western psychological theories about schizophrenia instead of taking Balinese thoughts and practices into serious consideration. That allows only one conclusion: Mead and Bateson failed to engage intellectually with the radical alterity of Balinese thought and life. Instead, they reified "the" Balinese as objects of psychological theories, and thus missed the chance to pursue anthropology in the sense of Foucault as a "contre-science" reflecting the limits of their own categories against the backdrop of radically different terms and practices.

My initial question was, "How did anthropology contribute to the schizophrenia discourse?" and my answer is, "In a highly ambiguous way" – by silencing Balinese thoughts about dissociation, personhood and emotion. Even though Mead and Bateson's fieldwork in Bali deeply influenced the critical Western discourse on schizophrenia, their emphasis on social or psychological rather than biological causes reflects the economic framework of their research and their inability to think radical alterity beyond their own psychological and ontological categories. Mead's explanation of the schizoid Balinese and Bateson's socio-psychological aetiology of schizophrenia remain "dans le vrai" – in the epistemological and ontological comfort zone – of a Western discourse and paradigm of reality according to which everything can either be explained in terms of natural laws or understood as a result of human society, psyche and culture – or more generally: of a universal human mind in its conscious and unconscious articulations.

That is why, even though "the" Balinese are paradigmatic and highly influential as the exotic "other" to Western subjects, they appear only as objects of the Western schizophrenia discourse. Their own ideas about trance remain silent and silenced.

Ethnographic Epilogue on Balinese Ideas About Mental Health and Dissociation

If physiological and socio-psychological explanations of schizophrenia are, as I have argued, only the complementary sides of a modern Eurocentric ontology and psychology that is currently imposed on a global scale – for example via the MGMH – what would an alternative to this Western discourse look like? And what could anthropology contribute if the question of global mental healing is not just the normalisation of an anthropological and ontological Western paradigm?

I suggest looking more closely at Balinese ideas and practices regarding human mind, madness and healing, and thus at exactly that dimension of radical alterity that Mead and Bateson excluded from their theories. I am not referring to a consistent Balinese theory about mental health, since I do not believe that such a thing exists. Rather, I make use of an example that shows an alternative way of dealing with madness, radical alterity and mental healing in relation to a local cosmology and understanding of possession: the story of Guru Mal.

Guru Mal was a kind and soft-spoken man in his late seventies when I first met him during a ritual in one of the mountain temples of the Kintamani region near Mead's field site of Bayung Gede. The temple where we met, Pura Bukit Mentik, is located in the Caldera of the Batur volcano next to a lake, which is home of a goddess, Dewi Danu, and associated with the irrigation of the rice terraces in South Bali. The Batur, one of Bali's most active volcanoes, erupted in 1929 and 1974 and left a dramatic landscape shaped by volcanic sand, ashes, and frozen waves of lava. Guru Mal's village community used to live in the caldera but after the disastrous eruption in 1926 had to move to the ridge of the caldera and found shelter in Bayung Gede and other villages nearby. At that time, the famous Batur temple was also moved up to its current position at the ridge of the caldera. In the same village of Kintamani Guru Mal sells clothes in the market, but despite the move, he and his community are still devout members of the temple Bukit Mentik in the Caldera, where he experienced the last eruption: his most lively memory is linked to an existential decision he had made during the eruption. During a temple festival, he showed me a wall of lava that was several metres high, and which seemed to have stopped right in front of the temple – a story that is famous among Balinese. He told me that at this time, the entire community was terrified that the volcano might destroy everything: the temple, the village and eventually all of Bali. The priest and the temple community felt strongly that they were responsible, not only for the place they lived, but also for the cosmic balance of Bali in general. Therefore, a high priest was called and decided not to leave but to stay in the temple, to perform a ritual and pray to god, begging him to spare the sacred place and the island. The priest announced to the temple community that he would stay in the temple, and asked who would dare to stay with him. Among the group of people that actually did risk their lives was Guru Mal, who is convinced that their prayers were heard and that this explains why the lava stopped short of the temple and started moving back down, as a frozen lava wall in front of the temple confirms.

Guru Mal did not tell this as a heroic story, but rather with a very modest tone and a smile, transporting his delight and surprise regarding this miracle that showed the presence of god in this place. He had trusted his life to god – and god had spared their lives and the temple. Could there be clearer evidence of his blessing?

During temple rituals, Guru Mal sometimes goes into deep trance possession, manifesting local deities who are, according to Balinese, only willing to enter spiritually pure human beings, no matter which religious doctrine they profess. Beyond this, he carries out administrative and practical tasks for the temple to which he is deeply devoted. In other words, he seems to be perfectly integrated in the community as one of the respected elders, and whenever I met him, he was particularly friendly and caring, inviting me to eat together with the temple community after the ritual, which is a special custom of the mountain area. Given his kind, serene and harmonious manners and his social position, I had never expected to hear another story that he told me one day when we were sitting after the temple ritual together with his wife and other members of the temple community.

He spoke of the greatest and life changing event of his biography, which was "the time when I was crazy (*gila*) – and was hospitalised in the psychiatric unit." According to Guru Mal, everything started in 1980 after a temple ritual in Pura Bukit Mentik when he suddenly felt overwhelmed with energy in front of the main shrine, and had all kinds of visions, clairvoyant experiences, and inspirations about everybody who happened to cross his way, as well as receiving "messages" about people in villages that lived hours away from his home. He did not understand what was happening to him but felt very strange and could not leave the temple. He followed a baying dog to a holy temple tree where he found an antique bottle of oil, with which he started healing people. He "saw" also what people were suffering from, and who performed witchcraft, and was forced in his highly energised state to run constantly and restlessly from one place to another, to tell people what he "saw" about them, and to heal them. In addition, he was told that a mystical *kris*, a ritual dagger, would be given to him, and it was! With this dagger, he continued to heal others. Yet, he felt he was going "mad" because despite all his truthfulness, others did not always believe him. He remained in this restless state for six months, followed by his wife who tried to take care of him. Yet he could not eat or sleep – and nor did he react to the efforts of the priest nor to holy water that would have brought him back to normality if he were possessed in the usual way, since the sprinkling of holy water over a possessed person is supposed to satisfy the deity and bring the human soul back. But Guru Mal did not "come back" – nor did a deity speak to the priest to communicate his or her wishes. It was therefore evident to everyone that this was not normal trance-possession (*kerauhan*) the arrival of a god, ancestor or a demon in his body, but something else, but what?

Guru Mal himself says that he felt highly energised, and that others perceived this as anger even though he did not feel angry but was able to see everything perfectly clearly and to foretell the truth about people he didn't even know. For example, he saw a man in the street and told him that he was going to die in four months, and sure enough, the man was dead four months later, and so forth. People became frightened of him. On the other hand, his wife and family were very concerned about him and his health because nobody could stop him from running around with the dagger. Finally, they called the police. But the policemen said that Guru Mal's behaviour did not fall within their area of responsibility, so they brought him to Bangli, the city with the first psychiatric hospital in Bali, founded by the Dutch Colonists. Up to this point, Guru Mal told his story (in front of nodding co-villagers) with pride and some amusement, because he insists that whatever he "saw" in his madness turned out to be true. He is convinced that his madness resulted only from the circumstance that others did not trust him enough, whereas he himself did not really believe he was crazy, but rather he felt that he was suddenly enabled to see and to reveal the normally hidden (*niskala*) dimension of the world in way that nobody understands. At the same time, he admits that he was unable to continue his normal life until he was hospitalised between many screaming persons. And yet, he remembers his transfer to psychiatry with the same shivers of horror as the huge injection that he was given and that made a traumatic impression on him: He was held and strapped down by several strong men and the injection left him unconscious for three whole days. After that he became calm, and after four weeks he could return to his family. He has never been "mad" again, but since this episode he would regularly go in trance possession during temple rituals.

While I was pondering the unusual connection Guru Mal made between madness and the revelation of truth, I asked him if it was the injection and the treatment in psychiatry that had "healed" him. But he only smiled at my confusion and shook his head, as did others from his community who had listened to his story just like me. He tried to explain what I had obviously mis-understood: "The injection and the hospital were a terrible experience! They stopped my extreme restlessness, but they made me numb, even unconscious. I was no longer myself, and I suffered from others who were truly mad and would stub out their cigarettes on me." Guru Mal emphasised that this was not healing. What he regarded as real mental healing took place only after he returned home, underwent several ritual purifications (*nuntun*) under the guidance of the priest, and was initiated to become a trance medium for temple rituals. To him, healing was obviously not the avoidance or repression of dissociation but quite the contrary, the integration of his dissociation as trance-possession in the service of the god and the temple community.

To ponder the significance of his idea about what it means to be mentally healed, it is important to understand that this community consists not only of living people but also and even more so of their divine ancestors and local gods, all of whom meet regularly during rituals. It turned out that the god who possessed Guru Mal was Batara Gede Motaring Jagat from Lempuhyang, one of Bali's most important direction temples. One could say that Balinese temple rituals are nothing other than celebrations of the communion and communication between visible and invisible persons to which humans contribute with beautiful offerings, dances and music, whereas the invisible guests contribute their blissful presence and sometimes communicate their recommendations, complaints, or wishes. In Bali's non-iconic religion, the adequate way to articulate this presence and communicate those messages is trance-possession. Possessed persons mediate and manifest the encounter between humans and gods or between the two dimensions of a world that does not consist of material objects and human subjects but of visible and invisible agents who need either a place in the environment or a temporary human "skin" in which to manifest.

But Guru Mal's story was slightly different because it involved a form of dissociation that, even from the perspective of him and his family, was not "normal" but rather crazy because it diverged from the common pattern of ritual possession. In the psychiatric hospital at Bangli it was obviously treated with antipsychotic drugs and Guru Mal might have been diagnosed as manic, psychotic or schizoid – all that he remembers is that they said he was "crazy". But it is also a story about Balinese ideas of mental health and a process of healing that is defined by the afflicted person and can only be understood in terms of Balinese ontology and lifeworld. Guru Mal says quite explicitly that the factual effect of the antipsychotic injection, did not "heal" him but only stopped his compulsorily manic behaviour. To him and to his community, dissociation is not a deviant state of the human mind or brain that must explained, controlled and avoided at any cost, nor is it, as Mead suggests, an outlet of his personal repressed feelings. On the contrary, dissociation indicates the presence of non-human agents, and supernatural truths that are potentially of public significance: a state of revelation to which the human mind normally has no access.

It is perhaps due to this conceptual framework that for Guru Mal the psychiatric aetiology and chemical or socio-psychological control of his condition is irrelevant to his healing. He accepts his own temporary "madness" as an event with spiritual significance that ultimately transcends human control and explanation. What matters is rather the creative process in which his radically altered behaviour was integrated as part of the communication between the visible and invisible agents of his community. There was no need to normalise him since his alterity was a blessing.

References

Aderibigbe, Yekeen A., D. Theodoridis, and W. Victor R. Vieweg. 1999. "Dementia Praecox to Schizophrenia: The First 100 Years." *Psychiatry and Clinical neurosciences* 53 (4): 437-48.

Arenz, Dirk. 2008. *Eine kleine Geschichte der Schizophrenie*. Bonn: Rabe.

Bateson, Gregory, Don D. Jackson, Jay Haley, and John Weakland. 1956. "Toward a Theory of Schizophrenia." *Behavioral Science* 1 (4): 251-64.

Bateson, Gregory, and Margaret Mead. 1942. "Balinese Character: A Photographic Analysis." *New York*, 17-92.

Belo, Jane. 1977. *Trance in Bali*. Greenwood Press.

Benedict, Ruth. 1934. *Patterns of Culture* (Vol. 8). Boston; New York: Houghton Mifflin Company.

Bleuler, Eugen. 1911. *Dementia Praecox: Oder Gruppe der Schizophrenien*. Leipzig; Wien: F. Deuticke.

—. 1950. *Dementia Praecox or the Group of Schizophrenias*. Madison: International Universities Press.

Böhlich, Walter. 1972. "Wildwuchs nicht länger geduldet." *Der Spiegel,* 31 January 1972. Accessed 8 July 2020. https://www.spiegel.de/spiegel/print/d-43019841. html.

Bogoras, Waldemar. 1909. *The Chukchee* (Vol. 11). Leiden: EJ Brill Limited.

Canguilhem, Georges. 1983. *Études d'Histoire et de Philosophie des Sciences*. Paris: Librairie Philosophique J. Vrin.

Chatterjee, Sudipto, Vikram Patel, Achira Chatterjee, and Helen A. Weiss. 2003. "Evaluation of a Community-Based Rehabilitation Model for Chronic Schizophrenia in Rural India." *The British Journal of Psychiatry* 182 (1): 57-62.

Cooper, David G. 1970. *Psychiatry and Anti-Psychiatry*. Paladin.

Deleuze, Gilles, and Félix Guattari. 1983 [1972]. *Anti-Oedipus: Capitalism and Schizophrenia*. Translated by Robert Hurley, Mark Seem, and Helen R. Lane. Minneapolis: University of Minnesota Press.

Falzeder, Ernst, ed. 2018. *History of Modern Psychology: Lectures Delivered at ETH Zurich, Volume 1, 1933-1934 by C.G. Jung*, 84-88. Princeton: Princeton University Press.

Foucault, Michel. 1963. *Naissance de la Clinique. Une Archeologie du Regard Medical*. Paris: Presses universitaires de France.

Foucault, Michel. 1966. Les mots et les chonses. Une archéologie des sciences humaines. Paris: Edition Gallimard.

—. 1975. *Surveiller et Punir. Naissance de la Prison*. Paris: Editions Gallimard.

Fromm-Reichmann, Frieda. 1948. "Notes on the Development of Treatment of Schizophrenics by Psychoanalytic Psychotherapy." *Psychiatry* 11 (3): 263-73.

Guloksuz, S., and Jim van Os. 2018. "The Slow Death of the Concept of Schizophrenia and the Painful Birth of the Psychosis Spectrum." *Psychological Medicine* 48 (2): 229-44.

Hacking, Ian. 1995. "The Looping Effects of Human Kinds." In *Symposia of the Fyssen Foundation. Causal Cognition: A Multidisciplinary Debate,* edited by Dan Sperber, David Premack, and Ann J. Premack, 351-94. Oxford: Clarendon Press/ Oxford University Press.

—. 1998. *Rewriting the Soul: Multiple Personality and the Sciences of Memory.* Princeton: Princeton University Press.

Hartwell, Carol E. 1996. "The Schizophrenogenic Mother Concept in American Psychiatry." *Psychiatry* 59 (3): 274-97.

Hornbacher, Annette. 2011. "The Withdrawal of the Gods: Remarks on Ritual Trance Possession and Its Decline in Bali. In *The Politics of Religion in Indonesia: Syncretism, Orthodoxy, and Religious Contention in Java and Bali*, edited by Michel Picard, and Rémy Madinier, 167-91. Abingdon: Routledge.

—. 2013. "A Mood of Crisis: Balinese Ritual Culture Between Creolization and Criticism." In *Faith in the Future*, edited by Thomas Reuter and Alexander Horstmann, 111-40. Leiden: Brill.

Jacknis, Ira. 1988. "Margaret Mead and Gregory Bateson in Bali: Their Use of Photography and Film." *Cultural anthropology* 3 (2): 160-77.

Johnston, Josephine. 2013. "The Ghost of the Schizophrenogenic Mother." *AMA Journal of Ethics* 15 (9): 801-05.

Kerner, Justinus. 1829. *Die Seherin von Prevorst* (Vol. 1). Tübingen: Cotta.

Leitner, Bernhard. 2014. "Zum Transfer von Psychiatrie: Narrative, Termini und Transkulturelle Psychiatrie in Japan." *NTM Zeitschrift für Geschichte der Wissenschaften, Technik und Medizin* 22 (3): 163-80.

Luhrmann, Tanya M. 2012. "Beyond the Brain." *The Wilson Quarterly* 36 (3): 28.

de Jesus Mari, Jair, Denise Razzouk, Rangaswamy Thara, Julian Eaton, and Graham Thornicroft, 2009. "Packages of Care for Schizophrenia in Low-And Middle-Income Countries." *PLoS Medicine* 6 (10): e1000165.

Mitrani, Philippe, 1992. "A Critical Overview of the Psychiatric Approaches to Shamanism." *Diogenes,* 40 (158): 145-64.

Pérez-Álvarez, Marino, José M. García-Montes, Oscar Vallina-Fernández, Salvador Perona-Garcelán, and Carlos Cuevas-Yust. 2011. "New Life for Schizophrenia Psychotherapy in the Light of Phenomenology." *Clinical psychology & psychotherapy* 18 (3): 187-201.

Podmore, Frank. 2011 [1908]. *Mesmerism and Christian Science: A Short History of Mental Healing.* Cambridge: Cambridge University Press.

Read, John, Richard Bentall, Loren Mosher, and Jacqui Dillon. 2013. "Genetics, Eugenics and the Mass Murder of 'Schizophrenics'." In *Models of Madness:*

Psychological, Social and Biological Approaches to Psychosis, edited by John Read, Richard Bentall, Loren Mosher, and Jacqui Dillon, 60-72. Abingdon: Routledge.

Read, John. 2013. "From Heresy to Certainty." In *Models of Madness: Psychological, Social and Biological Approaches to Psychosis*, edited by John Read, Richard Bentall, Loren Mosher, and Jacqui Dillon, 249. Abingdon: Routledge.

Rosenhan, David L. 1973. "On Being Sane in Insane Places." *Science* 179 (4070): 250-58.

Sax, William S. 2014. "Ritual Healing and Mental Health in India." *Transcultural Psychiatry* 51 (3): 829-49.

Schott, Heinz, and Rainer Tölle. 2006. *Geschichte der Psychiatrie: Krankheitslehren, Irrwege, Behandlungsformen.* München: CH Beck.

Silverman, Julian. 1967. "Shamans and Acute Schizophrenia 1." *American Anthropologist* 69 (1): 21-31.

Spandler, Helen. 1992. "To Make an Army Out of Illness: A History of the Socialist Patients' Collective Heidelberg 1970-2." *Asylum: A Magazine For Democratic Psychiatry* 6 (4): 4-16.

Szasz, Thomas S. 1960. "The Myth of Mental Illness." *American Psychologist* 15 (2): 113-18.

—. 1976. "Schizophrenia: The Sacred Symbol of Psychiatry." *The British Journal of Psychiatry* 129 (4): 308-16.

van Os, Jim. 2016. "'Schizophrenia' Does Not Exist." *British Medical Journal* 352: 375.

Walker, Elaine, Lisa Kestler, Annie Bollini, and Karen M. Hochman. 2004. "Schizophrenia: Etiology and Course." *Annual Review of Psychology* 55:401-30.

About the Author

ANNETTE HORNBACHER is professor of Cultural Anthropology at the University of Heidelberg. She received her PhD in philosophy (University of Tübingen) with a thesis on Friedrich Hölderlin's concept of poetic language as "higher enlightenment", and her *Habilitation* in Cultural Anthropology with a book on Balinese ritual dance as an alternative to modern Western paradigms of representation. She has conducted extensive fieldwork in Indonesia, particularly in Bali, where she worked on ritual dance drama as a kinaesthetic embodiment of cosmological knowledge. She has led several research projects: on *Religious Dynamics* in Post-Suharto Indonesia (funded by the German Ministry for Education and Research), on *Local Traditions and World Religions* (funded by the German Research Council), and on *Waterscapes* as interrelated nature-culture landscapes in Bali and Komodo (Heidelberg, Cluster of Excellence). In this context, she began working on competing concepts of ecology and human-animal relationships in the marine reserve of Komodo. Currently, she leads a research project on esoteric Balinese manuscripts in an interdisciplinary research area titled *"Material Textcultures"* (SFB933), and is conducting a comparative research project together with Prof. William Sax on tantric text practices in Bali and India.

4 Misdiagnosis

Global Mental Health, Social Determinants of Health and Beyond

Anindya Das and Mohan Rao

Abstract

We critically engage with the Movement for Global Mental Health (MGMH) through the lens of the Social Determinants of Health (SDH), suitably widened. We explore the socio-political context of Indian community mental health initiatives in order to elaborate the opportunities/impediments for a public programme. We critique the MGMH for being preoccupied with the burden of mental illness and its "treatment", while being inattentive to the social, economic, and political contexts shaping local/global ecologies of well-being/suffering. Hence the economic arguments of the MGMH fail to examine the realities of local contexts (poor public health funding and primary health care, lax pharmaceutical regulations, asymmetric power relations and indigenous knowledge systems). Using the concepts of globalisation and global health, and taking a population perspective, we describe a neo-materialistic version of SDH.

Keywords: global health, social determinants of health, neo-materialist, global mental health

Introduction

Since the publication of the call for Global Mental Health in *The Lancet* in 2007, followed by the renewed call in 2011, there has been a significant jump in research and publication in this field, with attendant funding. While the Movement for Global Mental Health (hereafter MGMH) movement purports to utilise a public health approach, it is one that is heavily influenced by individual health and clinical medicine. Our understanding of

Sax, William, and Claudia Lang (eds), *The Movement for Global Mental Health: Critical Views from South and Southeast Asia*. Taylor & Francis Group, 2021
DOI: 10.5117/9789463721622_CH04

public health depends upon a population-based approach that engages with supra-individual determinants, considers public health greater than just the sum of individuals' health, and considers health itself as context-dependent. For this, we employ the Social Determinants of Health approach to mental health, to critically evaluate Global Mental Health. We also problematise the so-called "treatment gap" which is purported to be a spectacular 90 per cent in the Low and Middle Income Countries (LMICs), thus creating a significant economic burden as calculated by the Disability Adjusted Life Years (DALY) metric. The proposed, purportedly "cost-effective" solution of task shifting supported by trials is essentially clinical, which, along with the attendant plan to "scale up" such services, effectively decontextualises population health.

In the following sections, we first present a case study of an Indian mental health programme that involved ideas similar to those of the MGMH but predated it by over two decades. In this way, we demonstrate how social and political contexts influence ideas around health and expansion of health services, in the case of mental health services. Next, we critically evaluate the MGMH and its recommendations, along with the research associated with it, showing that it fails to attend to the sociopolitical context of LMICs. In the final section, we clarify the concept of Social Determinants of Health as we understand it, and argue that it would be a much better foundation for mental health policy than the neoliberal foundation of the MGMH. Here we analyse the role of globalisation in global (mental) health to show that the "local" and the "global" are distinct, but directly linked. The chapter concludes by drawing upon the Social Determinants of Health theory to chart the way forward for Global Mental Health.

Community Mental Health and India

India can be considered a focus country in the MGMH. For one thing, it has been one of the leading sites for MGMH studies (Chatterjee et al. 2008; Patel et al. 2010a; Vellakkal and Patel 2015; Singla et al. 2014; Divan et al. 2015; Shidhaye et al. 2016; Nadkarni et al. 2015; Rajaraman et al. 2015), and in fact the idea of providing mental health care by non-mental health professionals/ Lay Health Workers (LHWs) was tried in India as long ago as the early 1980s (Jacob 2011). Recent MGMH studies have largely ignored local contexts, as these would pose problems for "scaling up" mental health care services (see *Introduction*, this volume). Moreover, neither the Indian experiment nor the MGMH studies take cognisance of the social determinants of health. We elaborate a much wider understanding of social determinants of health, unlike the limited scope with which the MGMH have engaged with (Patel et al. 2018). But before that, because what the MGMH proposes as task-shifting is so very similar to one of the major components of the National Mental Health Program of India, we take a look at the latter's history. In doing so, we intend to analyse the political and contextual circumstances that gave rise to it, which also have implications for the social determinants of health. Our analysis suggests that the conceptualisation of India's national mental health programme had its origin in a WHO recommendation in 1975 (World Health Organization 1975), following which the WHO established a multi-country project involving India, the Philippines, Brazil, Colombia, Egypt, Senegal, and Sudan, which sought to determine the efficacy of available general health service workers for the identification and treatment of "priority" psychiatric conditions (Sartorius and Harding 1983; see also Das 2014). This project was extended until 1986. During this period, a countrywide collaborative study funded by the Government of India was conducted by the Indian Council of Medical Research and the Department of Science and Technology, in which a cadre of LWHs (referred to as "Multipurpose Health Workers" in India) was involved in the provision of mental health care, in addition to the usual services such as the provision of comprehensive Primary Health Care (PHC) (Indian Council of Medical Research and Department of Science and Technology 1987). In the field, they were compelled to focus primarily on family planning and malaria control tasks due to priority being given to them and the under-resourced conditions of work (Priya 2005). Despite the limited success of this and other mental health programme related research in India (Wig et al. 1981), the National Mental Health Program was launched in 1982. By 2008-2009, only 127 out of 612 districts were covered, and of these only a few were functional (Mental Health Policy Group 2012). Although major investments in community care and the expansion of mental health training (integrating medical college departments of psychiatry with field sites, making them responsible for the provision of community mental health care, creating centres of excellence for training mental health professionals) were made, nothing much changed at the local, community mental health level (ibid.). Elsewhere, Das (2014) has argued that the initial idea of this national programme was much influenced by two important developments: first, the PHC movement leading up to the Alma-Ata Declaration in 1978; and second, the deinstitutionalisation movement in Europe and North America. Both of these had political ramifications for the social determinants of health approach. The Alma-Ata Declaration has been attributed, among other factors, to the disillusionment with post-war health sector developments centred on vertical programmes, and also with the politics of the Cold War and the example of Chinese public health achievements (including the so-called "barefoot doctors"), with China joining the WHO in 1975 (Rao 2010). This (re)oriented public health toward economic development, anti-poverty measures, food production, clean water, sanitation, housing, environmental protection, appropriate technologies and education. On the other hand, the deinstitutionalisation movement in the US and UK largely happened in a neoliberal political environment and a fiscal crisis that downsized psychiatric systems, although it was camouflaged as community care. But in Sweden in a social democratic political climate, and in Italy as part of left-wing political struggle, deinstitutionalisation and community-oriented services were considered to be basic rights (Scheper-Hughes and Lovell 1986; Carpenter 2000; Burti 2001). In India, the drive for community mental health care was rather ambiguous. Some advocated it for purposes of cost-cutting (Kapur 2004), others because of the shortcomings of institutional care (Srinivasa Murthy 2011). Thus PHC and the deinstitutionalisation movement, in different contexts, both created a potential opportunity to address the social determinants of mental health.

This was, however, the time when the world took a neoliberal turn with the election of Thatcher in 1979 and Reagan in 1980; PHC, which seemed to have promised something revolutionary in healthcare, was thus doomed at birth. The resultant politics of healthcare arm-twisted the international community into downsizing PHC into "*selective* PHC", an oxymoron. Selective PHC involved, again, a handful of vertical programmes that were deemed cost-effective. PHC it was argued, was utopian, with not enough resources to realise it. Moreover, the health sector reform post 1990s reduced funding and growth of public health services (particularly PHC). These factors played a significant part in the downward spiral of the community mental health movement in India since its services were designed to sink or swim with the success or failure of PHC.[1] The slow but sure degradation of the public health system made it even harder to address the social determinants of health. Because the national mental health programme had failed to deliver, it was re-strategised as a new programme known as the District Mental Health Programme for easy operationalisation. This made sense because the district

---

1   Two notable exceptions to this dilapidated state of PHC have been the states of Kerala and Tamil Nadu. Compared to the rest of the country, both these states have made significant progress in PHC (Gupta et al. 2010; Parthasarathi and Sinha 2016; Oommen 2018). As a result, the community mental health programme in these states is relatively well organised and functional (Gururaj et al. 2014; Lang 2019). A 2015-2016 nationwide survey suggested these states have the highest coverage under the district mental health programme (Gururaj et al. 2016).

is a basic territorial unit of administration throughout the country. But the programme was based on an experimental model (popularly known as the *Bellary* model) that relied heavily on experts for clinical identification and treatment, particularly by pharmacological means, and focused excessively on severe mental disorders. Jain and Jadhav's (2009) ethnographic study in one of Uttar Pradesh's district sites demonstrates both of these points. They concluded that the aims enshrined in the national mental health programme, such as community participation, play out at the periphery as machinery for distributing psychotropics. This important example of what happens to policies as they are actualised in practice is useful for our analysis of the MGMH, which seems not to recognise how the social environment contours community care, especially the care of the mentally ill in India. It shows the importance of incorporating social science models into the theory and practice of global mental health.

In 2011, the Indian Government established a Mental Health Policy Group. This group was tasked with identifying issues leading to the poor performance of the mental health programme and devise a national policy. But although the policy document that was produced (Ministry of Health & Family Welfare, Government of India 2014) seems to be much more aware of social constraints, and includes several lofty goals, it is shallow in depth and intent. This is primarily due to its ahistorical analysis, which does not address the political failure to address the social determinants of illness, which in turn all but guarantees the failure of the national mental health programme.

In fact, the latest financial plan of India (the Twelfth Five-Year Plan, 2012-2017) for mental health, with inputs from the influential Policy Group, continued financing the training of specialist mental health professionals but failed to conceptualise a comprehensive plan for training the primary or secondary level mental health care workers (particularly in areas of counselling techniques, social support and rehabilitation) who might have a far greater impact (Das 2018).

An important recent development is India's Mental Health Care Act 2017 (Mental Health Care Act 2017), which recommended that mental health conditions should also be covered by health insurance. While this might seem praiseworthy, we are concerned about the demand side financing of healthcare in India, the promotion of which is clearly regressive, amounting to a public subsidy to private medical care, often of dubious quality. The plan has already been rolled out in certain districts of the country where it has shown its ineffectiveness in benefitting the poor and protecting them from catastrophic health expenses (Selvaraj and Karan 2012; Karan et al. 2017). Moreover, the recent nationwide health insurance scheme, *Ayushman*

Bharat, has just made cosmetic changes and does not address the fact that it finances only hospitalisation costs resulting in the compartmentalisation of healthcare, which is no longer seen as a continuum that exists between primary, secondary, and tertiary care, the essence of PHC. Indeed, data from the country show that outpatient costs are more impoverishing than inpatient ones (Sengupta 2013). Additionally, insurance payments have drawn disproportionately on healthcare budgets rather than proportionately addressing healthcare needs (Sengupta 2013). Based on these facts, a recent analysis of health insurance models in India recommends improved financing of public healthcare institutions and services to develop them before a comprehensive regulatory framework is advanced for a public-private partnership such as this (Kurian 2015). Models of healthcare driven by private insurance are neither sustainable nor equitable. Indeed, in the Indian case, in particular, it is seen that such models are associated with increased healthcare costs due to unnecessary and costly investigations and surgical procedures.

Problematising the Movement for Global Mental Health

We believe that the premises of the MGMH are problematic in theory and especially in practice. This can be seen by taking a close look at the above described India's community mental health programme, which adopted the strategies espoused in the *Lancet* call.

The formulation of the global mental health problem by the MGMH is encapsulated in the term "treatment gap" in Low and Middle Income Countries (LMICs) (Patel et al. 2010b); that is, the percentage difference between the number of people assumed to require treatment for mental illness and the actual number receiving it from medical or professional service providers (Kohn et al. 2004). This "gap" is estimated to be from 75 to 90 per cent (Patel et al. 2010b, World Health Organization 2010) and is linked to assumptions regarding an "epidemic" of untreated mental illness (see *Introduction*, this volume). Formulating an appropriate response to this "epidemic" is said to be the main motivation for the MGMH and its subsequent work of raising awareness and developing solutions (Whitley 2015). The solutions proposed by the MGMH are twofold: task-shifting/-sharing and scaling-up. The logic for task-shifting is the acute scarcity of biomedically-trained mental health professionals[2] in LMICs. The proposal thus involves utilising Lay Health

2   The term "biomedically trained mental health professionals" have been specifically used to imply professionals who are considered to have received sufficient training to manage clinical

Workers (LHWs) for the job, with advocates of the MGMH arguing that existing evidence suggests that they will be able to efficiently complete their assigned tasks (Dias et al. 2008; Araya et al. 2003; Chatterjee et al. 2003; Rahman et al. 2008). At the systemic level, however, the evidence can be questioned because most of it focuses on single diseases with pre-existing structural support or separate internal monitoring mechanisms. Nevertheless, the use of LHWs may be a key ingredient for the success of global mental health (Das and Rao 2012). Even if LHWs are effective, more difficult is the proposal for scaling-up. For this, the leaders of the MGMH have planned, and in some cases initiated, multicentred cluster randomised control trials (e.g. the Indian MANAS and COPSI trial, Zimbabwean Friendship Bench Project, the Nigerian EXPONATE trial, Ethiopian RAISE and TASCS trial, and Brazil's PROGRAVIDA trial). Such trials use the concept of community based intervention by LHWs for screening, case management, compliance management for psychotropics and administration of psychotherapy/psychoeducation/individualised rehabilitation with the support of available primary health care doctors or private general practitioners, who in turn are supervised by specialised psychiatric services. This has been referred to as the "stepped-care approach". The unit of randomisation in most studies is the primary health centre/general practitioners, representing an attempt to generate evidence at the health service level. Published studies have shown a modest positive effect when LHWs provide care for milder conditions. But even cursory look at these trials suggests major problems. Some of these are the poor uptake of Western forms of group (Chatterjee et al. 2008, 43) or individual (Patel et al. 2010a, 2093) psychotherapy with costly mechanisms for monitoring LHWs (Chatterjee et al. 2014, 1390). There has been no effect on psychiatric symptoms of community interventions in participants attending private (probably urban) healthcare practitioners (Patel et al. 2011, 462) or specialist (probably private and urban) psychiatric services (Chatterjee et al. 2014, 1389). Further, community interventions (and psychoeducation) have not made any difference to stigma or discrimination (Chatterjee et al. 2014, 1390). Besides, the above studies prove only that LHWs are effective at sites that are not resource-scarce (Gupta and Srinivasamurthy 2014) but have an opportunity for collaborative care with specialists in a supervisory and referral role.

Strangely, none of these trials reported the socio-economic profile of the sample or the sites, nor did they control for socio-economic status. They

---

situations in India. And most often psychologists and social workers in India are certified to treat/manage people with mental illness when they undergo training in a biomedical environment.

did not include the characteristics of the LHWs in their interpretation of the findings. The LHWs in the published trials were mostly local women, and it is apparent from the varied publications of the MGMH that the concept of LHW is intricately linked to gendered thinking, although this bias is not acknowledged. To advance the argument: one link in the logic of task-shifting (for cheaper alternatives and unavailable skilled professionals) is to bank on the traditional idea of the women's caregiving role with the mentally ill. Thus, the idea of LHWs becomes tied to cheaper labour and the structural location of women in a subordinate position within the health structure. Moreover, in the real world, for mental health professionals (read psychiatrists) in public health settings, the meaning of treatment gap and the nature of service users' needs are deeply informed by the biomedical paradigm and its associated Eurocentric epistemologies of modernity, science and medicine (see Introduction and Sax's chapter; also Cooper 2016).

The other major problem is the economic argument put forth by the MGMH. We have discussed this issue in an earlier publication (Das and Rao 2012). To summarise the arguments: The first problem is the unidimensional biomedical use of the concept of disability in the metric DALY to the exclusion of social support structures available in the LMICs. The second problem is that expectations of formal economic output from individuals are not realistic. The third is the problematic assumption that life expectancy is influenced by medical measures alone. DALYs have been critiqued for favouring biomedical models of healthcare and also for distorting epidemiological priorities (Anand and Hanson 2004). The fourth argument is that the calculation of disease burden is based on poor quality epidemiological evidence (especially for LMICs), that accounts neither for co-morbidity (especially for mental disorders) nor for the contribution of mental illness to early mortality (Vigo et al. 2016). Scholars have also critiqued the epidemiological basis of the calculation of disease burden of depression (Brhlikova et al. 2011). Moreover, disability, generically defined, is ill-suited to capture essential issues that are more important for the patients and carers (Cooper 2017). A miscalculation of the burden of illness eventually distorts the cost-effectiveness of proposed treatments.

A critical evaluation of the papers on cost-effective interventions (Chisholm 2005a, 2005b; Chisholm et al. 2004a, 2004b, 2005, 2008; Chisholm and Saxena 2012) shows that the MGMH's calculations are based on many questionable/unreal assumptions that gloss over nuances and amplify perceived benefits. Some of these are: (1) the reference point is the Global

Burden of Disease study, which itself has its own problems;[3] (2) the calculation of treatment benefits is in comparison to no treatment (null set); (3)
the calculation of population-level health gain is based on comparison
with an epidemiological situation representing the natural history of
disease (with zero intervention); (4) costing is based on an "ingredient
approach", meaning valuation of inputs in terms of personnel salary, the
price of pharmaceutical agents, cost for in-patient days, out-patient visits,
lab services, and so on, while ignoring investment in a satisfactory level of
hospital beds and out-patient clinics (overhead costs), thereby assuming
an optimal availability of these in all world regions while at the same time
implicitly comparing intervention against the null set; (5) the target treatment coverage for each mental health condition has been estimated based
on the severity of symptoms along with challenges of case identification
and medical treatment seeking behaviour while absolutely ignoring the
effect of community services available (which is assumed to be zero at
the beginning) and ignoring the plethora of non-medical services; (6) opportunity costs for patients and caregivers in attending services, especially
in chronic conditions where this requires repeated contact with the service
system, are not computed; (7) the assumption is that a "basic mental health
package" will address the needs of the mentally ill, whereas this group
suffers from many physical problems which also require treatment; (8)
the care provider's need for support in order to manage chronic illness at
home is ignored; and (9) there is a failure to account for investments in
structures, programmes, and practices to avoid human rights violations in
treatment settings and outside them. Moreover, for cost calculations, the
population-level effectiveness of interventions is based on compliance data
of high-income countries (HIC) (Chisholm 2004b; Chisholm et al. 2005b).
Effectiveness of treatment is dependent on compliance rates (i.e. efficacy
of a treatment that is evaluated under a strict experimental condition
such as controlled trials) and is particularly important when dealing with
chronic conditions. Compliance rates in particular illnesses in high income
countries are usually thought to be higher than those in LMICs. Aware of
this, the authors adjusted compliance rates by a factor of two-thirds for
LMIC based on data of high income countries, which seems arbitrary. In
addition, the baseline "no treatment scenario" is particularly remarkable
and is compounded by the fact that the authors ignore non-medical and

---

3   Some of these have been discussed above, such as the interlinked problem of the DALY
metric, inadequate epidemiological evidence for robust calculation, and methodological flaws
that do not account for comorbidity and early mortality in mental illness.

traditional support and services widely available in LMICs – one of the primary arguments in this volume. All these assumptions might inflate the cost-effectiveness ratio for the LMIC and bias policy makers.

As a result of such analyses, and because of not accounting for overhead costs, caring for certain conditions such as epilepsy appears to be more cost-effective than for schizophrenia, whereas the inclusion of overhead costs and accounting for these assumptions may bring these differences down.

More recently, the goal for the MGMH has shifted to research on capacity-building and an attempt at multi-country, multi-institutional partnership in the scaling-up of low-cost mental health interventions for specific high burden disorders (Lund et al. 2015; Mangezi et al. 2014; Semrau et al. 2015) together with other research hubs such as the Latin American Treatment and Innovation Network in Mental Health (Latin-MH) and South Asian Hub for Advocacy, Research and Education on Mental Health (SHARE). The attempt is to broaden the geographical reach of this research agenda and achieve synchronisation between researchers and trials tackling different diseases. An uncritical approach to the above research has resulted in greatly increased funding, mostly from rich donor countries as part of their development budgets, on research to integrate the above models in a scaled-up manner (Lund et al. 2012). The PRIME project is one such endeavour to develop, deliver, scale-up, and evaluate evidence-based mental health programmes in five African and Asian countries (De Silva et al. 2016). Similarly, the EMERALD programme (which somewhat complements the PRIME project, but is much broader) is working towards the strengthening of health systems in delivering mental health care in six African and Asian countries (Semrau et al. 2015) and should be seen as a more system-wide approach that attempts to involve policies, legislations, governance systems, inter-sectoral linkages and service users' participation to mental health care. The latter approach has greater potential than the former to address the social determinants of mental health.

The MGMH also over-relies on randomised control trials of the complex they plan to scale up. The methodology designed for complex interventions depends upon an atomistic understanding of specific and non-specific therapeutic elements as potentially separable. There are numerous active components of the intervention in the above-mentioned cluster randomised control trials involving multiple levels such as: (1) modification of organisation of health services by introduction of LHWs for community based service delivery; (2) alteration of health professional behaviour in terms of mental health condition evaluation and referral by physicians; and (3) direct individual patient multi-component intervention including psychotherapy/psychoeducation/adherence management. As the level of complexity of a system increases (or better, when a system is understood in all its complexity) the ostensibly separable parts can no longer be grasped atomistically, but only as parts of a whole in a well-defined state. Thus, trials for complex interventions are compromised by their inherent atomism. However, the analysis of complex social phenomena including demographic background, organisation of health services, individual circumstances, distress and lived experience, help and help-seeking, treatment, physician behaviour and healing requires a holistic methodology that explains social phenomena by involving the properties of entities that are irreducibly supra-individual (Yadavendu 2013). In other words, the elements investigated in cluster randomised controlled trials viz., the "patient", the LHW, the place of administering the treatment, the treatment, and the interpreter of the results are intricately entangled with each other, and knowledge of such entanglements is essential to properly understand the results. Moreover, certain adverse implications of such services, such as stigma or undermining local coping mechanisms, maybe outside the ambit of evaluation.

It is primarily the problems associated with the assumption of mental illness that drives the MGMH, its research and actions. Mental illnesses are regarded in the MGMH literature as primarily biological and only somewhat psychological. Hence the "effective treatment strategies" are overwhelmingly biomedical, while secondary consequences like stigma and human rights have only modest social implications and these are largely addressed by psychological and pharmacological treatment and health education to the community. The MGMH has systematically built up its evidence base, presumably to influence policy makers and health bureaucracies in those countries where it seeks to establish its programmes. As a result of the increasing criticism levelled at the assumptions informing the MGMH, a *Lancet* Commission recently reoriented its agenda in the context of Sustainable Development Goals (Patel et al. 2018). As a result, the MGMH plans certain positive shifts, but these fall short of addressing the social determinants of mental health in any comprehensive way, for example by addressing mental illness as part of a spectrum including physical health. This has potential in addressing the social determinants of mental health if population-level interventions are prioritised.

At a more general level, the leaders of the MGMH are trained psychiatrists and so their support for a biomedical model is understandable (Harland et al. 2009). Though the interest of "Big Pharma" (Fernando 2011) may not be obvious in the MGMH, the research agendas (Das and Rao 2012) and research outcomes (Healy and Cattell 2003) within psychiatry and worldwide (Petryna et al. 2006) have led many commentators to suggest bias due to big pharma influence. For example, an analysis of evidence in *The Lancet*'s 2007 article concerning (Patel et al. 2007) effective treatment and prevention methods for depression shows 80 per cent of trials in LMICs were for psycho-pharmaceuticals alone. Moreover, the recommendation of Selective Serotonin Reuptake Inhibitors in the foregoing publication and the WHO mhGAP Intervention Guide among the antidepressants is in itself controversial in the wake of research that questions their efficacy (Kirsch et al. 2008) as well as the efficacy of other, newer antidepressants (Turner et al. 2008). Though the WHO mhGAP Intervention Guide recommends the use of generics and preparations that are outside patent protection, it would be naïve to assume the commercial interests do not adapt to and transform such well-intentioned plans. Thus, in markets like India where control and regulation of the production, marketing, prescription and availability of pharmaceutical products are lax (Ecks and Basu 2009), while consumption is based on partial knowledge (or a different knowledge system), a whole new meaning is ascribed to such recommendations (Ecks 2005). As ethnographic work in Kolkata by Ecks and Basu (2009) suggests, the common use of antidepressants (and even psychotropics) by general practitioners and unlicensed practitioners occurs through "floating prescriptions" (i.e. prescriptions modelled on those written by psychiatrists that are carried around by patients). Personal experience of working in India also suggests that such prescriptions are often used beyond the prescribed duration to avoid the difficulties of consulting a specialist again; a practice that is facilitated by lax regulation at retail pharmacy counters. Moreover, although biomedical professionals tend to assume that psychopharmaceuticals uniformly act on humans despite cultural and historical variation, medical anthropologists have been able to show that such drugs are ingested in a complex context which influences their use and the patient's experience of them (Schlosser and Ninnemann 2012).

Although the MGMH agenda is to get health ministries on board, the movement seems unconcerned with the social and political contributors to "global" mental ill-health and instead push for low-cost strategies for disseminating psychiatric treatments within primary care. However, the physical and institutional infrastructure of primary care is in many LMICs are underdeveloped or under threat (due to conflict) (Rohde et al. 2008). It is widely accepted, for example, that primary health care in most of India is in its death throes (Rao 2010). Despite the lack of any comprehensive plan for primary health care in countries like Nigeria and Zimbabwe and the involvement of researchers in these countries, no serious engagement with its sociopolitical principles (Cueto 2004; Carpenter 2000) informs the movement. On the other hand, the involvement of the policy makers could be used to leverage health system strengthening for mental health through financial support, human resource management, inter-sectoral coordination and civil society participation (Jenkins et al. 2011) and finally rally for the social determinants of mental health.

A deeper concern that the MGMH glosses over is the monotonous bio-medical and evidence-based paradigm that it attempts to propagate. The great speed with which the movement has managed to establish itself and build a group of scientists and practitioners who share its ideology while excluding critical voices, is cause for alarm, as is its ongoing programme for indoctrinating young researchers in the name of "capacity building". Such rapid success is, in our view, not simply due to the power of ideas (which have been roundly criticised from many directions), but also because of global politics where dominant Western epistemologies are supported through development funds, bringing us back to the question; "whose globalisation?" (Navarro 1998).

Social Determinants of Health: The Theoretical Backdrop

Social Determinants of Health is a theoretical framework recognising the non-medical and non-behavioural determinants of health and illness (Raphael 2009), primarily the socio-economic conditions in which people are born, grow, live, work, age, and die. Its history has been drowned by a shift in the concept of health itself, from one encompassing broadly social factors – availability of food, regularity and security of employment, wages, hours and conditions of work, the structure of the family and work for women, leisure time and care of infants and children, a more nebulous sense of solidarity and community – to the mere absence of disease (Hamlin 1992).

The Social Determinants of Health approach focuses on the health, not merely of individuals, but rather of communities, regions, nations, and even the globe. Whereas individual-centred approaches focus on individual biology and health behaviour, the population perspective seeks to identify health determinants beyond these. While the former implies that health is largely governed by an individual's actions and personal choices, the latter asserts that such choices are largely context dependent. The Social Determinants of Health approach's focus on context emerged from a recognition of certain patterns in the health achievements of populations when grouped by socio-economic category. The *Black Report* in the UK, for example, showed the differential mortality and morbidity patterns in differing occupational groups (Gray 1982). A comprehensive synthesis by Raphael (2006, 7), who focused on Canada, but whose work has important worldwide implications, suggests twelve key social determinants of health: "Aboriginal status, early life, education, employment and working conditions, food security, gender, healthcare services, housing, income and its distribution, social safety net, social exclusion, and unemployment and employment security".

While these determinants are largely transparent, differing schools of thought exist on how they "get under the skin" to influence health. A *materialistic* framework emphasises how the material aspects of people's life (e.g. their socio-economic position in the country they live in) influence physical and social health. A *psychosocial* framework, on the other hand, points towards people's perception of inequality, working either through varied "individual" psychobiological mechanisms or through social capital (support, trust and shared norms of cooperation between groups), influencing health (Szreter and Woolcock 2004). We believe that a *neo-materialistic* framework goes further and best explains the relationship between material conditions and aspects of social capital (intermediary determinants) and health by offering a more nuanced, inclusive, and holistic framework in terms of describing the complex, varied and inter-linked mechanisms that influence the intermediary determinants. Such an approach focuses on the overarching context including political, economic and social forces that shape the quality of the various social determinants of health. It leads directly to policies and thereby politics that can influence the societal infrastructure and how resources are distributed in society and can transform social institutions and their practices.

Social Determinants of Mental Health: A Vital Element for Global Mental Health

In this section we use the concept of social determinants of health developed in the previous section to analyse two documents where the MGMH engages with the social determinants of health: First, the World Health Organization (WHO) document entitled *Social Determinants of Mental Health* (World Health Organization and Calouste Gulbenkian Foundation 2014) and second, *The Lancet Commission on Global Mental Health and sustainable development* (Patel et al. 2018).

We ascribe special importance to the World Health Organization document because we assume that it is a key stakeholder in the Global Mental

Health movement. WHO's recommendations such as the mhGAP: Mental Health Gap Action Program (World Health Organization 2008) make significant references to the MGMH. The WHO publication reviews the evidence and reaches certain conclusions with respect to social determinants of health and common mental disorders (including sub-threshold conditions). It applies a multilevel framework for strategies and interventions to tackle the social determinants of mental health including the individual, the family, the community and its services and, finally, the nation in terms of the policies that define social care. In addition, it employs a life course perspective to gain an understanding of the effects of socio-economic factors acting throughout the lifespan in influencing health outcomes in the future. The life course perspective has also been discussed in great depth in the social determinants of health approach (but not adequately in the WHO report) in terms of examining latent effects (critical period exposure that manifests only later with some other, exposure in later life) or pathways effects (where exposures add together, cluster or cause chains of risk) (Ben-Shlomo and Kuh 2002) which interact in a complex and inter-related manner (Hertzman et al. 2001).

Two additional aspects that do not find a place in the WHO report should be mentioned. First, social determinants of mental health influence not only common mental disorders and sub-threshold conditions (such as anxiety and depressive disorders, which are the main preoccupation and subjects of research of the MGMH) as suggested by the report, but also severe mental disorders like schizophrenia and bipolar disorder. Consider the well-known fact that amongst the mentally ill, mortality rates not directly attributable to mental illness (e.g. suicide or mortality secondary to substance use problems) is greater than those of the general population (Das et al. 2015). In the case of serious mental disorders, this is more apparent, especially when one considers the historical evidence of excess mortality in lunatic asylums (residents of which were probably more severely mentally ill) (Esqliirol 1838: Farr 1841) and findings of increased mortality in hospitalised long-stay psychiatric patients (Räsänen et al. 2003). In one study, mentally ill persons with histories of hospitalisation had higher mortality compared to the out-patient sample (Crump et al. 2013). There are similar findings among those in specialised psychiatric care versus primary care (Kisely et al. 2005). Assuming that serious mental disorders are overrepresented in psychiatrically hospitalised patients and patients in specialised psychiatric care, what is apparent from all the foregoing studies is that excess mortality is a *sine qua non* of serious mental disorders. Although this excess mortality has been attributed to adverse health behaviours, iatrogenic effects of psychotropics and discrimination in general health services, such factors are still inadequate to describe the whole picture. Furthermore, much of these factors are also patterned by social determinants of health such as smoking, obesity, stress, poor diet (i.e. lacking in fruits and vegetables) or lack of exercise and importantly availability/accessibility to general health services. It has also been noted that in particular country mental health settings, the life expectancy of people with mental disorders improved in association with deinstitutionalisation (even when taking into account an improvement in the mortality rates among the general population). This had occurred in Denmark, Finland, and Sweden, in the context of progressive community care, strong and stable socio-economic protective factors and social care policies (Wahlbeck et al. 2011). Clearly, the social and economic environment strongly influences the course of serious mental disorders, especially when considering determinants more broadly having influence throughout the lifespan and not just as aetiological entities. Moreover, social policy clearly influences aspects of (mental) health, as argued by the neo-materialistic approach to the social determinants of health. Recent research on the economic crisis in the European Union has also proved this point. Unemployment during the crisis was found to be related to all-cause mortality, particularly marked for suicide, violence, and death due to alcohol misuse. But this effect was much buffered in countries/regions where prevailing labour market programmes supported the unemployed during this phase (Stuckler et al. 2009). In short, by emphasising the political economy of mental illness, the social determinant of disease approach would appropriately and fruitfully broaden the framework for global mental health.

A second and more important aspect, absent in the WHO report, is that of the relationship of the social determinants of health to *mental* as well as physical *health*. Though there are well-established indicators for clinically defined mental disorders, there are no parallel indicators of mental health. In this context let us look into early child development, particularly focusing on cognitive development. It is commonly understood that childhood experiences during the early years are critical for the entire life course and are a powerful predictor of not only later physical and mental health outcomes but also of particular importance for social and economic achievement as adults (World Health Organization 2015). Among mental health outcomes, those with poor cognitive development in their early years are more likely to develop lifetime depression, anxiety disorders, schizophrenia spectrum disorders, and severe personality impairment (Der et al. 2009; Koenen et al. 2009; Moran et al. 2009; Martin et al. 2007). Evidence suggests gaps in all domains of development (viz. socio-emotional, cognitive, language, and motor) and educational achievement between the richest and the poorest economic categories (defined variously by family income, household wealth [Shanks 2007] or parental income) in a given region, consistently in the high-income countries and also in the LMICs (Cueto et al. 2009; Paxson and Schady 2007; Fernald et al. 2012), where there is also evidence to suggest a socio-economic gradient in the developmental achievement of children (Dearden et al. 2011; Schady et al. 2015). Moreover, it is seen that the gap widens from infancy to middle childhood (Rubio-Codina et al. 2015; Fernald et al. 2011). Early childhood development has been related not only to the socio-economic status of the family but also directly to the socio-economic characteristics of the neighbourhood (Kershaw et al. 2005). Other social factors influencing developmental achievements, though not divorced from the socio-economic circumstances of child's environment, include quality of stimulation, support and nurturance in the family (Power and Hertzman 1999), parental (maternal) education status [and cognitive skills (Korenman et al. 1995; Blau 1999)], the capacity to provide an enriching and responsive environment for language, the degree of organisation in the family environment (Hart and Risley 1995), opportunities for play and degree of hospitality in the neighbourhood environment (Hertzman and Boyce 2010). This holds not only within countries but also between countries at the macro-social level, as the evidence suggests that steeper of the socio-economic gradients between countries adversely influence cognitive development of adolescents in the lower socio-economic strata. And consistent with a neo-materialistic approach to the social determinants of health, the socio-economic gradient is dependent on the social care policies of the country, implying that in a country where the welfare state is less well developed compared to the countries with a long history of welfare state regimen, the socio-economic gradient is steeper (Siddiqi et al. 2007).

The second document by the *Lancet* Commission is, in effect, a review by leading figures in the MGMH of their own movement in relation to Sustainable Development Goals. It attempts to engage with the social determinants of health approach by expanding its agenda from reducing the so-called treatment gap to also addressing preventive, quality, and social care gaps. To achieve these goals, the commission proposes a staged approach that recognises the spectrum from mental well-being to mental illness, addresses both biological and social determinants, and shows a willingness to engage with service user voices. This reorientation is encouraging in many respects, but we expect more from the commission's operationalisation of the above principles. Rather than elaborating upon population-level interventions for mental health/well-being and considering that well-being can be achieved despite suffering from mental disorders, it refers to a staging model to identify mental disorder prodromes and propose individual level solutions (e.g. trans-diagnostic psychological interventions). The social care gap for the commission is to be addressed through individualised treatment (rehabilitation or supported employment). The commission considers five key domains of social determinants of health viz., demographic, economic, neighbourhood, environmental, and social or cultural, but forgets to explicitly mention the political domain, with just a passing mention of the distal structural arrangements of society.

In what follows, we attempt to clarify this need for an explicit engagement with the political determinants of health and to expand the meaning of "global" in global health so as to include political processes.

Global (Mental) Health and Globalisation

To understand global mental health, we must understand what is meant by globalisation and how this is related to mental health. Globalisation since the early 1990s has been referred to as the second wave, the first of course being colonialism. With the lowering of trade barriers, opening up of developing economies, liberalisation of foreign exchange restrictions, and removal of capital controls, cross-border financial flows have not only increased in absolute terms, but also undergone a transformation: where once they were largely between national governments, they are now dominated by private transnational corporations and metropolitan speculative finance (Woodward et al. 2001; Patnaik 2003). The factors that brought these changes are the 1970s recession in the industrialised world, the "oil crisis" and policies that increased interest rates on loans to the developing world; the consequent setting up of overseers like the International Monetary Fund and World Bank, which imposed policies like the Structural Adjustment Programmes. These policies were designed to cut social spending in order to repay debts and create markets for international finance in the developing world. The development model for these nations in this period was strongly shaped by transnational speculative finance. Globalisation consists not only of economic and political forces and their attendant institutions, agents and ideas, but also involves the redefinition of social connections and association between people, circulating global values, and images (Burawoy 2000) facilitated by innovations in communication technology. The supranational character of global forces, connections, and imaginations are essential aspects of the definition of global health (Janes and Corbett 2009). This, too, has facilitated the shift from an earlier conceptualisation of "international health" to the current notion of "global health" (Rowson et al. 2012). Thus the "global" in global health denotes "supra-territorial" space, processes and connections, irreducible to smaller units like the nation state, although having local (territorial) health implications (Bozorgmehr 2010). "Global" also denotes the political space that houses the playing field of power, contouring global processes, connections and images. These global factors and pathways are mutually interrelated and are not conceived as distant or acting at different levels, but directly through complex pathways to influence health. Domestic factors viz. policy, politics, and social structures also have essential interrelations with such global determinants and mediate effects on health.

Mental health, on the other hand, has long been at the periphery, both during the "tropical medicine" era in the heyday of colonialism, and the "international health" era (Whitley 2015) of the Cold War and neocolonial years, largely shaped by the WHO. The call for global mental health and its associated "movement" (Patel et al. 2011) have successfully brought the agenda of mental health to the global level. In this chapter, we have consistently argued that the MGMH should make a greater effort to link globalisation to the social determinants of health (Labonte and Torgerson 2005; Labonté and Schrecker 2007a, 2007b), giving due importance to political and social aspects. The "asymmetrical" expression of contemporary globalisation and its impacts might then be related to the asymmetrical distribution of mental health and disease, in relation to the increasingly unequal distribution within and across national borders of gains, losses, and ability to influence globalisation's outcomes" (ibid., 3). In fact, these issues should be central to the conception of global mental health; nevertheless, the MGMH has not enthusiastically engaged with them, preferring to employ a limited set of theoretical tools to tackle the problem of global mental health. Yet the MGMH has studiously avoided the fact that contemporary globalisation is a new form of imperialism. Indeed, it could be argued that global mental health and the MGMH are themselves deeply neo-imperial (see the Introduction). To illustrate, the agrarian crisis of the neoliberal order has spread throughout the world, and in India, more than 150,000 farmers have committed suicide in the last fifteen years (Patnaik and Moyo 2011). A substantial number of these suicides occurred in the more "developed" states of Maharashtra, Andhra Pradesh and Karnataka. When regional variations in suicide are taken into account, factors such as state withdrawal from financing and consequent increase in the power of private moneylenders, indebtedness, cash crop cultivation, and marginal landholdings explain 74 per cent of the variability of farmer suicides (Kennedy and King 2014), showing how neo-imperial globalisation created the groundwork for the epidemic of farmer suicides in India. Some commentators argue that this is largely due to mental illness requiring psychiatric treatment (Rai 2015). This seems eerily to reflect MGMH recommendations, brushing aside the political economic crisis in which peasant agriculture in the so-called Third World is mired.

Conclusion

It is time for the global health community to engage with mental health, and therefore the MGMH is admirable. But its theory and practice are unsatisfactory due to their narrow, biomedical bias while engaging with a very constricted view of the social determinants of health. Such a limited approach falls short of engaging with the contextual determinants of mental health. The social determinants approach to mental health, as we see it, brings us face to face with the sociopolitical aspects of globalisation, not only for determining the economic and social policies of LMICs, but also in terms of their influence on intermediary determinants of mental health such as employment, housing, income equity, social exclusion, and healthcare services. In other words, the dominant discourse of the MGMH is shaped by the power dynamics of globalisation, where the Western individualistic conception of mental health, along with the corporate interests of the pharmaceutical industry, insurance industry, and private healthcare services intersect. Despite the best intentions in the MGMH, an ignorance of links between local suffering and global power dynamics are implicit in a neocolonial enterprise. Despite their good intentions, the advocates of the MGMH largely ignore global power dynamics and their role in the production of mental suffering. In that respect, they are complicit with the neocolonial aspects of globalisation. There is however a way to avoid this trap, and that is to take seriously the social determinants of health approach, and include the political, economic and epistemic dimensions of global mental health.

References

Anand, Sudhir and Kara Hanson. 2004 "Disability-Adjusted Life Years: A Critical Review." In *Public Health, Ethics, and Equity*, edited by Sudhir Anand, Fabienne Peter, and Amartya Sen, 183-200. Oxford: Oxford University Press.

Araya, Ricardo, Graciela Rojas, Rosemarie Fritsch, Jorge Gaete, Maritza Rojas, Greg Simon, and Tim J. Peters. 2003. "Treating Depression in Primary Care in

Low-Income Women in Santiago, Chile: A Randomised Controlled Trial." *Lancet* 361 (9362): 995-1000.

Ben-Shlomo, Yoav, and Diana Kuh. 2002. "A Life Course Approach to Chronic Disease Epidemiology: Conceptual Models, Empirical Challenges and Interdisciplinary Perspectives." *International Journal of Epidemiology* 31 (2): 285-93.

Blau, David M. 1999. "The Effect of Income on Child Development." *The Review of Economics and Statistics* 81 (2): 261-76.

Bozorgmehr, Kayvan. 2010. "Rethinking the 'Global' in Global Health: A Dialectic Approach." *Globalization and Health* 6: 19. https://doi.org/10.1186/1744-8603-6-19.

Brhlikova, Petra, Allyson M. Pollock, and Rachel Manners. 2011. "Global Burden of Disease Estimates of Depression-How Reliable Is the Epidemiological Evidence?" *Journal of the Royal Society of Medicine* 104 (1): 25-34.

Burawoy, Michael. 2000. "Conclusion: Grounding Globalization." In *Global Ethnography: Forces, Connections, and Imaginations in a Postmodern World*, edited by Michael Burawoy, Joseph A. Blum, Sheba George, Zsuzsa Gille, Teresa Gowan, Lynne Haney, Maren Klawiter, Steven H. Lopez, Sean O. Riain, and Millie Thayer, 337-50. Berkeley: University of California Press.

Burti, Lorenzo. 2001. "Italian Psychiatric Reform 20 Plus Years After." *Acta Psychiatrica Scandinavica* 104 (s410): 41-46. https://doi.org/10.1034/j.1600-0447.2001.104s2041.x.

Carpenter, Mick. 2000. "Health for Some: Global Health and Social Development since Alma Ata." *Community Development Journal* 35 (4): 336-51.

Chatterjee, Sudipto, Neerja Chowdhary, Sulochana Pednekar, Alex Cohen, Gracy Andrew, Gracy Andrew, Ricardo Araya, et al. 2008. "Integrating Evidence-Based Treatments for Common Mental Disorders in Routine Primary Care: Feasibility and Acceptability of the MANAS Intervention in Goa, India." *World Psychiatry* 7 (1): 39-46.

Chatterjee, Sudipto, Smita Naik, Sujit John, Hamid Dabholkar, Madhumitha Balaji, Mirja Koschorke, Mathew Varghese, et al. 2014. "Effectiveness of a Community-Based Intervention for People with Schizophrenia and Their Caregivers in India (COPSI): A Randomised Controlled Trial." *Lancet* 383 (9926): 1385-94.

Chatterjee, Sudipto, Vikram Patel, Achira Chatterjee, and Helen A. Weiss. 2003. "Evaluation of a Community-Based Rehabilitation Model for Chronic Schizophrenia in Rural India." *The British Journal of Psychiatry* 182: 57-62.

Chisholm, Dan, Oye Gureje, Sandra Saldivia, Marcelo Villalón Calderón, Rajitha Wickremasinghe, Nalaka Mendis, Jose-Luis Ayuso-Mateos, and Shekhar Saxena. 2008. "Schizophrenia Treatment in the Developing World: An Interregional and Multinational Cost-Effectiveness Analysis." *Bulletin of the World Health Organization* 86 (7): 542-51.

Chisholm, Dan, Jürgen Rehm, Mark Van Ommeren, and Maristela Monteiro. 2004a. "Reducing the Global Burden of Hazardous Alcohol Use: A Comparative Cost-Effectiveness Analysis." *Journal of Studies on Alcohol* 65 (6): 782-93.

Chisholm, Dan, Kristy Sanderson, Jose Luis Ayuso-Mateos, and Shekhar Saxena. 2004b. "Reducing the Global Burden of Depression: Population-Level Analysis of Intervention Cost-Effectiveness in 14 World Regions." *British Journal of Psychiatry* 184 (5): 393-403.

Chisholm, Dan, and Shekhar Saxena. 2012. "Cost Effectiveness of Strategies to Combat Neuropsychiatric Conditions in Sub-Saharan Africa and South East Asia: Mathematical Modelling Study." *BMJ* 344:e609. https://doi.org/10.1136/bmj.e609.

Chisholm, Dan, Mark van Ommeren, Jose-Luis Ayuso-Mateos, and Shekhar Saxena. 2005. "Cost-Effectiveness of Clinical Interventions for Reducing the Global Burden of Bipolar Disorder." *The British Journal of Psychiatry* 187: 559-67.

Chisholm, Dan. 2005a. "Choosing Cost-Effective Interventions in Psychiatry: Results from the CHOICE Programme of the World Health Organization." *World Psychiatry* 4 (1): 37-44.

—. 2005b. "Cost-Effectiveness of First-Line Antiepileptic Drug Treatments in the Developing World: A Population-Level Analysis." *Epilepsia* 46 (5): 751-59.

Clark, Jocalyn. 2014. "Medicalization of Global Health 2: The Medicalization of Global Mental Health." *Global Health Action* 7:24000. https://doi.org/10.3402/gha.v7.24000.

Cooper, Sara. 2015. "Prising Open the 'Black Box': An Epistemological Critique of Discursive Constructions of Scaling up the Provision of Mental Health Care in Africa." *Health* 19 (5): 523-41.

—. 2016. "'How I Floated on Gentle Webs of Being': Psychiatrists Stories About the Mental Health Treatment Gap in Africa." *Culture, Medicine and Psychiatry* 40 (3): 307-37.

Crump, Casey, John P. A. Ioannidis, Kristina Sundquist, Marilyn A. Winkleby, and Jan Sundquist. 2013. "Mortality in Persons with Mental Disorders Is Substantially Overestimated Using Inpatient Psychiatric Diagnoses." *Journal of Psychiatric Research* 47 (10): 1298-303.

Cueto, Marcos. 2004. "The Origins of Primary Health Care and Selective Primary Health Care." *American Journal of Public Health* 94 (11): 1864-74.

Cueto, Santiago, Juan Leon, Gabriela Guerrero, and Ismael Muñoz. 2009. "Psychometric Characteristics of Cognitive Development and Achievement Instruments in Round 2 of Young Lives." *Young Lives Technical Note* 15. Accessed 4 August 2020, http://repositorio.minedu.gob.pe/handle/123456789/4134.

Das, Anindya, Mohan Rao, and Mercian Danial. 2015. "Early Mortality and Mental Illness: 'Fatal' Discrimination." *Bengal Journal of Psychiatry* 20: 14-19.

Das, Anindya, and Mohan Rao. 2012. "Universal Mental Health: Re-Evaluating the Call for Global Mental Health." *Critical Public Health* 22 (4): 383-89.

Das, Anindya. 2014. "The Context of Formulation of India's Mental Health Program: Implications for Global Mental Health." *Asian Journal of Psychiatry* 7 (1): 10-14.

—. 2018. "Primary (Mental) Health Care and the National Mental Health Program." *Indian Journal of Psychological Medicine* 40 (6): 503-06.

De Silva, Mary J., Sujit D. Rathod, Charlotte Hanlon, Erica Breuer, Dan Chisholm, Abebaw Fekadu, Mark Jordans, et al. 2016. "Evaluation of District Mental Healthcare Plans: The PRIME Consortium Methodology." *British Journal of Psychiatry* 208 (s56): s63-70.

Dearden, Lorraine, Luke Sibieta, and Kathy Sylva. 2011. "The Socio-Economic Gradient in Early Child Outcomes: Evidence from the Millennium Cohort Study." *Longitudinal and Life Course Studies* 2 (1): 19-40.

Der, Geoff, G. David Batty, and Ian J. Deary. 2009. "The Association between IQ in Adolescence and a Range of Health Outcomes at 40 in the 1979 US National Longitudinal Study of Youth." *Intelligence* 37 (6): 573-80.

Dias, Amit, Michael E. Dewey, Jean D'Souza, Rajesh Dhume, Dilip D. Motghare, K. S. Shaji, Rajiv Menon, Martin Prince, and Vikram Patel. 2008. "The Effectiveness of a Home Care Program for Supporting Caregivers of Persons with Dementia in Developing Countries: A Randomised Controlled Trial from Goa, India." *PloS One* 3 (6): e2333. https://doi.org/10.1371/journal.pone.0002333.

Divan, Gauri, Syed Usman Hamdani, Vivek Vajartkar, Ayesha Minhas, Carol Taylor, Catherine Aldred, Kathy Leadbitter, Atif Rahman, Jonathan Green, and Vikram Patel. 2015. "Adapting an Evidence-Based Intervention for Autism Spectrum Disorder for Scaling up in Resource-Constrained Settings: The Development of the PASS Intervention in South Asia." *Global Health Action* 8: 27278. https://doi.org/10.3402/gha.v8.27278.

Ecks, Stefan, and Soumita Basu. 2009. "How Wide Is the 'Treatment Gap' for Antidepressants in India? Ethnographic Insights on Private Industry Marketing Strategies." *Journal of Health Studies* 2: 68-80.

Ecks, Stefan. 2005. "Pharmaceutical Citizenship: Antidepressant Marketing and the Promise of Demarginalization in India." *Anthropology & Medicine* 12 (3): 239-54.

Esqliirol, Étienne. 1838. *Des Maladies Mentales*. Paris: Chez J.-B. Baillière.

Farr, William. 1841. "Report on the Mortality of Lunatics." *Lancet* 36 (926): 332-35.

Fernald, Lia C. H., Patricia Kariger, Melissa Hidrobo, and Paul J. Gertler. 2012. "Socioeconomic Gradients in Child Development in Very Young Children: Evidence from India, Indonesia, Peru, and Senegal." *Proceedings of the National Academy of Sciences of the United States of America* 109 (s2): 17273-80.

Fernald, Lia C. H., Ann Weber, Emanuela Galasso, and Lisy Ratsifandrihamanana. 2011. "Socioeconomic Gradients and Child Development in a Very Low Income Population: Evidence from Madagascar." *Developmental Science* 14 (4): 832-47.

Fernando, Suman. 2011. "A 'Global' Mental Health Program or Markets for Big Pharma." *Open Mind* 168: 22. http://www.sumanfernando.com/Global%20 Program%20&%20Big%20Pharma.pdf.

Government of India. 2017. *The Mental Health Care Act 2017*.

Gupta, Monica Das, B. R. Desikachari, Rajendra Shukla, T. V. Somanathan, P. Padmanaban, and K. K. Datta. 2010. "How Might India's Public Health Systems Be Strengthened? Lessons from Tamil Nadu." *Economic & Political Weekly* 15 (10): 46-60.

Gupta, Nitin, and R. Srinivasamurthy. 2014. "The COPSI Trial: Additional Fidelity Testing Needed." *Lancet* 384 (9954): 1572-73.

Gray, Alastair McIntosh. 1982. "Inequalities in Health. The Black Report: A Summary and Comment." *International Journal of Health Services* 12 (3): 349-80.

Gururaj, G., C. Ramasubramanian, N. Girish, V. Mathew, and S. Sunitha. 2014. *Tamil Nadu Mental Health Care Assessment: Review of District Mental Health Programme, 2013*. Publication No. 106, Bangalore: National Institute of Mental Health and Neuro Sciences.

Gururaj G., M. Varghese, V. Benegal, G.N. Rao, K. Pathak, L.K. Singh, R.Y. Mehta, et al., and NMHS collaborators group. 2016. *National Mental Health Survey of India, 2015-16: Mental Health Systems*. Publication No. 130, Bengaluru: National Institute of Mental Health and Neuro Sciences.

Hamlin, Christopher. 1992. "Predisposing Causes and Public Health in Early Nineteenth-Century Medical Thought." *Social History of Medicine* 5 (1): 43-70.

Harland, Robert T., Elena Antonova, Gareth S. Owen, Matthew R. Broome, Sabine Landau, Quinton Deeley, and Robin Murray. 2009. "A Study of Psychiatrists' Concepts of Mental Illness." *Psychological Medicine* 39 (6): 967-76.

Hart, Betty, and Todd R. Risley. 1995. *Meaningful Differences in the Everyday Experience of Young American Children*. Baltimore, MD: Brookes Publishing Company.

Healy, David, and Dinah Cattell. 2003. "Interface between Authorship, Industry and Science in the Domain of Therapeutics." *British Journal of Psychiatry* 183: 22-27.

Hertzman, Clyde, and Tom Boyce. 2010. "How Experience Gets under the Skin to Create Gradients in Developmental Health." *Annual Review of Public Health* 31: 329-47.

Hertzman, Clyde, Chris Power, Sharon Matthews, and Orly Manor. 2001. "Using an Interactive Framework of Society and Lifecourse to Explain Self-Rated Health in Early Adulthood." *Social Science & Medicine* 53 (12): 1575-85.

Indian Council of Medical Research and Department of Science and Technology. 1987. "A Collaborative Study of Severe Mental Morbidity. A Report." ICMR and DST: New Delhi.

Jacob, K. S. 2011. "Repackaging Mental Health Programs in Low- and Middle-Income Countries." *Indian Journal of Psychiatry* 53 (3): 195-98.

Jain, Sumeet, and Sushrut Jadhav. 2009. "Pills That Swallow Policy: Clinical Ethnography of a Community Mental Health Program in Northern India." *Transcultural Psychiatry* 46 (1): 60-85.

Janes, Craig R., and Kitty K. Corbett. 2009. "Anthropology and Global Health." *Annual Review of Anthropology* 38 (1): 167-83.

Jenkins, Rachel, Florence Baingana, Raheelah Ahmad, David McDaid, and Rifat Atun. 2011. "How Can Mental Health Be Integrated into Health System Strengthening?" *Mental Health in Family Medicine* 8 (2): 115-17.

Karan, Anup, Winnie Yip, and Ajay Mahal. 2017. "Extending Health Insurance to the Poor in India: An Impact Evaluation of Rashtriya Swasthya Bima Yojana on Out of Pocket Spending for Healthcare." *Social Science and Medicine* 181: 83-92. https://doi.org/10.1016/j.socscimed.2017.03.053.

Kapur, Ravindra L. 2004. "The Story of Community Mental Health in India." In *Mental Health: An Indian Perspective 1946-2003,* edited by S.P. Agarwal, D.S. Goel, R.L. Ichhpujani, R.N. Salhan, and S. Shrivastava, 92-100. New Delhi: Directorate General of Health Services, Ministry of Health and Family Welfare.

Kennedy, Jonathan, and Lawrence King. 2014. "The Political Economy of Farmers' Suicides in India: Indebted Cash-Crop Farmers with Marginal Landholdings Explain State-Level Variation in Suicide Rates." *Globalization and Health* 10: 16. https://doi.org/10.1186/1744-8603-10-16.

Kershaw, Paul W., and Human Early Learning Partnership 2005. *The British Columbia Atlas of Child Development,* 1st ed. Canadian Western Geographical Series, v. 40. British Columbia: Human Early Learning Partnership.

Kirsch, Irving, Brett J. Deacon, Tania B. Huedo-Medina, Alan Scoboria, Thomas J. Moore, and Blair T. Johnson. 2008. "Initial Severity and Antidepressant Benefits: A Meta-Analysis of Data Submitted to the Food and Drug Administration." *PLoS Medicine* 5 (2): e45. https://doi.org/10.1371/journal.pmed.0050045.

Kisely, Stephen, Mark Smith, David Lawrence, and Sarah Maaten. 2005. "Mortality in Individuals Who Have Had Psychiatric Treatment: Population-Based Study in Nova Scotia." *British Journal of Psychiatry* 187: 552-58.

Koenen, Karestan C., Terrie E. Moffitt, Andrea L. Roberts, Laurie T. Martin, Laura Kubzansky, HonaLee Harrington, Richie Poulton, and Avshalom Caspi. 2009. "Childhood IQ and Adult Mental Disorders: A Test of the Cognitive Reserve Hypothesis." *The American Journal of Psychiatry* 166 (1): 50-57.

Kohn, Robert, Shekhar Saxena, Itzhak Levav, and Benedetto Saraceno. 2004. "The Treatment Gap in Mental Health Care." *Bulletin of the World Health Organization* 82 (11): 858-66.

Korenman, Sanders, Jane E. Miller, and John E. Sjaastad. 1995. "Long-Term Poverty and Child Development in the United States: Results from the NLSY." *Children and Youth Services Review* 17 (1): 127-55.

Kurian, Oommen C. 2015. *Financing Healthcare for All in India: Towards a Common Goal.* New Delhi: Oxfam India. Accessed 14 July 2020, https://oxfamilibrary. openrepository.com/bitstream/handle/10546/556476/wp-financing-healthcare-for-all-india-290515-en.pdf;jsessionid=C0984A7B1A17AFE38D63C48D72FB51 7E?sequence=1.

Labonté, Ronald, and Ted Schrecker. 2007a. "Globalization and Social Determinants of Health: Introduction and Methodological Background (Part 1 of 3)." *Globalization and Health* 3: 5. https://doi.org/10.1186/1744-8603-3-5.

—. 2007b. "Globalization and Social Determinants of Health: The Role of the Global Marketplace (Part 2 of 3)." *Globalization and Health* 3: 6. https://doi.org/10.1186/1744-8603-3-6.

Labonté, Ronald, and Renee Torgerson. 2005. "Interrogating Globalization, Health and Development: Towards a Comprehensive Framework for Research, Policy and Political Action." *Critical Public Health* 15 (2): 157-79.

Lang, Claudia. 2019. "Inspecting Mental Health: Depression, Surveillance and Care in Kerala, South India." *Culture, Medicine and Psychiatry* 43 (4): 596-612. https://doi.org/10.1007/s11013-019-09656-3.

Lund, Crick, Atalay Alem, Marguerite Schneider, Ccharlotte Hanlon, Jen Ahrens, Chiwoza Bandawe, Judith K. Bass, et al. 2015. "Generating Evidence to Narrow the Treatment Gap for Mental Disorders in Sub-Saharan Africa: Rationale, Overview and Methods of AFFIRM." *Epidemiology and Psychiatric Sciences* 24 (3): 233-40.

Lund, Crick, Mark Tomlinson, Mary De Silva, Abebaw Fekadu, Rahul Shidhaye, Mark Jordans, Inge Petersen, et al. 2012. "PRIME: A Programme to Reduce the Treatment Gap for Mental Disorders in Five Low- and Middle-Income Countries." *PLoS Medicine* 9 (12): e1001359. https://doi.org/10.1371/journal.pmed.1001359.

Mangezi, Walter O., Sekai M. Nhiwatiwa, Frances M. Cowan, Dixon Chibanda, James Hakim, Crick Lund, and Melanie A. Abas. 2014. "Improving Psychiatric Education and Research Capacity in Zimbabwe." *Medical Education* 48 (11): 1132. https://doi.org/10.1111/medu.12554.

Martin, Laurie T., Laura D. Kubzansky, Kaja Z. LeWinn, Lewis P. Lipsitt, Paul Satz, and Stephen L. Buka. 2007. "Childhood Cognitive Performance and Risk of Generalized Anxiety Disorder." *International Journal of Epidemiology* 36 (4): 769-75.

Mental Health Policy Group. 2012. "XIIth Plan District Mental Health Programme." Accessed 14 July 2020, https://mhpolicy.files.wordpress.com/2012/07/final-dmhp-design-xii-plan2.pdf.

Ministry of Health & Family Welfare, Government of India. 2014. *New Pathways, New Hopes. National Mental Health Policy of India.*

Moran, Paul, Britt A. F. Klinteberg, G. David Batty, and Denny Vågerö. 2009. "Childhood Intelligence Predicts Hospitalization with Personality Disorder in Adulthood: Evidence from a Population-Based Study in Sweden." *Journal of Personality Disorders* 23 (5): 535-40.

Nadkarni, Abhijit, Richard Velleman, Hamid Dabholkar, Sachin Shinde, Bhargav Bhat, Jim McCambridge, Pratima Murthy, Terry Wilson, Benedict Weobong, and Vikram Patel. 2015. "The Systematic Development and Pilot Randomized Evaluation of Counselling for Alcohol Problems, a Lay Counselor-Delivered Psychological Treatment for Harmful Drinking in Primary Care in India: The PREMIUM Study." *Alcoholism, Clinical and Experimental Research* 39 (3): 522-31.

Navarro, Vicente. 1998. "Comment: Whose Globalization?" *American Journal of Public Health* 88 (5): 742-43.

Oommen, Suby Elizabeth. 2018. "Growth of Primary Health Care System in Kerala: A comparison with India." *International Journal of Interdisciplinary Research and Innovations* 6 (2): 481-90.

Parthasarathi, R., and S. Sinha. 2016. "Towards a Better Health Care Delivery System: The Tamil Nadu Model." *Indian Journal of Community Medicine* 41 (4): 302-04. https://doi.org/10.4103/0970-0218.193344.

Patel, Vikram, Ricardo Araya, Sudipto Chatterjee, Dan Chisholm, Alex Cohen, Mary De Silva, Clemens Hosman, Hugh McGuire, Graciela Rojas, and Mark van Ommeren. 2007. "Treatment and Prevention of Mental Disorders in Low-Income and Middle-Income Countries." *Lancet* 370 (9591): 991-1005.

Patel, Vikram, Pamela Y. Collins, John Copeland, Ritsuko Kakuma, Sylvester Katontoka, Jagannath Lamichhane, Smita Naik, and Sarah Skeen. 2011. "The Movement for Global Mental Health." *British Journal of Psychiatry* 198 (2): 88-90.

Patel, Vikram, Helen A. Weiss, Neerja Chowdhary, Smita Naik, Sulochana Pednekar, Sudipto Chatterjee, Mary J. De Silva, et al. 2010. "Effectiveness of an Intervention Led by Lay Health Counsellors for Depressive and Anxiety Disorders in Primary Care in Goa, India (MANAS): A Cluster Randomised Controlled Trial." *Lancet* 376 (9758): 2086-95.

Patel, Vikram, Mario Maj, Alan J. Flisher, Mary J. De Silva, Mirja Koschorke, Martin Prince, and WPA Zonal and Member Society Representatives. 2010. "Reducing the Treatment Gap for Mental Disorders: A WPA Survey." *World Psychiatry* 9 (3): 169-76.

Patel, Vikram, Shekhar Saxena, Crick Lund, Graham Thornicroft, Florence Baingana, Paul Bolton, Dan Chisholm, et al. 2018. "The Lancet Commission on Global Mental Health and Sustainable Development." *Lancet* 392 (10157): 1553-98.

Patel, Vikram, Helen A. Weiss, Neerja Chowdhary, Smita Naik, Sulochana Pednekar, Sudipto Chatterjee, Bhargav Bhat, et al. 2011. "Lay Health Worker Led Intervention for Depressive and Anxiety Disorders in India: Impact on Clinical and Disability Outcomes over 12 Months." *British Journal of Psychiatry* 199 (6): 459-66.

Patnaik, Prabhat. 2003. *The Retreat to Unfreedom: Essays on the Emerging World Order.* New Delhi: Tulik.

Patnaik, Utsa, and Sam Moyo. 2011. *The Agrarian Question in the Neo-Liberal Era: Primitive Accumulation and the Peasantry.* Cape Town: Fahamu Books and Pambazuka Press.

Paxson, Christina, and Norbert Schady. 2007. "Cognitive Development among Young Children in Ecuador: The Roles of Wealth, Health, and Parenting." *Journal of Human Resources* 42 (1): 49-84.

Petryna, Adriana, Andrew Lakoff, and Arthur Kleinman. 2006. *Global Pharmaceuticals: Ethics, Markets, Practices.* Durham: Duke University Press.

Power, Chris, and Clyde Hertzman. 1999. "Health, Well-Being and Coping Skills." In *Developmental Health and the Wealth of Nations: Social, Biological, and Educational Dynamics,* edited by Daniel P. Keating, Clyde Hertzman, 41-54. New York: Guilford.

Priya, Ritu. 2005. "Public Health Services in India. A Historical Perspective." In *Review of Healthcare in India,* edited by Leena V Gangolli, Ravi Duggal, and Abhay Shukla, 41-73. Mumbai: Centre for Enquiry into Health and Allied Themes.

Rahman, Atif, Abid Malik, Siham Sikander, Christopher Roberts, and Francis Creed. 2008. "Cognitive Behaviour Therapy-Based Intervention by Community Health Workers for Mothers with Depression and Their Infants in Rural Pakistan: A Cluster-Randomised Controlled Trial." *Lancet* 372 (9642): 902-09.

Rai, Pronoy. 2015. "Matters of the Mind and the Agrarian Political Economy in Eastern Maharashtra." Kafila on WordPress.com. Accessed 14 July 2020, https://kafila.online/2015/11/03/matters-of-the-mind-and-the-agrarian-political-economy-in-eastern-maharashtra-pronoy-rai/.

Rajaraman, Divya, Sandra Travasso, Achira Chatterjee, Bhargav Bhat, Gracy Andrew, Suraj Parab, and Vikram Patel. 2012. "The Acceptability, Feasibility and Impact of a Lay Health Counsellor Delivered Health Promoting Schools Programme in India: A Case Study Evaluation." *BMC Health Services Research* 12: 127. https://doi.org/10.1186/1472-6963-12-127.

Rao, Mohan. 2010. "Health for All and Neo-liberal Globalisation: An Indian Ropetrick." In *Morbid Symptoms: Health Under Capitalism (Socialist Register, 2010),* edited by Leo Panitch and Colin Leys, 262-78. New York: Monthly Review Press.

Raphael, Dennis. 2009. "Social Determinants of Health: An Overview of Key Issues and Themes." In *Social Determinants of Health: Canadian Perspectives,* 2nd ed., edited by Dennis Raphael, 2-19. Toronto: Canadian Scholars' Press.

Raphael, Dennis. 2006. "Social Determinants of Health: Present Status, Unanswered Questions, and Future Directions." *International Journal of Health Services* 36 (4): 651-77.

Räsänen, Sami, Helinä Hakko, Kaisa Viilo, V. Benno Meyer-Rochow, and Juha Moring. 2003. "Excess Mortality among Long-Stay Psychiatric Patients in Northern Finland." *Social Psychiatry and Psychiatric Epidemiology* 38 (6): 297-304.

Rohde, Jon, Simon Cousens, Mickey Chopra, Viroj Tangcharoensathien, Robert Black, Zulfiqar A. Bhutta, and Joy E. Lawn. 2008. "30 Years after Alma-Ata: Has Primary Health Care Worked in Countries?" *Lancet* 372 (9642): 950-61.

Rowson, Mike, Chris Willott, Rob Hughes, Arti Maini, Sophie Martin, J. Jaime Miranda, Vicki Pollit, Abi Smith, Rae Wake, and John S. Yudkin. 2012. "Conceptualising Global Health: Theoretical Issues and Their Relevance for Teaching." *Globalization and Health* 8 (1): 36. https://doi.org/10.1186/1744-8603-8-36.

Rubio-Codina, Marta, Orazio Attanasio, Costas Meghir, Natalia Varela, and Sally Grantham-McGregor. 2015. "The Socioeconomic Gradient of Child Development: Cross-Sectional Evidence from Children 6-42 Months in Bogota." *Journal of Human Resources* 50 (2): 464-83.

Sartorius, Norman, and Timothy W. Harding. 1983. "The WHO Collaborative Study on Strategies for Extending Mental Health Care, I: The Genesis of the Study." *American Journal of Psychiatry* 140 (11): 1470-73.

Schady, Norbert, Jere Behrman, Maria Caridad Araujo, Rodrigo Azuero, Raquel Bernal, David Bravo, Florencia Lopez-Boo, et al. 2015. "Wealth Gradients in Early Childhood Cognitive Development in Five Latin American Countries." *Journal of Human Resources* 50 (2): 446-63.

Scheper-Hughes, Nancy, and Anne M. Lovell. 1986. "Breaking the Circuit of Social Control: Lessons in Public Psychiatry from Italy and Franco Basaglia." *Social Science and Medicine* 23 (2): 159-78. https://doi.org/10.1016/0277-9536(86)90364-3.

Schlosser, Allison V., and Kristi Ninnemann. 2012. "Introduction to the Special Section: The Anthropology of Psychopharmaceuticals: Cultural and Pharmacological Efficacies in Context." *Culture, Medicine and Psychiatry* 36 (1): 2-9.

Selvaraj, Sakthivel, and Anup K. Karan. 2012. "Why Publicly-Financed Health Insurance Schemes are Ineffective in Providing Financial Risk Protection." *Economic and Political Weekly* 47 (11): 61-68.

Semrau, Maya, Sara Evans-Lacko, Atalay Alem, Jose L. Ayuso-Mateos, Dan Chisholm, Oye Gureje, Charlotte Hanlon, et al. 2015. "Strengthening Mental Health Systems in Low- and Middle-Income Countries: The Emerald Programme." *BMC Medicine* 13: 79. https://doi.org/10.1186/s12916-015-0309-4.

Sengupta, Amit. 2013. "Universal Health Care in India: Making It Public, Making It a Reality." Occasional Paper No. 19, Municipal Services Project, International

Development Research Centre. Accessed 14 July 2020, http://uhc-india.org/up-loads/Sengupta_Universal_Health_Care_in_India_Making_it_Public_May2013. pdf.

Shanks, Trina R. Williams. 2007. "The Impacts of Household Wealth on Child Development." *Journal of Poverty* 11 (2): 93-116.

Shidhaye, Rahul, Sanjay Shrivastava, Vaibhav Murhar, Sandesh Samudre, Shalini Ahuja, Rohit Ramaswamy, and Vikram Patel. 2016. "Development and Piloting of a Plan for Integrating Mental Health in Primary Care in Sehore District, Madhya Pradesh, India." *British Journal of Psychiatry* 208 (s56): s13-20.

Siddiqi, Arjumand, Ichiro Kawachi, Lisa Berkman, S. V. Subramanian, and Clyde Hertzman. 2007. "Variation of Socioeconomic Gradients in Children's Developmental Health across Advanced Capitalist Societies: Analysis of 22 OECD Nations." *International Journal of Health Services* 37 (1): 63-87.

Singla, Daisy R., Benedict Weobong, Abhijit Nadkarni, Neerja Chowdhary, Sachin Shinde, Arpita Anand, Christopher G. Fairburn, et al. 2014. "Improving the Scalability of Psychological Treatments in Developing Countries: An Evaluation of Peer-Led Therapy Quality Assessment in Goa, India." *Behaviour Research and Therapy* 60: 53-59.

Murthy, R. Srinivasa. 2011. "Mental Health Initiatives in India (1947-2010)." *National Medical Journal of India* 24 (2): 98-107.

Stuckler, David, Sanjay Basu, Marc Suhrcke, Adam Coutts, and Martin McKee. 2009. "The Public Health Effect of Economic Crises and Alternative Policy Responses in Europe: An Empirical Analysis." *Lancet* 374 (9686): 315-23.

Szreter, Simon, and Michael Woolcock. 2004. "Health by Association? Social Capital, Social Theory, and the Political Economy of Public Health." *International Journal of Epidemiology* 33 (4): 650-67.

Turner, Erick H., Annette M. Matthews, Eftihia Linardatos, Robert A. Tell, and Robert Rosenthal. 2008. "Selective Publication of Antidepressant Trials and Its Influence on Apparent Efficacy." *New England Journal of Medicine* 358 (3): 252-60.

Vellakkal, Sukumar, and Vikram Patel. 2015. "Designing Psychological Treatments for Scalability: The PREMIUM Approach." *PloS One* 10 (7): e0134189. https://doi.org/10.1371/journal.pone.0134189.

Vigo, Daniel, Graham Thornicroft, and Rifat Atun. 2016. "Estimating the True Global Burden of Mental Illness." *Lancet Psychiatry* 3 (2): 171-78.

Wahlbeck, Kristian, Jeanette Westman, Merete Nordentoft, Mika Gissler, and Thomas Munk Laursen. 2011. "Outcomes of Nordic Mental Health Systems: Life Expectancy of Patients with Mental Disorders." *British Journal of Psychiatry* 199 (6): 453-58.

Whitley, Rob. 2015. "Global Mental Health: Concepts, Conflicts and Controversies." *Epidemiology and Psychiatric Sciences* 24 (4): 285-91.

Wig, Narendra N., R. Srinivasa Murthy, and Timothy W. Harding. 1981. "A Model for Rural Psychiatric Services-Raipur Rani Experience." *Indian Journal of Psychiatry* 23 (4): 275-90.

Woodward, David, Nick Drager, Robert Beaglehole, and Debra Lipson. 2001. "Globalization and Health: A Framework for Analysis and Action." *Bulletin of the World Health Organization* 79 (9): 875-81.

World Health Organization and Calouste Gulbenkian. 2014. *Social Determinants of Mental Health*. Geneva: World Health Organization.

World Health Organization. 1975. *Organization of Mental Health Services in Developing Countries: 16th Report of the WHO Expert Committee in Mental Health*. Geneva: World Health Organization.

—. 2010. *mhGAP Intervention Guide for Mental, Neurological and Substance Use Disorders in Non-Specialized Health Settings: Version 1.0*. Geneva: World Health Organization.

—. n.d. "Social Determinants of Health. Early Child Development." Accessed 19 October 2015, http://www.who.int/social_determinants/themes/earlychilddevelopment/en/.

Yadavendu, Vijay Kumar. 2013. *Shifting Paradigms in Public Health. From Holism to Individualism*. New Delhi: Springer India.

About the Authors

ANINDYA DAS is currently Consultant Psychiatrist and Associate Professor of Psychiatry at All India Institute of Medical Sciences, Rishikesh, India. He has an MD in Psychiatry from Central Institute of Psychiatry, Ranchi, and a Master's in Public Health from Jawaharlal Nehru University. He is a full time clinician responsible for training graduate medical students and postgraduate residents of psychiatry. He has established and manages a tele-training psychiatry service. He has a particular interest in community and social psychiatry, and is working with the state government to establish a community mental health programme at the local level.

MOHAN RAO was, till recently, a Professor at the Centre of Social Medicine and Community Health (CSMCH), School of Social Sciences, Jawaharlal Nehru University, New Delhi. A medical doctor specialising in public health, he has written extensively on health and population policy, and on the history and politics of health and family planning. He is the author of *From Population Control to Reproductive Health: Malthusian Arithmetic* (Sage, 2004) and has edited *Disinvesting in Health: The World Bank's Health Prescriptions*

(Sage, 1999) and *The Unheard Scream: Reproductive Health and Women's Lives in India* (Zubaan/Kali for Women, 2004). He has edited, with Sarah Sexton of Cornerhouse, UK, the volume *Markets and Malthus: Population, Gender and Health in Neoliberal Times* (Sage, 2010); and with Sarah Hodges, *Public Health and Private Wealth: Stem Cells, Surrogacy and Other Strategic Bodies* (Oxford University Press, 2016). His latest work is the edited volume *The Lineaments of Population Policy in India: Women and Family Planning* (Routledge, 2018). He has been a member of the National Population Commission, as well as several Working Groups of the National Rural Health Mission of the Government of India. He has worked on the Committee established by the National Human Rights Commission to examine the two-child norm in population policy, and is a member of the Executive Committee of the Centre for Women's Development Studies. He is also actively involved in the Jan Swasthya Abhiyan (People's Health Movement).

The Limits of Global Mental Health

5   Jinns and the Proletarian Mumin Subject

Exploring the Limits of Global Mental Health in Bangladesh

Projit Bihari Mukharji

Abstract
This article describes an epidemic of jinn attacks on schoolchildren in contemporary Bangladesh. It explores the ways in which the psychiatric and state health establishment of the country has repeatedly labelled these outbreaks 'mass psychogenic illness' and dismissed the widespread local use of kobirajes in these cases. By exploring strategies through which the biomedical establishment has, notwithstanding its own failure to understand or treat these outbreaks, sought to assert the authority of its own frameworks and discredit jinn-based frameworks, I argue that we can glimpse deeper differences between how the two competing frameworks conceptualise the subject of suffering.

Keywords: hysteria, psychosocial, Islam, ritual therapy, ontology

Rumi Khatun died on 19 May 2015. She was only eleven years old the time of her death and studied in Class Five at the Bordanagar Government Primary School in the Pabna district of Bangladesh. She had been admitted to the government health centre at Chatmohar the day before. Doctors at the Chatmohar Upazila Health Complex tried their best to save her life, but were unable to determine exactly what ailed her and she eventually passed away (Ranju 2016).

Less than two years later on 13 February 2017, another young girl, Rani Khatun, died under very similar circumstances. Rani was a student of Class Nine at the Dr. Hanif Uddin High School in Dari Hamidpur in the Jamalpur district of Bangladesh. Rani had come back from school on 26 January and

Sax, William, and Claudia Lang (eds), *The Movement for Global Mental Health: Critical Views from South and Southeast Asia.* Taylor & Francis Group, 2021
DOI: 10.5117/9789463721622_CH05

immediately fallen mysteriously ill. She had lost all sensation in both her legs and had begun to speak incoherently. She was taken to the hospital, but her unexplained and mysterious symptoms persisted. Though Rani had been in hospital for close to a month, the doctors remained unsure about precisely what had ailed her. (Jamalpur Correspondent 2017).

The only silver lining in this otherwise tragic loss of two young lives was the fact that the death toll was limited in each case to a single individual. The mysterious illnesses from which the girls died had, unfortunately, not afflicted them alone. A number of their classmates had also fallen ill and been hospitalised at the same time. The illness, often described vaguely as "mass psychogenic illness" [MPI] or "mass hysteria," has erupted repeatedly throughout Bangladesh in recent years. Schools seem particularly vulnerable to outbreaks. But Bangladesh's numerous garment manufacturing factories, catering to an ever-growing export market, have also been susceptible to this type of illness (Anon. 2015b; Ahmed 2016; Representative 2016).

The cases rarely fail to bring about a clear and public clash of rival models of explanation. News reports detail how friends and family of those afflicted insist that jinns, or more rarely ghosts (*bhut*), haunt these spaces. Yet both government and media reject such explanations as products of "ignorance", preferring instead the vague and under-defined categories of "mass hysteria", "mass psychogenic illness" or even simply "Psychiatric Problems". One police officer investigating one of the cases explicitly said, "I cannot say jinns killed someone while wearing a government uniform" (Comilla News Desk 2018).

The sources of the popularity and authority of such psychiatric models of explanation are not difficult to locate. Apart from a long history of such "medical" models being regarded as modern and progressive (Pringle 2013; Eneborg 2013; Attewell 2004), recent efforts by state, non-state, and international organisations participating in the Movement for Global Mental Health (MGMH) have also been hugely influential in establishing (or undermining) the authority of various models of mental health and illness. Television and other forms of mass media have played a significant role in disseminating medicalised models of psychiatric distress through programmes such as the animated series *Meena* (Hasan and Thornicroft 2018). No less a person than the Bangladeshi Prime Minister's own daughter, Saima Wazed Putul – a licensed school psychologist in her own right, has become WHO-SEARO's Goodwill Ambassador for Autism. She is also a member of the WHO Expert Advisory Panel on Mental Health. These two positions have led to WHO's mental health initiatives receiving wide coverage in the Bangladeshi media. Many of these media reports refer to Ms. Putul simply as a "Global Mental Health advocate" or even a "Global Mental Health champion". (Anon. 2017a;

Anon. 2017b; Senior Correspondent n.d.). Such coverage no doubt adds to the power and prestige of both Global Mental Health in particular and psychiatric models more generally.

The authority of biomedical paradigms also builds on the simple belief amongst those who consider themselves fully modern (as opposed to their more "ignorant" or "backward" countrymen) that biomedicine "works" (Sax 2014; Callan 2012) whereas the actions that follow from explanations involving jinns simply do not work. Much of the extant anthropological literature on possession has therefore tried to explore alternative models of efficacy. They have, in the process, advanced perceptive and novel explanations that show that possession-based frameworks of healing work by pathways distinct from biomedical pathways. Amongst such proposed alternative pathways are mechanisms involving aesthetics (Desjarlais 2011), narrative (Bellamy 2011) and collective social action (Sax 2009) etc. But what has been, in the process, largely ignored is the reverse question – does biomedicine really work?

Biomedicine's cultural authority is partly sustained by repeated and lurid airings of every failing of every non-biomedical institution. But failings of biomedical institutions are somehow carefully managed so as to prevent the incident from tarnishing the authority or image of biomedicine per se. Consider for instance the comparative framings of two tragic fires. A 2001 fire at Erwadi, a Sufi shrine in southern India that cared for the possessed, which resulted in 30 deaths was used to great effect to attack the alleged "barbarity" and "primitiveness" of all types of "religious" therapies (Davar 2015). By contrast, a fire at the super-specialty AMRI Hospital in 2011 that led to 89 deaths was consistently framed as an issue of corruption and negligence on the part of those running the hospital. But the latter discourse did not singe the image of biomedicine per se (Pal and Ghosh 2014).

In order to look beyond these power-laden rhetorical strategies and approach a more balanced and equitable comparison of biomedical and non-biomedical therapeutics, I believe we need to look more seriously at biomedicine's limits: at how it manages uncertainty and even outright failure. That is what I will do in this article, by focusing on the phenomenon of collective jinn possession, viz. the possession of entire groups, rather than individuals, by jinns in Bangladesh. I will commence by describing the phenomenon. Since statistical data is not available, I will provide a basic list of the cases I have been able to locate through perusal of the local media to convey some sense of the magnitude of the issue. In this section, I will also give some examples of the kind of symptoms demonstrated by those afflicted. In the second section I will describe the way those afflicted and their families and neighbours explain the phenomena. Third, I will explore the Mental Health establishment's response, including a brief sketch of categories such as "mass psychogenic illness" through which the psychiatrists speak of the phenomenon. Finally, I will explore why the mental health paradigm might be out of its depth when dealing with phenomena like "mass possession". In the concluding section, I shall pull the strings of the discussion together and offer a historically grounded paradigm to understand the phenomenon.

Collective Jinn Possession

Most of the extant literature on jinn possession, whether amongst medical professionals or anthropologists, deals with individual patients/ victims. The phenomenon that I want to discuss here is quite different. These are cases when an entire group is affected by jinn possession.

Let us begin with the case of Rumi Khatun who, along with her four classmates Ankhi Khatun (aged eleven), Arjina Khatun (ten), Murshida Khatun (ten) and Swarna Khatun (ten), required hospitalisation. Several other girls of the same school were also affected. Likewise, in Rani's case, two other classmates – Sadia Khatun and Ishrat Jahan – were also severely ill. Such instances could easily be multiplied. The numbers vary, from a minimum of five or six students, to cases where over a hundred students have been affected. Table 5.1 lists all the cases over the last decade that I have been able to find. It is based on survey of local newspapers, television channels, medical articles and government reports. It is far from being comprehensive or exhaustive, but it does indicate the simple fact that the phenomenon afflicts groups rather than individuals.

In speaking of the afflicted subject as a "group", it is important to distinguish them from the "mass" of the psychiatric literature. "Mass" connotes a much less cohesive and more serendipitous collection of rather faceless persons than does the notion of a "group". When I speak of a group, I mean to indicate a set of individual persons, each with his or her own particular characteristics, but also with a certain number of characteristics shared by other members of the group. Classmates at particular rural schools, in my view, are much more a "group" than a "mass". This is a distinction that I shall develop further in the concluding sections of this article.

The symptoms exhibited by those afflicted by these episodes, notwithstanding substantial variations from case to case, also demonstrate some regularities. A disproportionately high percentage of those effected

Table 5.1 List of jinn possession in schools

Date	Place	Number effected
11 July 2007	Adiabad Islamia High School and College, Narsingdi	50
4 August 2007	Jaforabad High School, Chittagong	15
27 October 2010	Kalitola Durgapur Govt. Primary School	
30 October 2010	Barokona Govt. Primary School	
30 October 2010	Sabajerpara Govt. Primary School	
30 October	Shujalpur Govt. Primary School	
1 March 2015	Collectorate School and College, Pabna	25
13 May 2015	Boradnagar Govt. Primary School, Pabna	8
11 August 2015	Haritana Model High School, Barguna; Taslima Memorial Academy, Barguna	16; 2
30 August 2015	Shailamari Girls High School, Meherpur	45
19 January 2016	Shibram Road Academy, Faridpur; Khalilpur High School	100 +
5 March 2016	Jorpukuria Govt. Primary School, Gangni, Meherpur	4
22 March 2016	Kalidas Kalim Uddin High School, Sakhipur, Tangail	14
4 March 2017	Nursing Institution, Ad-Din Sakhina Medical College, Chachra, Jessore	30
21 March 2017	Nandidumuria Govt. Primary School, Jhikargachha, Jessore	7
8 July 2017	Purba Kachuakhali Govt. Primary School, Lalmohan, Bhola	51
7 August 2017	KGS School and College, Bakarganj	20

are young girls. Though several boys too have suffered, there is a clear preponderance of girls in the reported cases. Several of those who fall ill lose consciousness for varying periods of time. Some of them, especially the more serious cases, also complain of severe abdominal pain. Another regularly reported symptom is extreme muscle spasms, especially in the limbs, and the limbs becoming insensate. Confused speech, dizziness and nausea are also common (Tarafder et al. 2016).

In most cases the phenomenon begins with one or a small number of individuals falling ill. This is rapidly followed by the symptoms spreading to other individuals. The actual sight of a classmate suffering is said to convey the symptoms to others. In several instances, those affected also smelt noxious or powerful odours before they fell ill. In some cases, they heard unusual sounds just prior to their illness. The senses, especially sight but also hearing and smelling, seem to play a key role in the transmission of symptoms from one sufferer to another.

In every outbreak the phenomenon seems to be spatially clearly limited. The victims all fell prey at school. Many of them carried the distress back when they returned home and continued to be ill, but it is important to note that the point of origin was unambiguously at school. In some cases, the spatial grid of affliction was so specific that people who usually did not enter the vulnerable area remained unaffected until and unless they happened to do so. Thus, when the phenomenon broke out at the Purba Kachuakhali Govt. Primary School, a madrasa located almost immediately next to it was entirely unaffected. But when, upon hearing of the strange phenomenon one of the madrasa's staff members Rahima Begum entered the neighbouring school out of curiosity, she was immediately taken ill (Anon. 2017d). Moreover, even within the effected premises not all areas are usually equally effected. It is usually a specific room or area of the school building that is affected. Interestingly, toilets in particular seem to be really vulnerable spots and several cases were reported to have started in a particular school toilet (Anon. 2016).

Aside from the school children, another group seems particularly vulnerable to such group illnesses: workers in garment factories. Over the past decades, Bangladesh has emerged as a key producer of cheap textiles for western markets. As a result, many sweatshops have emerged with poor working conditions and oriented almost entirely towards the export market. Most workers at such factories are low-skilled, socio-economically disadvantaged women. The sweatshops are mostly located in Dhaka and other urban centres. Most of the women actually hail from rural backgrounds or from the numerous slums on the outskirts of the city. They are only slight less vulnerable to such collective diseases than the schoolgirls. Table 5.2 gives details of some of these outbreaks that I have compiled.

The symptoms amongst the garment factory workers seem to closely resemble those of the students, though the workers are generally older. I would especially like to draw attention to the fact the factory workers also associate their illness with a specific work environment and are invariably affected in a group, rather than as individuals.

Though I will not be discussing the garment factory cases in this article these cases are interesting because they provide valuable comparative material. Aihwa Ong's illuminating study of spirit possession amongst female factory workers in Malaysia provides a very good comparative benchmark for the situation in Bangladesh (Ong 1987). There is however, one major area where my approach differs from Ong's. In the latter's account "capitalist discipline" is constantly juxtaposed with "noncapitalist morality" (xiv). As a historian, I am uncomfortable with hitching "discipline" entirely and exclusively to "capitalism" and juxtaposing it to "morality". There is for instance, a wealth of excellent scholarship by intellectual historians of

Table 5.2 Partial list of jinn possession in garment factories

Date	Place	Number effected
18 March 2015	Norf Knitting Garments, Gajipur Sadar	
24 January 2016	DNB Clothing, Adamji EPZ, Narayanganj	20
27 August 2016	Deco Design, Ashulia	50

Islamic and Islamicate societies who describe the classical Islamic notion of *hisba* according to which every pious Muslim was meant to be "commanding right and forbidding wrong" (*al-amr bi'l-ma'rūf wa'l-nahy 'an al-munkar*) (Agrama 2012; Fahmy 2018). Effectively, this meant that the moral community itself became the locus of disciplining. Discipline was not necessarily something external to the moral order that had to be enforced by a political or economic process.

The choice of schools rather than factories as the site of analysis reveals these complex genealogies more fully. Pedagogical institutions in many cultures, with or without capitalist regimes of work, have enforced some form of discipline. The fact that some of the schools in Bangladesh where so-called MPI cases have occurred are either themselves madrasas (Islamic schools) or situated close to such madrasas, highlights these mixed genealogies of pedagogically oriented disciplinary institutions.

Another point where my analysis diverges from Ong's is that I refuse to reduce the jinns and spirits that patients and their neighbours speak of mere "metaphors" (Ong 1987, xv). Metaphorisation, for me, is a problematic analytic move that preserves the ontological privilege afforded to entities recognised by modern scientific disciplines. To push my point, I might question why "capital", a category recognised by modern political economic discourse, should be considered more real than the Malay *hantu* (spirit) that Ong considers to be merely "images" and "metaphors" (1).

Caught by Jinns

Overwhelmingly those afflicted by the illness and their families tend to invoke jinns as the cause. In the incident that led to the death of young Rumi Khatun for instance, several of the students and their relatives mentioned that the events began when a disused toilet that had long been kept shut was reopened. Those who used the toilet, claimed to have seen a red doll inside. Some even said that the doll was smiling at them. Some of the schoolgirls also said that they had witnessed bloody palm prints on the walls. Rumi's mother reported that her daughter had returned ill from school and said that it begun after she had seen the smiling doll in the new school toilet. One of Rumi's classmates, Alpana Khatun, who was also taken ill, said that the troubles started after she saw a doll in the toilet. A *kobiraj,* a practitioner of "traditional" Bangladeshi therapeutics who uses a combination of spiritual and herbal therapies,[1] who examined Alpana diagnosed her illness as a case of jinn possession (Pabna Correspondent 2015). He recommended the sacrifice of a goat at the school along with the offering of *milad* prayers. *Milad,* which derives from the Arabic term *maulid,* is the celebration of the Prophet Muhammad's birth. Though it is mainly celebrated on a specific day, viz. the twelfth day of the Islamic month of Rabi al-Awwal, in Bangladesh *milad* celebrations are also held on several occasions such as the commencement of a new business, the birth of a child, entering a new house etc. The celebrations entail the recounting of the events of the Prophet's life, recital of Quranic verses in praise of the Prophet, discussion of the Islamic code of ethics etc. On occasion, the Islamic view of death is explicated at length (Ali n.d.). The school's principal, Rafiqul Islam, after some slight hesitation asked the parents of the students for subscriptions. The money raised allowed for two goats to be sacrificed rather than just one, along with the organisation of a *milad mehfil* (*milad* celebrations) (Pabna Correspondent 2015).

In the incident leading to the death of Rani Khatun, classmates and their relatives once again insisted that the school was being haunted by jinns. Lokman Hossain, the elder brother of one of the first girls to be affected, explained that there had been an old gooseberry tree behind the school building that had reputedly been haunted. Recently, the school authorities cut down the tree. It was believed that the jinns haunting the tree were vexed by this and moved into the school building itself. In fact, it was the guardians of the students who met with the school authorities and insisted that a *kobiraj* be called in and propitiatory rites be performed. They even called in a *kobiraj,* Masud Miah, who confirmed the presence of jinn and advised that particular rites be performed to secure the building (Jamalpur Correspondent 2017). Silimarly, at schools in Lalmohan and Nandidumuria too, outbreaks were attributed to jinns and a *kobiraj* called in. At the former school, Students said that usually the attacks commenced precisely at noonday when a mysterious black cloud arose outside a certain classroom

---

1   The word *kobiraj* is mostly used to refer to practitioners of Ayurvedic medicine. In contemporary rural Bangladesh, however, it refers to practitioners who use a mix of herbal and spiritual therapeutics with no putative or professed connection to Ayurveda. Unlike the majority of Ayurvedic practitioners, most of the rural Bangladeshi *kobirajes* are Muslims.

window. A breeze blew into the classroom from this cloud and whoever the breeze touched instantly fell ill and began to behave in ways that were entirely out of character. A *kobiraj* called in by the principal insisted that the school had been built on a site where something malignant had once happened and that is why the jinns were preying upon the students (Anon. 2017d, Anon. 2017e). Whilst at Nandidumuria, students said a strange man beckoned them from just outside their classroom window. When they stepped out, the man disappeared and the students immediately felt unwell. The *kobiraj*, Abdus Sattar Munshi, said that the school buildings and its immediate surroundings were infested with over 200 jinns, and performed rites of propitiation and protection. Village elders also assembled and prayed on the site. The outbreak seemed to die down after that (Alamgir 2017).

Anwarul Karim, writing in 1988, had described the rural Bangladeshi *kobiraj* as a "shaman" akin to the *ojha, fakir,* or *khundker* (Karim 1988). A more focused study of what kind of healing the *kobiraj* actually practices remains missing. The fact that the same word is used to refer to the much-better studied practitioners of Ayurvedic medicine has meant that the rural Bangladeshi *kobiraj* has usually been seen through the same prism. This, however, is incorrect, and a fuller study of the actual therapeutic repertoire of the *kobiraj* is much needed.

Though details of the actual treatments, leave alone the explanatory frameworks, used by the *kobirajes* are missing, we can get a sense of their outlook from a perusal of the several cheap Bengali books that deal with the topic of jinns and the treatment of jinn-possession. Most of these books reorganize Islamic lore culled from a diverse array of Perso-Arabic and Urdu texts into a series of new chapters aimed at explicating the characteristics of jinns, their effect on humans and recommended treatments. One such text published in 2015 describes *jinne pawa* as the entrance of Jinns and, sometimes, Shoitan ['Satan'] himself, into the human body and circulate in the victim's blood. The symptoms attributed to such jinn-possessions included, 'madness' (*paglamo*), insanity (*unmad*), speaking in tongues, ability to withstand beatings that would make even a camel flinch, ability to read languages the victim does not know (Al-Madani 2015, 110-112). Other books further expanded upon these symptoms. A text published in 2001 for instance, said that speaking in tongues often meant speaking in languages such as English, Hindi, Arabic, Persian, Urdu and German. It also added that young boys and girls who were possessed by jinns could often state many facts about faraway lands that even adults did not know. jinn-possessed people could also rapidly and easily climb trees or get on to the roofs of houses (Islam 2001, 204-205).

Sheikh Abdul Hamid Faizi Al-Madani gives three reasons for jinns attacking humans. First, he said Jinns often fell in love with humans of the opposite sex and thus attached themselves to the humans. Second, if humans inadvertently offended a jinn, by acts such as throwing water or urinating on them, the jinns sought vengeance. Finally, some jinns were simply malicious and sought to make humans fight amongst themselves or pray to idols (Al-Madani 2015, 227-228). Al-Madani also outlined a number of moments of vulnerability in one's life when Jinn's were particularly likely to attack. Amongst these, the foremost was when one went to the toilet. Other moments of vulnerability included moments of anger, sexual intercourse, when one heard a donkey braying etc. (185-191). A.N.M. Sirajul Islam states that, jinns have subtle bodies and therefore can be inhaled along with air. They can also enter the body via one of the other orifices of the body, such as the ears, mouth, genitals, anus etc. (Islam 2001, 205), Once inside the body they exist within the body just as "germs or bacteria" (204). They can also reside in the stomach in the way certain 'insects' (*poka*) are known to exist and even multiply in the stomach (205).

When it comes to the actual treatement of jinn-possession, we find authors adopting one of two broad strategies. Some authors, such as Islam and Al-Madani adopt a philosophical and scripturalist approach. They lay down the broad philosophical approach to be adopted and describe a number of incidents of jinn-possession and cure narrated in various Islamic works of the past, focussing especially on *hadith* literature. Al-Madani for instance, advised the physician (*chikitshok*) to begin by making the jinn aware of the will of Allah by citing the appropriate scriptural passages, before explaining to the jinn the error of their ways (Al-Madani 2015, 229-230). Islam went a step further and described the physician dealing with jinns as a *mujahid* (holy warrior) and the treatment itself as a *jihad* (holy war). The physician's own piety and purity of faith was thus supremely important to the success of the treatment. Islam particularly recommended the reciting of the powerful Throne Verse (*ayatul kursi*) of the Quran by the physician at the beginning of the treatment (Islam 2001, 211). Unlike these broader philosophical discussions, other authors writing in Bengali give more specific practical instructions. Many of these describe the use of specific magical diagrams for use. One remedy in a book allegedly first published in 1830 but still in print, for instance, enjoins the victim of a jinn-possession to write out a specific magical diagram and wear it in an amulet on the patient's arm. Another remedy in the same book advises writing out another specific magic diagram, rolling it into a wick and using it to light a lamp. This lamp was then to be placed in front of the victim/patient along with some flowers and incense. On so doing, the jinn would appear on top of the patient and talk to the physician before leaving forever (Fakir 1830, 38-39).

Several of these authors also explicitly outlined the distinction between their treatments and biomedical doctors. Quoting an incident mentioned by the medieval philosopher Ibne Taymiyyah, Al-Madani described how some intellectuals belonging to the medieval Mu'tazila school refused to believe in Jinns, before adding that, "just as the scientifically inclined and the realists [today] think of all this as baseless ideas" (Al-Madani 2015, 111). Islam was even more forthright and wrote that, "the insane are of two types, a) physical (*sharirik*) and b) spiritual (*atmik*)". The first type of insanity, he posited, developed when "due to the derangement (*bikriti*) of the brain (*mastishka*) causing an electric current to pass through the cells (*kosh*) of the brain...consequently the symptoms of diseases such as hysteria etc.". The second type of insanity however, was entirely distinct from such physical causes and arose from the machinations of jinns. This latter type thus, could only be dealt with by dealing with jinns (Islam 2001, 212).

Notwithstanding the refusal of the mainstream media or the state to attach any importance to the insistence of the schoolgirls, their families and in some cases even the school authorities, that the affliction was caused by jinns, a systematic, complex and clearly demarcated discourse on Jinn-possessions continue to flourish in Bangladesh. Moreover, far from being the idiosyncratic ideas of isolated, rural individuals, the exponents of these jinn-based explanations have developed a discourse that clearly outlines its difference and distance from the biological, scientific and realist models of disease-causation.

Mental Health

A number of reports have recently appeared in Bangladeshi and foreign medical journals about these cases (Tarafder et al. 2016; Anon. 2011; Farhana Haque et al. 2013; Kendall E.A et al. 2012; Mamun et al. 2018). All the reports seem to follow two general strategies. First, they confess to their inability to actually detect any causal mechanism or reason for what has happened. Second, they insist with great confidence that what has occurred is an instance of "mass psychogenic illness".

The combination of these two strategies would seem odd at first – that is, the confession of failure together with an insistence on a label. But this precisely what Michelle Murphy (2006) has described in her fascinating account of Sick Building Syndrome, the label whose history is also tied up with "mass psychogenic illness". Murphy notes that sciences operate by creating "regimes of perceptibility" that are twinned with "domains of imperceptibility". What can be seen and evidenced is always rendered in terms of what is wilfully not seen. In her account when western feminist workers began to first articulate anxieties about low-level chemical exposures in the workplace, the scientific establishment cultivated new technologies of evidencing exposure whose own, constitutive uncertainties were wilfully overlooked. Murphy argues that "'unknowing', ignorance, and imperception were not just accidentally but purposefully generated in the history of knowledge practices" (9). Perceptibility and imperceptibility were twinned modes of knowledge. Chemical exposure was measured in specific ways that excluded many other forms of bodily discomfort. These latter were then plotted within the domain of imperceptibility by labelling them as symptoms of "mass psychogenic illness" (MPI). Murphy details how researchers of the National Institute of Occupational Safety and Health (NIOSH) in the United States in the 1970s, insisted on the diagnosis of MPI when their specific techniques for measuring chemical exposure failed to detect any "physical" cause for the distress many office workers complained of. The NIOSH inspectors also insisted on the gendered nature of the complaints and argued that the allegedly greater emotional volatility of women made them susceptible to "patholog[ies] of perception misconnected to concrete matters of environment" (95). A diagnosis of MPI was therefore precisely what allowed NIOSH's protocols of measuring discomfort in terms of chemical exposure to appear "real". Murphy is clear that the diagnosis of MPI was resented by the women office workers and that MPI was a way in which the reality of their physical discomfiture was rendered "nonexistent". In fact, she describes it as a mode of "gendered nonexistence" (92-95).

   Another comparable account of how a diagnosis of MPI allowed for the simultaneous privileging of certain forms of knowing and delegitimising others has been provided by Yolana Pringle in her study of an epidemic of "mass madness" in postcolonial Uganda. Pringle describes how a series of extremely invasive physical examinations, including lumbar punctures and pushing of one-inch-long needles into the skin (Pringle 2013, 122), were used to rule out any "physical" cause for the symptoms and arrive at a diagnosis of "mass hysteria", which then in turn delegitimised the multiple frameworks within which the affected Gisu tribespeople sought to make sense of the afflictions. Especially ignored were the accounts of patients to be able to see and speak directly with spirits and dead ancestors (Pringle 2013, 123). Moreover, just as the NIOSH investigators had reinforced their delegitimation of women's experiences by invoking sexist tropes of female emotional volatility, the Ugandan psychiatric establishment framed its own dismissal of Gisu knowledge and experience by invoking a racialised tropology of primitivism (Pringle 2013, 126).

The label MPI is, therefore, simultaneously both underdefined and over-determined. Its underlying patho-physiological mechanisms are confessedly absent and yet it is made to appear solidly "objective" by overdetermin-ing it with older, established tropes about gender, race, and primitivity. Socially, epistemologically and professionally, this curiously vacuous and yet oft-repeated category helps to privilege certain ways of making sense of suffering, certain types of expertise and particular forms of therapies, while delegitimising others.

In the Bangladeshi instance we notice the same interplay of under- and overdetermination. It is much more a place holder than a robust category with well-worked out explanatory models of causation, aetiology etc. This twinning of confident assertions about the label's validity and its actual underdetermination is illustrated by a series of strategies. One of the key strategies is individuation. Published reports are at pains to isolate a so-called "index case" (i.e. identifying the first person to fall ill). Often this person is then said to have some kind of a "psychological illness". The details of what this "psychological illness" might be or how it was detected or indeed what were its distinctive symptoms are never mentioned. At best, vague references to "conversion disorders", where social or emotional problems or anxiety are allegedly erroneously "converted" into non-existent somatic problems, are used to describe the "psychological illness" of the "index case". Having thus isolated the person and rendered her into a mentally ill patient, it is alleged that her illness affects others around her through "hysteria". Once again, no explanation is offered to explain how seeing someone else in pain might bring on the same pain in a friend or neighbour.

A second strategy that reinforces the first involves adding a long historical section that provides a laundry list of instances from around the world, especially in the West, where "mass psychogenic illnesses" have been diagnosed. In constructing these historical prefaces, "mass psychogenic illnesses" are also seamlessly aligned with a number of other designations that have been offered over the centuries, such as "Mass Sociogenic Illness", "Mass Hysteria", "Conversion Disorder", and the like. Historical prefaces in general have increasingly become rare in contemporary professional medical journals and hence their inclusion in these reports about MPI is worthy of note. As Pringle has pointed out in her study of postcolonial Uganda, the mere linking of medieval European anecdotes to contemporary schoolchildren or members of other gendered, raced or exoticised groups, itself builds upon older ideas about cultural recapitulation founded upon a framework of primitivism. It also assumes, and implicitly establishes, that MPI as an objective category has persisted throughout a universalisable historical time (Pringle 2013, 126).

A third and final strategy seen in the medical articles on the subject involves the use of demographic data. The reader is overwhelmed by the seeming wealth of data that populate these articles. From age tables to gender ratios of incidence, from income charts to bar graphs showing levels of academic performance of the students who fell ill, there is a literal flood of data. The presentation of these data sets in striking visual formats – tables, charts, graphs, and so on – adds to their seeming incontrovertibility. It recalls Theodore Porter's (1996) observation regarding "trust in numbers". He argues that numbers are a "technology of distance", they work to supply the trust deficit that mars impersonal communications at a distance. The numbers in these articles, I would argue, attempt to win the reader's trust, precisely because there is a perceived deficit in biomedicine's claims to deal with the phenomenon. More recently, Vincanne Adams has written about the "metrics work" that is central to the new regime of Global Health. She argues that number crunching and metrics work need to be reconceptualised as forms of storytelling, which tells stories about "what those who produce them and those who rely on them care about most" (Adams 2016, 16).

The use of demographic data also needs to be seen within the longer history of a notion of "psychosocial" phenomenon. The Bangladeshi doctors who write about MPI, frequently invoke the term to explain the epidemic proportions the affliction often achieves (Amin 2009). Though the notion of the "psychosocial" originated in the last decade of the nineteenth century, it was during the interwar years that the development of a range of statistical techniques gave it a new reality. After the WWII, the development of the welfare state and the wealth of demographic data it collected made a certain kind of psychosocial phenomenon legible. Though some of the early deployments of the concept of the psychosocial had indeed hinted at the limits of biological models, as Rhodri Hayward points out, by the 1960s such attempts had failed (Hayward 2012, 9). As Nikolas Rose argues, this was the period when what he dubs the "neurochemical self" began to emerge (Rose 2017). From our perspective two points are worth underlining. First, the post-WWII history of the concept of the psychosocial is intimately tied up to psychology becoming a tool of statecraft and government. Indeed, its very legibility is grounded in its dependence on the statistical processes of statecraft. Second, in this post-WWII the psychosocial is a concept that does not transcend the individual as such. Instead, it further reinforces the individual as a unit of therapeutic action.

Over and above all these strategies there are of course the usual allegations that devious *kobirajes* are preying on the poor and hapless by propagating spurious ideas about jinns. It is remarkable how little interest is taken in how the *kobirajes* detect or deal with the phenomenon. Given their ubiquity, one would think that at least some of the public health workers to have at least a perverse and ironic interest in the methods of the *kobirajes*. But neither the public health literature nor the mainstream media that zealously participates in the construction of the divide between "modern" and "superstitious" demonstrate the slightest interest in their methods. The *kobiraj* appears in the public health literature on mass psychogenic illnesses uniformly as a shady charlatan out to fleece his simple, rustic neighbours.

To comprehend the larger politics of these strategies however, we need to locate them within the actual set of institutions and actors who mobilise them. While some proponents of the Movement for Global Mental Health have sought to incorporate MPIs into their ever-expanding calls for the psychiatrisation of "mental health" and the scaling up of biomedically oriented interventions, most of the writers I have been citing above do not directly affiliate with the Global Mental Health Movement. Instead, they are overwhelmingly Bangladeshi psychiatrists working within the government health service. One of the earliest studies of the topic, for instance, was published in 2009 in the Journal of the Dhaka Medical College by a team led by Dr. Mohammad Robed Amin, a Junior Medical Consultant at the Hathazari Medical Complex in Chittagong. Other co-authors included Dr. S. Mahmood, the Upazila Health and Family Planning Officer and Dr. S.F. Rabbi, Medical Officer, both located at the Hathazari Medical Complex along with the headmaster of the high school where the outbreak happened and the executive office of the sub-division (*upazila*) (Amin 2009). Another, much more recent study, was authored mostly by faculty in psychiatry departments of several Bangladeshi medical colleges, led by Dr. Abdullah Al Mamun of the Department of Psychiatry at the Dhaka Medical College. The study was published in the Bangladesh Journal of Psychiatry (Mamun 2016). Both the journals and the affiliations of the authors therefore implicate these studies broadly within the state health services, rather than any matrix of Global Mental Health. Neither do these authors invoke the language of Global Mental Health directly. The only international institution in Bangladesh to address the issue is the International Centre for Diarrhoeal Disease Research, Bangladesh (ICDDR, B): a flagship medical institution that owes its origin to the era of International, rather than Global, Health in the 1960s. The ICDDR, B had started out in 1962 as the Cholera Research Laboratory, but has evolved over the politically tumultuous decades of Bangladeshi history since then while retaining much of its International Health era focus on broad Public Health and state involvement rather than embrace the Global Health mantra of privatisation and targeted interventions (On the comparison of International Health and Global Health see Birn et al. 2017). It is the ICDDR, B that published a lengthy report on MPI in its health bulletin for 2011.

Beyond the Bangladeshi context exponents of Global Mental Health have been asking for the inclusion of MPIs into their ambit. Lancet Psychiatry for instance, carried an article in 2018 citing MPIs as a key type of psychiatric complaint that is "communicable" or "infectious" (Wainberg 2018). The research, which is partly funded by the Global Mental Health Research Fellowship, argues Global Health institutions such as the WHO need to rethink their definitions of "communicable" or "infectious diseases". They propose three pathways – infectious and ecological, familial, and sociocultural – by which psychiatric disorders become communicable. While on the face of it these authors seem to be challenging the traditional individualistic approach in psychiatry towards mental health issues, their proposals are mainly to scale up surveillance and interventions by standard psychiatric methods while also promoting educational programs to popularise a psychiatric framework for such afflictions. There is absolutely no concern for the ways in which the patients conceptualise these afflictions or the kinds of remedies they seek out in the absence of a psychiatrist. In fact, they state that while patients might attribute such cases to witchcraft or environmental toxicity, they can be reproduced in "psychology laboratory settings", thereby implying that they are mainly psychological.

The 2018 article led to a lively discussion on the pages of Lancet Psychiatry in 2019. Two researchers from the Neuropsychiatric Institute in Salt Lake City, Utah wrote in to suggest a fourth pathway by which psychiatric disorders might become communicable: iatrogenesis. While broadly supportive, they also feared that enhanced surveillance might inadvertently produce more "false positives" and encourage greater consumption of psychiatric drugs (Kious et al. 2019). Two of the original authors responded accepting the likelihood of iatrogenic communication, while reiterating their earlier call for enhanced screening and psychiatric education of the public (Wainberg 2019). Notwithstanding the minor differences of opinion, none of the participants in the debate seemed to care much for non-psychiatric models for explaining or alleviating the distress of their patients. In fact, the researchers from Utah baldly stated that part of the problem was that "Psychiatric illnesses are more likely than physical illnesses to be subject to unreliable report because diagnosis is often based on symptom reports" (Kious et al. 2019).

Very different historical ontologies inform the mental health professional and those who invoke jinns. One recent study published mostly by researchers based in the Netherlands have drawn attention to both the extensive prevalence of jinn-based afflictions amongst Muslim populations as well as the dearth of proper understanding of this framework amongst health policy makers (Lim et al. 2018). Even without challenging the framework of biomedicine and psychiatry, these researchers argue that it is essential for psychiatrists to have a proper understanding of these frameworks before they can successfully offer treatment. Besides outlining a symptomatology based on interviews the team had conducted, these researchers also described some of the fundamental ontological incompatibility between the jinn-based frameworks and the psychiatric ones. For instance, contrary to much popular media writing that calls jinns "spirits", according to the Quran jinns are a species of living beings created by Allah. This attribution of their symptoms not to bodily or mental causes, but rather to independent, agential entities shaped views about what kinds of treatment were necessary and what kind of outcomes were possible. In fact, Sudhir Kakar has argued that whether we accept the reality of jinns or not, it is precisely this externalisation of the cause that is often instrumental in the greater therapeutic success of physicians who accept Jinn-based frameworks than psychiatrists (Kakar 1991). My point here is more straightforward. Unlike Kakar, I am not arguing that jinn-based frameworks are necessarily more successful in ameliorating the symptoms and distress of patients. My point is simply this that we first need to understand how exactly the jinn-based frameworks differ from the psychiatric ones, especially the different ways they understand patient subjectivity, aetiology etc. In other words, the different historical ontologies that undergird each framework.

As Murphy explains "historical ontology" is a conceptual tool intended to "describe historical accounts of how objects, such as germs, immune systems, subatomic particles, diseases, and so on, came into being as recognisable objects via historically specific circumstances" (2006, 7). "Mass psychogenic illness" as an object obviously differs amply from jinns. Not only do these two objects emerge through very different historical trajectories but they also require very specific ways of knowing to become perceptible or remain imperceptible to those who invoke them. Furthermore, they are embedded within very different social, cultural, and intellectual assemblages. Everything from discourses about tradition and modernity, to different forms of social power and authority as well as divergent supporting intellectual assumptions make up these assemblages. The relationship between these two ontological objects, especially the decision of which one is recognised in which context, is essentially a political choice. This is what I am calling *ontopolitics*.

My thinking on ontopolitics has been influenced by a number of recent interventions. Most powerful of these has been the recent "Ontological Turn" in anthropology and its call pluralise our view of "nature" has done much put provincialise scientifically designated objects. Scholars such as Eduardo Viveiros de Castro have argued that instead of a facile "multiculturalism" that preserves the epistemic authority of modern science, we need a robust "multinaturalism" whereby the ontological objects recognised by various "modern" scientific disciplines are placed on the same level as ontological objects recognised by various other traditions of knowledge (Viveiros de Castro 2004). More specifically, in the context of medicine, Stacey Langwick's excellent account of how biomedical and jinn-based aetiologies of disease co-exist and occasionally contradict each other in Tanzania has demonstrated how jinns, as ontological objects, can be treated on a par with such biomedically authorised ontological objects as germs (Langwick 2011). Also illuminating has been Ruy Blanes and Diana Espirito Santo's call for an anthropology of "nonthings". They argue that instead of taking the non-existence of entities such as ghosts and spirits, we ought to critically engage with the very epistemic procedures through which existence and non-existence are produced (Blanes and Santo 2013).

To unpack this ontopolitics further it is important to dissect the two relevant historical ontologies a little further. While the concept of historical ontologies has mostly been used to designate the historical emergence of objects and categories within specific scientific disciplines, I want to deliberately push it another step so as to be able to posit the objects of "modern science" on the same footing as those posited by "Islamic theology". Such a usage, I think, is already hinted at in Murphy's pitting of chemical expertise against the embodied knowledge of female office workers and Pringle's account of how Ugandan psychiatrists systematically ignored Gisu ideas about angered ancestors. Two features of the mental health paradigm and its historical ontologies are particularly significant in this regard. First, there is the strict dichotomy between the mind and the body that continues to inform psychiatric knowledge and practice. As William Sax helpfully points out, "While this observation is trite, even hackneyed, it bears constant repetition because mind-body dualism is so persistent and deep-rooted in the culture of academia in general, and medicine and psychiatry in particular" (2014, 834). The insistence for example that "mass psychogenic illness" is in fact emotional or social distress that has been mistakenly "converted" into a somatic one, is clearly premised on the fundamental understanding of there being a clear divide between what is "really" somatic and what is essentially "mental".

This divide in turn allows for mass psychogenic illness to be understood as a "pathology of perception, a form of misperception" (Murphy 2006, 92). As Pringle's study points out, such delegitimising techniques acquire a particular set of resonances in colonial and postcolonial contexts (Pringle 2013). Discourses of "backwardness" and "modernity" provide the scaffolding upon which the idea of "pathologies of perception" rest. Moreover, "backwardness" frequently gets mapped onto explanations involving deities, spirits and ancestors, whilst "modernity" is engendered in biomedical frameworks. What is most striking is the way racialised notions of "perception" often retain their grip in the work of postcolonial psychiatrists (Pringle 2013). In South Asia, David Arnold's pioneering work has demonstrated both the colonial roots of such delegitimatising techniques, as well as its uptake by nationalist elites (Arnold 1993).

This specifically colonial and postcolonial history builds however, with a broader movement within the history of what we today call biomedicine wherein the physician's frameworks has progressively been divorced and privileged over the patient's frameworks of illness. The redoubtable Charles Rosenberg describes the "therapeutic revolution" that led to the very emergence of biomedicine towards the end of nineteenth century as a process by which the physicians' understanding of the body became clearly demarcated from the layperson's view of the body (Rosenberg 1977). Robert Aronowitz, drawing on linguistic theory, has described this nineteenth-century transition as one from a symptom-based approach to a sign-based approach in medicine (Aronowitz 2001). The general de-legitimation of the patient's own understanding of her body and the exclusive privileging of the physician interpretation of specific bodily signs was especially onerous for patient's from socially disenfranchised groups (Aronowitz 1991). The recent trend towards metricisation under the regime of Global Health, which I have alluded to earlier, has further contributed to this way of delegitimising the embodied experiences of marginalised populations (Adams 2016).

One of the key aspects of such alleged misperception is the claim that patients are not able to sufficiently or adequately distinguish the suffering of their friend or neighbour from their own, personal suffering. Put differently, this allegation essentially castigates the patient for being incapable of sufficiently individualising herself. As a result, the individual is unquestionably naturalised as the only plausible subject of suffering. Once again Sax is insightful on this point. He approvingly cites Clifford Geertz' comment that the idea of the individual is a "rather peculiar idea within the context of the world's cultures", before adding that, "individualism is better characterised as an ideology than a description" (2014, 435). We have already seen how mental health professionals in Bangladesh are at pains to identify "index cases" that allow them to disaggregate and reduce a group phenomenon to an individual's malady. In fact Jocalyn Clark, a researcher who worked in Dhaka, points out that individualism, along with reductionism and a penchant for technological solutions, are the three most prominent characteristics of the process of medicalisation (Clark 2014a). Medicalisation is, amongst other things, also the process through which biomedical professionals assert their authority over a particular aspect of life or society. Life events such as pregnancy, childbirth, ageing, losing or gaining weight, and so on, for instance, over which physicians had had little authority in the past have increasingly become matters over which they claim and exercise authority. Recoding jinn attacks as MPIs is clearly also an effort to medicalise a form of social suffering and bring it under the control of psychiatrists, rather than *kobirajes*.

Global Mental Health, Clark points out, has become a powerful new vehicle for medicalisation of social suffering. With it therefore has also come a new push towards individualism and individualisation (2014b). This push is engendered not only by the ways that mental health professionals conceptualise the suffering of patients, but also in the solutions they prescribe. In every case in Bangladesh, the health establishment recommended early hospitalisation, communication of biomedical information and medication. Naturally, the isolation of index cases was also a priority. The thrust therefore was clearly to individualise, and then treat the individuals with therapies focused on them as individual persons rather than considering, say, the social context in which the problem arose. As Clark points out,

> While there is recognition on the part of GMH advocates of the social drivers of poor mental health – poverty, social inequalities, injustice – and that the human rights of those suffering must be promoted and protected this stands at odds with the main focus on scaling-up of health care services – that is, medical treatments including medication targeted towards individuals[.] (2014b, 3)

The victims of jinn attacks at schools and garment factories in contemporary Bangladesh are clearly not individuals as such. By claiming that they are "not individuals as such", I mean that their individuality is intimately tied up with their membership of a specific group. They all fall ill because they belong to a certain group and not others. One might think of this kind of an individual as an individual-in-a-group. The subject that is affected by jinn-possession is not simply a series of isolated, corpuscular individuals, but rather an members within a specific group whose minds and bodies seem to be connected in ways that defy psychiatric notions of individuality. It is important therefore to investigate the nature of this particular subject a little further. In South Asian Studies, the main figure of the non-individual subject that has been invoked has been that of the "dividual". Proposed first by McKim Marriott and popularised mostly by scholars connected to the University of Chicago, the dividual has been imagined as a dynamic and socially embedded subject whose substance is constantly reshaped by her interactions with her surroundings (Marriott 1990). Everything, from whom she meets or marries to what she eats and what gifts she receives, constantly transforms her.

The subjects of my cases are, however, not dividuals. For one, Marriott had been clear that the dividual was a Hindu category. It was never quite clear in his framework what happened to non-Hindu South Asians. Were they to be entirely understood with reference to Hindu categories? Was their distance from Hinduism entirely inconsequential? The overwhelming majority of the sufferers I have mentioned were non-Hindus, mostly Muslims, many of them devout. I am therefore sceptical about how far they may be understood through "Hindu categories".

Moreover, unlike the dividual, we are not dealing here merely with a shifting, dynamic personhood. Rather, we are faced with a situation where an entire group seems to be attacked at the same time and *as a group*. If we resist the psychiatric obsession with 'index cases' that seeks to reorganize the suffering into a number of individualized incidents, we see both the attack and the religious therapeutics used to deal with it, treat the entire group as being the victim. Theorists of human genocide, have in recent years, been deeply engaged with the issue of group suffering. They have pointed out that our modern medical paradigms as well as the simple structures of language that express what we can write or say tend to decompose group suffering into the suffering of individuals. Yet there is increasing evidence that some forms of suffering and injury cannot be conceptualised as essentially operating upon an isolated individual. The group character of such suffering is not incidental or secondary to the suffering of the individual. It is absolutely central (Winter 2006).

Another reason I find the dividual inadequate to describe the phenomena here is its lack of historicity. The dividual seems to be grounded in structures of thought and practice that leave little room for historical change. It would be well nigh impossible to pinpoint when the dividual actually emerged and how it may have changed. By contrast, there are enough historical studies now that seek to historically locate the emergence of the modern individual subject (e.g. Chakrabarty 1992).

I will argue that the subject that suffers at these schools and garment factories needs to be theorised on its own terms. It is a subject that is deeply entangled with the history of the emergence of quintessentially modern spaces such as girl's schools and modern textile factories. Its character is also overwhelmingly Islamic. The faith in jinn, which itself is grounded in Koranic learning, as well as the sort of remedies prescribed, embed the subject within an Islamicate tradition. We might go further and insist that the particular scripturalist version of Islam that underpins these incidents is a fairly modern one in the content of the history of Bengal. (For transformations of Bengali Islam see, Ahmed 1998; Roy 2016; Harder 2011; Irani 2011). Finally, it is worth reiterating the ways in which the suffering is disseminated by a kind of sensory contagion whereby seeing or smelling things, including another group member's suffering, makes one fall ill. This consolidates a sense of the subjects being a somatically integrated with each other.

Indeed, this sense of interpellated, pious subjects suffering from jinn-attacks is directly theorized in some of the Bengali Islamic theological discussions on jinns. Such psychic imbrications between pious Muslim subjects during attacks by the Shoitan is theorized through the difficult-to-define notion of *asasa*. Derived from the Arabic word *waswas*, and sometimes translated as 'whispering', the notion of *asasa* explains how the Shoitan can infiltrate one's innermost thoughts and feelings. One of the modalities through which Shoitan articulates his *asasa* is by revealing the deepest thoughts of one Muslim to another. This means troubling doubts, fears and selfish desires of an individual buried deep in their own minds can be suddenly and completely revealed or transmitted to their neighbours. An encyclopaedic Bengali text on jinns, based on the Arabic writings of the fifteenth century Egyptian scholar, Jalaluddin Suyuti, lists a number of anecdotes from the *hadith* literature on this kind of mutual interpellation of psyches whereby the secrets in one's mind are mysteriously communicated to all his neighbours by the Shoitan through the medium of *asasa* (Hadiujjaman 2001, 120-122). The same text also describes how devout Muslims, that is the 'mumin', are particularly vulnerable to such *asasa* (118).

Asasa provides therefore a very different model of psychic entanglement within a pious and localized group, from that of the psychiatric theories of psychic contagion from a single 'index case'. Unlike the latter, *asasa* does is not a form of 'contagion' but rather a way in which psyches – and, in some readings, bodies too – become entangled by the deliberate agency of the Shoitan, thereby giving rise of a quasi-unified subject that is more expansive than the individual.

I will describe this subject as a "proletarian mumin". The Bengali word "mumin", derived from the Arabic "momin", designates a believing Muslim. It is frequently used in Bengali books on jinns to describe the average Muslim subject who encounters them. It therefore accents the moral and spiritual dimensions of this form of subjectivity and locates it within an Islamic cosmology. By itself however, it would fail to refer to the collective aspect that derives from particularly modern character of the suffering subject and its implication in spaces like schools and factories. Coupling "mumin" with the word "proletarian" not only alludes to this modern, corporate and emplaced feature of the suffering subject I have been describing but also signals towards the ways that government schools in rural areas become conduits that pull young children out of a rural, agrarian milieu and into the modern workforce. Taken together the words "proletarian mumin" therefore evoke a subject of suffering who is both a proletarian (or on the way to becoming a member of the proletariat), and a believing Muslim with access to its world of unseen jinn.

Proletarian mumins, rather than either dividuals or individuals, are the subject of the jinn possessions that Bangladeshi mental health professionals insist in recasting as "mass psychogenic illness". The process of recasting entails the ontopolitical confrontation of the individual subject of modern psychiatry, with its strict mind-body dichotomy, with the proletarian mumin subject, with its corporate, pious, and emplaced character.

Conclusion

In this article I have shown how the Global Mental Health Movement's push for the scaling up of mental health facilities is being stretched and thwarted at its limits by the phenomena dubbed "mass psychogenic illness" by public health officials. Such forms of suffering have become widespread in Bangladesh in recent times, and mental health professionals struggle both to make sense of them and to assert their authority over them by delegitimising alternative frameworks of jinn-possession. In some cases, they have also failed to save the lives of those afflicted, resulting in at least two documented deaths.

Notwithstanding such failures, the mental health establishment continues its attempt to establish its hold over the phenomena by individualising, quantifying, and labelling it, as ways of deflecting attention away from its failure to actually deal with the suffering. They also continue to disregard, disparage and demonise the *kobirajes* to whom most sufferers tend to turn for alternative therapies.

The ontopolitical confrontation between mental health professionals and *kobiraji* models of explanation are crucially played out around the fundamental assumptions regarding the nature of the suffering subject. The former assume that the subject of suffering is always an individual and that her suffering can be adequately classified as either mental or somatic. Moreover, they argue that the sufferer is herself misled about the true nature of her suffering, thus mistakenly "converting" a mental affliction to a somatic one. By contrast, the subject who suffers from jinn possessions in these group outbreaks is a proletarian mumin; that is, a subject who is corporate, piously Muslim, and emphatically non-individual, while also being either in or on the way to becoming proletarianised.

My efforts to conceptualise the proletarian mumin subject are intended to illuminate ontopolitical conflicts that continue to challenge and limit GMH's relentless push to appropriate the phenomenon of group jinn possessions. In the process it is my ambition to explore both the facts and foundations of biomedicine's continued failures to address certain types of suffering, despite all the resources and social legitimacy that accrue to those speaking in the idiom of biomedicine in general and GMH in particular.

References

Adams, Vincanne. 2016. "Introduction." In *Metrics: What Counts in Global Health*, edited by Vincanne Adams. Durham, NC: Duke University Press.

Agrama, Hussein Ali. 2012. *Questioning Secularism: Islam, Sovereignty, and the Rule of Law in Modern Egypt*. Chicago: University of Chicago Press.

Ahmed, Nasir. 2016 "Hotath Asustho 25 Sramik, Karkhanaye Chhuti [25 Workers Suddenly Ill, Factory Closed]." *Ntv Online*, 24 December 2016. Accessed 20 November 2018, https://www.ntvbd.com/bangladesh/100997/.

Ahmed, Rafiuddin. 1998. *The Bengal Muslims, 1871-1906: A Quest for Identity*. Delhi: Oxford University Press.

Alamgir, M. 2017. "Jhikargachhar Nandidumuria Prathomik Bidyaloye Kothita Jin Atonko! Akranta 7 [Alleged Jin Terror at the Nandidumuria Primary School in Jhikargachha! 7 Attacked]." *Bangladesh Banee*, 27 March 2017. Accessed 25 November 2018, http://www.bangladeshbani24.com/varieties/2017/03/21/26084/print.

Ali, Syed Ashraf. 2015. "Milad." *Banglapedia: National Encyclopedia of Bangladesh*. Accessed 5 August 2019, http://en.banglapedia.org/index.php?title=Milad&oldid=18587.

Al-Madani, Sheikh Abdul Hamid Faizi. 2015. *Quran-Sunnar Aloke Jinn O Shoitan Jogot* [The World of Jinns and Satan in Light of the Quran and Sunnah]. Rajshahi: Wahidiya Islamiya Library.

Anonymous. 2015a. *Femili Gaid Boi: Manoshik Rog O Madokasokti* [Family Guide Book: Mental Illness and Intoxicant Addiction]. Dhaka: National Institute of Mental Health.

—. 2015b. "Rupganje Poshak Karkhanaye Jin Atonko [Jinn Terror in Garment Factory at Rupganj]." *Samakal*, 27 August 2015. Accessed 20 November 2018, https://samakal.com/whole-country/article/1508158120.

—. 2016. "Pabna School Closed over 'Toilet Ghost' Panic." *The Daily Star*, 16 May 2015. https://www.thedailystar.net/country/pabna-school-closed-over-toilet-ghost'-panic-82618.

—. 2017a. "Ms. Saima Wazed Hossain Champions for Autism Spectrum Disorder. WHO-SEARO." *News Center*. Accessed 11 August 2019, http://www.searo.who.int/mediacentre/sear-in-the-field/autism-spectrum-disorder-interview/en/.

—. 2017b. "Saima Wazed New WHO Champion for Autism." *Dhaka Tribune*, 2 April 2017. Accessed 11 August 2019, https://www.dhakatribune.com/bangladesh/nation/2017/04/02/saima-wazed-new-champion-autism.

—. 2017c. "Joshor Ad-Dween Narsingye Jin Atonke Asustho 30. Bondho Ghoshona. [30 Ill from Jinn terror at Jessore's Ad-Din Nursing. Closure Announced]." *Dainik Janakantha*, 5 March 2017. Accessed 25 November 2018, http://web.dailyjanakantha.com/details/article/253421/যশোরে-আদ-দ্বীন-নার্সিংয়ে-জিন-আতঙ্কে-অসুস্থ-৩০-বন্ধ-ঘোষণা/print/.

—. 2017d. "Lalmohon O Bakerganje Shikshikasaha 60 Shiksharthi Akoshmik Asustho [60 including a lady teacher suddenly ill in Lalmohan and Bakerganj]." *Jago Barishal*, 8 August 2017. Accessed 25 November 2018, http://jagobarisal.com/2017/08/08/লালমোহন-ও-বাকেরগঞ্জে-শকি/.

—. 2017e. "Lalmohane Jin Atonke Schoole Jachhe Na Chhatrira [Girl Students Avoiding School at Lalmohan Due to Fear of Jinns]". *Jugantar*, 6 August 2017. Accessed 25 November 2018. https://www.jugantor.com/news-archive/today-print-edition/bangla-face/2017/08/06/145862

Arnold, David J. 1993. *Colonizing the Body: State Medicine and Epidemic Disease in Nineteenth Century India*. Berkeley: University of California Press.

Aronowitz, Robert A. 2001. "When Do Symptoms Become a Disease?" *Annals of Internal Medicine* 134 (9 Part 2): 803-08.

—. 2008. "An Underappreciated Mechanism for the Social Pattering of Health."
    Social Science & Medicine 67 (1): 1-9.

Attewell, Guy N. A. 2004. "Authority, Knowledge and Practice in Unani Tibb in India,
    c. 1890-1930." Diss., School of Oriental and African Studies, University of London.

Bellamy, Carla. 2011. *The Powerful Ephemeral: Everyday Healing in an Ambiguously
    Islamic Place.* Berkeley: University of California Press.

Blanes, Ruy, and Diana E. Santo. 2013. *The Social Life of Spirits.* Chicago: University
    of Chicago Press.

Callan, Alyson. 2012. *Patients and Agents: Mental Illness, Modernity and Islam in
    Sylhet, Bangladesh.* New York: Berghahn Books.

Chakrabarty, Dipesh. 1992. Postcoloniality and the Artifice of History: Who Speaks
    for "Indian" Pasts? *Representations* 37:1-26.

Clark, Jocalyn. 2014a. "Medicalization of Global Health 1: Has the Global Health
    Agenda Become Too Medicalized?" *Global Health Action* 7 (1): 23998.

—. 2014b. "Medicalization of Global Health 2: The Medicalization of Global Mental
    Health." *Global Health Action* 7 (1): 24000.

Comilla News Desk. 2018. "Kumillaye Skul Chhatrake Jweene Merechhe: Sambad
    Tolpar [School Student Killed by Jinn in Comilla: Breaking News]. *Kumillar Barta*,
    29 January 2018. Accessed 24 November 2018, https://comillarbarta.com/?p=2889.

Davar, Bhargavi. 2015. "Justice in Erwadi: A Case Study." In *The Law of Possession:
    Ritual, Healing, and the Secular State*, edited by William S. Sax and Helene Basu,
    117-37. New York: Oxford University Press.

Desjarlais, Robert R. 2011. *Body and Emotion: The Aesthetics of Illness and Healing
    in the Nepal Himalayas.* Philadelphia: University of Pennsylvania Press.

Eneborg, Yusuf M. 2013. "Ruqya Shariya: Observing the Rise of a New Faith Healing
    Tradition Amongst Muslims in East London." *Religion & Culture* 16 (10): 1080-96.

Fahmy, Khaled. 2018. *In Quest of Justice: Islamic Law and Forensic Medicine in
    Modern Egypt.* Berkeley: University of California Press.

Harder, Hans. 2011. *Sufism and Saint Veneration in Contemporary Bangladesh: The
    Maijbhandaris of Chittagong.* Abingdon, UK: Routledge.

Hadiujjaman, Muhammad. 2001. *Jin Jatir Bismoykor Itihas* [The Wonderous History
    of the Jinn Nation]. Dhaka. Medina Publications.

Hasan, M. Tasdik, and Graham Thornicroft. 2018. "Mass Media Campaigns to
    Reduce Mental Health Stigma in Bangladesh." *The Lancet Psychiatry* 5 (8): 616.

Hayward, Rhodri. 2012. "The Invention of the Psychosocial: An Introduction."
    History of the Human Sciences 25 (5): 3-12.

Haque, Farhana, Subodh K. Kundu, Md S. Islam, S. M. Murshid Hasan, Asma Khatun,
    Partha S. Gope, Zahid H. Mahmud, et al. 2013. "Outbreak of Mass Sociogenic
    Illness in a School Feeding Program in Northwest Bangladesh, 2010." *PLoS ONE*
    8 (11).

Irani, Ayesha A. 2011. *Sacred Biography, Translation, and Conversion: The "Nabivamsa" of Saiyad Sultan and the Making of Bengali Islam, 1600-Present.* Philadelphia: University of Pennsylvania Press.

Islam, A.N.M. Sirajul. 2001. *Jin O Shoitaner Itikotha* [The Origin Story of Jinns and Satan]. Dhaka: Biswo Prokashoni.

Jamalpur Correspondent. 2017. "Jamalpure Jiner Bhoy Shiksharthi Shunya Dui Bidyaloy [Two Schools in Jamalpur Empty after Jinn Scare]." *Dainik Shiksha*, 17 March 2017. Accessed 25 November 2018, http://www.dainikshiksha.com/জামালপুরে-জিনের-ভয়ে-শিক্ /77013/.

Jessore Representative. 2017. "Jin Atonke Joshore Ad Dween Sakhina Medical Haspataler Shiksharthira [Students of the Ad Din Sakina Medical Hospital in Fear of Jinns]." *Bangla Tribune*, 5 March 2017. Accessed 25 November 2018, http://www.banglatribune.com/country/news/186155/জিন-আতত-যশোরে-আদ--ীন-সথিনা-মডিক্ল?print=1#jadewits_print.

Kakar, Sudhir. 1991. *Shamans, Mystics and Doctors: A Psychological Inquiry into India and its Healing Traditions.* Chicago: University of Chicago Press.

Karim, Anwarul. 1988. "Shamanism in Bangladesh." *Asian Folklore Studies* 47 (2): 277-309.

Kendall, Emily A., Rashid Uz Zaman, Ruchira T. Naved, Muhammed W. Rahman, Mohammed A. Kadir, Sahila Arman, Eduardo Aziz-Baumgartner, and Emily S. Gurley. 2012. "Medically Unexplained Illness and the Diagnosis of Hysterical Conversion Reaction (HCR) in Women's Medicine Wards of Bangladeshi Hospitals: A Record Review and Qualitative Study." *BMC Women's Health* 12 (1): 38.

Kious, Brent M., and Benjamin R. Lewis. 2019. "Correspondence: Classifying Psychiatric Disorders as Communicable Diseases." *Lancet Psychiatry* 6 (1): 13-14.

Langwick, Stacey A. 2011. *Bodies, Politics and African Healing: The Matter of Maladies in Tanzania.* Bloomington: Indian University Press.

Lim, Anastasia, Hans W. Hoek, Samrad Ghane, Mathijs Deen, and Jan D. Blom. "The Attribution of Mental Health Problems to Jinn: An Explorative Study in a Transcultural Psychiatric Outpatient Clinic." *Frontiers in Psychiatry* 9:89.

Mamun, Abdullah A., Mohammad M. Maruf, Avra D. Bhowmik, Khaleda Begum, and Zulfiquer Ahmed Amin. 2016. "Mass Psychogenic Illness: Comparison on Selected Variables between Cases and Non-cases." *Bangladesh Journal of Psychiatry* 30 (1): 14-19.

Marriott, McKim. 1990. *India through Hindu Categories*. New Dehli: Sage Publications.

Murphy, Michelle. 2006. *Sick Building Syndrome and the Problem of Uncertainty.* Durham, NC: Duke University Press.

Ong, Aihwa. 2010. *Spirits of Resistance and Capitalist Discipline: Factory Women in Malaysia.* Albany: State University of New York Press.

Pabna Correspondent. 2015. "Atonke Bidyaloyer Shikshok-Shiksharthira. [Students and Teachers of School Terrorized]." *Ajker Patrika*, 18 May 2015. Accessed 24 November 2018, http://ajkerpatrika.com/last-page/2015/05/18/34495/print.

Pal, Indrajit, and Tuhin Ghosh 2014. "Fire Incident at AMRI Hospital, Kolkata (India): A Real Time Assessment for Urban Fire." *Journal of Business Management & Social Sciences Research* 3 (1): 9-13.

Porter, Theodore M. 1996. *Trust in Numbers: The Pursuit of Objectivity in Science and Public Life.* Princeton: Princeton University Press.

Pringle, Yolana. 2013. "Investigating 'Mass Hysteria' in Early Postcolonial Uganda: Benjamin H. Kagwa, East African Psychiatry, and the Gisu." *Journal of the History of Medicine and Allied Sciences.* 70 (1): 105-36.

Ranju, Abdul Latif. 2016. "Chatmohare Prathomik Bidyaloye Jween Atonko; Skul Chharchhe Chhatrira [Terror of Jinns at Chatmohar Primary School; Girl Students Leaving School]." *bd24live.com*, 9 May 2016. Accessed 25 November 2018, https://www.bd24live.com/bangla/article/90300/index.html.

Representative. 2016. "Sripure Bhut Atonke Gyan Harachhen Karkhanar Sramikra [Workers Falling Unconscious from Fear of Ghosts at Sripur]." *Bhorer Kagaj*, 11 October 2016. Accessed 20 November 2018, http://www.bhorerkagoj.com/print-edition/2016/10/11/110927.php.

Rosenberg, Charles E. 1977. "The Therapeutic Revolution: Medicine, Meaning, and Social Change in Nineteenth-Century America." *Perspectives in Biology and Medicine* 20 (4): 485-506.

Roy, Asim. 2016. *Islamic Syncretistic Tradition in Bengal.* Princeton: Princeton University Press.

Sax, William S. 2009. *God of Justice: Ritual Healing and Social Justice in the Central Himalayas.* New York: Oxford University Press.

—. 2014. Ritual Healing and Mental Health in India. *Transcultural Psychiatry* 51 (6): 829-49.

Senior Correspondent. 2018. "Address Mental Health Issues during Emergencies: Saima Wazed." *bdnews24*, 30 August 2018. Accessed 30 December 2018, https://bdnews24.com/health/2018/08/30/address-mental-health-issues-during-emergencies-saima-wazed.

Tarafder, Binoy K., Mohammad A. I. Khan, Md. Tanvir Islam, Sheikh A. Al Mahmoud, Md. Humayun K. Sarker, Imtiaz Faruq, Md. Titu Miah, and S. M. Yasir Arafat. 2016. "Mass Psychogenic Illness: Demography and Symptom Profile of an Episode." *Psychiatry Journal* 2016:1-5.

Viveiros de Castro, Eduardo. 2004. "Perspectival Anthropology and the Method of Controlled Equivocation." *Tipiti: The Journal for the Anthropology of Lowland South America* 2 (1): 3-22.

Wainberg, Milton L., and Francine Cournos. 2019. "Correspondence: Author's Reply." *Lancet Psychiatry* 6 (1): 14.

Wainberg, Milton L., Liat Helpman, Cristiane S. Duarte, Sten H. Vermund, Jennifer J. Mootz, Lidia Gouveia, Maria A. Oquendo, Karen McKinnon, and France Cournos. 2018. "Curtailing Communicability of Psychiatric Disorders." *Lancet Psychiatry* 6 (11): 940-44.

Winter, Stephen. 2006. "On the Possibilities of Group Injury." *Metaphilosphy* 37 (3-4): 393-413.

About the Author

PROJIT BIHARI MUKHARJI is an Associate Professor at the University of Pennsylvania. He was educated at the Presidency College, Calcutta, Jawaharlal Nehru University, New Delhi, and the School of Oriental and African Studies, London. He is the author of *Nationalizing the Body: The Medical Market, Print and Daktari Medicine* (London, 2009) and *Doctoring Traditions: Ayurveda, Small Technologies and Braided Sciences* (Chicago, 2016). He is also the Editor-in-Chief of *History Compass,* Associate Editor of *South Asian History & Culture* and Book Review Editor of *Isis.*

6   Psychedelic Therapy

Diplomatic Re-compositions of Life/Non-life, the Living and the Dead

Harish Naraindas

Abstract

This chapter, which is an ethnography of a psychosomatic department in a German hospital, functions as a foil to the rest of the volume. It allows us to ask the following: Why is the movement for global mental health preoccupied with the Global South? Why does mental health in the Global South primarily revolve around the psycho-pharmaceutical, while psychosomatic medicine, which in the German context is a separate discipline divorced from psychiatry, is normatively built on eschewing psycho-pharmaceuticals? Why is mental health in the Global South built on the distinction between superstition (past lives, trance, possession – in short, 'rituals' invoking the spirits and the dead) and science (psychiatry, rational diagnosis, asylums, drugs), while in Germany the two are often fused?

Keywords: animism, family-constellation, global mental health, psychiatry, psychosomatic

Introduction

This chapter is an ethnography of a psychosomatic department in a German Hospital (*Klinik*),[1] where past-life aetiologies are invoked and addressed through art, body work, breathwork, exotic music, trance, and collective

---

1   I will hereafter use *Klinik* instead of Hospital, and the abbreviated word *Therme* instead of *Thermalbad* (spa), following popular usage, throughout the essay. The meaning of both these terms will become increasingly clear as the essay unfolds.

Sax, William, and Claudia Lang (eds), *The Movement for Global Mental Health: Critical Views from South and Southeast Asia*. Taylor & Francis Group, 2021
DOI: 10.5117/9789463721622_CH06

psychotherapeutic journeys that meld the past and the present, the living and the dead, East and West. This is played out against a large mountain park (*Bergpark*) and a *Thermalbad* (spa) on either side of the *Klinik*, each of which sport Greek, Roman, and Anglo-Chinese motifs in their architecture and landscape. Together, these function as a formal and para-formal therapeutic resource for patients, who may draw energy through divination techniques from spots in the park, or do aqua gymnastics with their ailing bodies in the *Therme*. This ensemble is enabled by the therapists, some of whom traverse these several worlds literally and figuratively by interning with Brazilian shamans and Hindu gurus, and fusing them with New Age psychotherapies from California invented by Germans, along with an initial training in Protestant theology.

This psychedelic and "panpsychic world" (Jonas 1982; Goff 2019), paid for by mandatory German health insurance, is the perfect foil to the "movement for global mental health" (MGMH), whose claim to being global is belied by its preoccupation with the Global South. This preoccupation is predicated on the notion of a "treatment gap" because of rudimentary and inadequate mental health facilities and personnel in the Lower and Middle Income Countries (LMICs).[2] It advocates closing the "treatment gap" by making mental health a fundamental right for the millions of undiagnosed, under or misdiagnosed persons suffering from mental pathologies (Patel et al. 2007, 2011, 2012). And it offers Western psychiatry and pharmaceuticals as the primary mode of redemption, although it makes appropriate noises about adapting it to local contexts, including making it broad-based by, for example, "task shifting to non-specialist health workers" (Patel et al. 2012), including training general practitioners (GPs) to address mental health.

It has its share of critics. They have pointed out, as do several papers in this volume, that (a) the Global South may have its own way of approaching mental health (Bracken et al. 2016); (b) exporting Western psychiatry may be inappropriate (Summerfield 2008) and smacks of medical imperialism (Summerfield 2013); (c) the single largest mental pathology that seems to be addressed is depression (Misra et al. 2019), and the treatment for it is primarily advocated through psychopharmaceuticals; (d) for this reason there is a synergy if not a collusion between the MGMH and the pharmaceutical industry (Bracken et al. 2016); and (e) such a pharmaceuticalisation precludes the possibility of addressing the social determinants of health (Whitley 2015), which are often the root cause of mental distress. Finally,

---

2   The "treatment gap" is ostensibly 50 per cent in the Global North and 90 per cent in the LMICs (Patel et al. 2013).

asking poor countries to allocate limited health budgets to mental health so conceived may be at the cost of other programmes and societal health broadly conceived (Freeman 2016), with an example being asking GPs to address mental health in "out-patient departments" (OPDs). This may not only be impractical but, if implemented, given the amount of time required to address a mental health patient, it may be at the cost of several other patients in extremely overcrowded OPDs.

While the above is not an exhaustive list, what perhaps unites the critics of global mental health is that *they, too*, appear to be preoccupied with the Global South. While the most trenchant may go to the extent of pointing out the existence of alternative ways of conceptualising "mental health" with their attendant epistemologies, the Global North, which is the tacit point of reference, is not brought into an explicit and relational play with the Global South.[3] It is readily understood that the healing modalities of the Global South, under the sign of "belief" and "culture", may bring into play religion, deities, demons, the dead, the spirits and the ancestors, both as aetiological and therapeutic agents. But it is tacitly presumed that in the Global North the cognitive and therapeutic institutions are premised upon a clear separation between life and non-life, and the living and the dead; and if the dead or non-life are invoked, they are seen not as "real" aetiological or therapeutic agents (as they nominally are in the Global South), but rather as symbols or metaphors. Nature and culture stay apart, and the dead do

---

3   I have tried to show the importance and necessity of such a "relational" constituting of objects of enquiry in three other instances. I attempted to demonstrate, with reference to "tropical medicine", that counter to then and current modes of explanation, which had "reduced" its advent to colonialism and imperialism, its birth could be neither fully nor correctly understood by focusing solely on the tropics (Naraindas 1996). I chose to focus primarily on the temperate world, and argued that its preoccupation with the weather and climate as part of its "medical history" was cardinal in understanding the discourse on the tropics. I then showed that the eighteenth-century British understanding of smallpox in India was at the same time, if not principally, a conversation that British medical practitioners in India were having with their peers about their practice in Britain (Naraindas 2003), and how such a perspective could provide us with a different vantage point from which to understand the advent of vaccination in the nineteenth century (Naraindas 1998). And the third, to a lesser extent, is the homebirth movement in the US, Europe, and India in a comparative perspective (Naraindas 2014), which I partly reprise at the end of this chapter. This, unfortunately, is not the way that Anglo-European South Asian scholars usually constitute their objects of enquiry. And as for South Asian historians and anthropologists, their fate is to be nothing other than "informants of their own society", as their objects of enquiry, with some exceptions, are their own grandmothers – that is, they usually study their own linguistic and/or religious communities, and often their own caste, village, neighbourhood, or state. Some of my own work is no exception to this.

not even nominally[4] metamorphose into the living as they do in the Global South. Or, to put it differently, Germans no longer literally tie their dead down in their coffins because the dead no longer wake up at night and insist on having a beer with the living, as they did in the past.[5] In other words, we (the Global North – which is also found in the Global South) no longer inhabit a world that is macabre – where the dead, too, are alive – but a world that is morbid, where even the living are presumed to be dead, except for that strange thing called the mind or consciousness.

I offer my contribution to this volume as a foil to such a premise. I believe that my ethnography of a psychosomatic department in a German *Klinik* will allow us to rethink, with Povinelli (2019), the binary of life/non-life, and, with Stengers (2012), the "sad nature devoid of life" that is the provenance of science, and the metaphoric rather than the metamorphic world of culture that is the provenance of all other disciplines including anthropology. I hope to show that ancestors and the dead may not merely be part of "culture", "belief", and the "metaphoric", but metamorphose into aetiological and therapeutic agents in the Global North as they do in the Global South, albeit in not quite the same way; and that "sad nature", rather than being "devoid of life", may well be animated and/or panpsychic, especially in the hands of geriatric female German patients and their therapists. And it is these "intangible-tangibles", rather than "tangible psychopharmaceuticals" that appear to be the therapeutic mainstay in the psychosomatic department.

Such a methodological move allows us to ask, from a completely different vantage point to the critiques we have listed above, why "mental health" in the Global South appears to revolve around the material substance of the psychopharmaceutical, while psychosomatic medicine – which in the German context is a separate discipline, divorced from psychiatry – is normatively built on eschewing psychopharmaceuticals; why "mental health" in the Global South is built on the distinction between superstition (past lives, trance, possession, or in short, "rituals" invoking the spirits and the dead) and science (psychiatry, rational diagnosis, asylums, drugs), while in Germany (exemplary of the Global North?) the two are often fused. In

---

4   I say nominally because, in the last instance, the *explanation* that anthropologists in-variably offer for a phenomenon such as possession, even in the Global South, is metaphorical and functional, despite disclaimers to the contrary. I call such anthropological explanations "sacramental" (Naraindas 2017) in so far as anthropology is genuinely unable to countenance theurgy and supplants the divine by the human. Both the "ontological turn" and the "animistic turn" are symptoms of this quandary.

5   For those who may be interested, the Museum of Sepulchral Culture in Kassel, Germany, offers a wonderful display of these practices.

other words, what does a politics of life/non-life, which is a politics of "us" versus "them" (Povinelli 2019, 2016), have to say to what appears to be an "evangelical" movement for global mental health – a movement that is not only preoccupied with the Global South but one that appears to be predicated on redeeming the millions of "under-diagnosed" and "misdiagnosed" patients through psychiatry and psychopharmaceuticals? By contrast, in the Global North (the tacit if not the explicit point of reference) the redemption for a large class of mental problems seems ironically to involve renouncing psychopharmaceuticals and supplanting them by the diplomatic composing of a "common world" (Latour 2004) that blurs, if not altogether abrogates, the distinction between human/non-human and life/non-life, but not quite "us" and "them".

I   Triptych: The Park, the *Klinik*, and the *Therme*

Roughly in the centre of Germany is a city that was razed to the ground during the Allied bombing. Unlike Dresden, artfully rebuilt to its medieval proportions with moss, lichen, and patina-covered walls, this West German city, not too far from the erstwhile East German border, was rebuilt as a "featureless" industrial city. This, in any case, is the general sense that many Germans seem to have of it. But I found it rather lovely, surrounded as it is by low, verdant hills nestled in a valley, with a baroque *Orangerie* by the river at its eastern end, and perhaps the largest mountain park in Europe to its West. Begun in the early eighteenth century in the French baroque style, it metamorphosed by the end of the century – unlike the *Orangerie* – into an *Anglo-Chinois* landscape-garden with sham ruins, Chinese pagodas, winding gravel paths, grottoes, pavilions, hot houses and footbridges. But the centrepiece of the park is the waterworks that runs from a Greek demi-god at the summit to a large pond halfway down. Twice a week in the summer, large crowds gather to witness the water show, when the water flows from the foot of the demi-god to the pond and spectacularly erupts into one of the tallest gravity-induced fountains in the world.

Declared a UNESCO World Heritage site a few years ago, the park is increasingly home to its share of tourists, especially in the summer. Occasionally, one may see a mock eighteenth-century German princess in full regalia, chaperoned by her eighteenth-century mother, sauntering down a gentle slope, and once a year it may be overrun by a horde of adolescents from around the world, dressed up as manga characters from Japanese comic books. But the park is also home to a more quotidian presence: a quasi-geriatric and largely female clientele that comes from a *Klinik* at the foot of the park. Some of them come to see the Renaissance paintings in the Castle museum, while others come to stroll or gaze at the geese in the lotus and lily pond, or have cake and coffee at the museum cafe. Some come in well-heeled groups for a brisk walk and body work led by a physical therapist, or for a session of Nordic walking in full gear. Some come to wade in shallow step wells in what the Germans call a *Kneippkur* (hydrotherapy). There are others who come, often alone in the wee hours of the morning, or at high noon, to hug and talk to their chosen tree, or to silently and intensely converse with giant sized sunflowers. Still others come with their water dowsing sticks to find energy spots on which they stand to get charged. And finally, for some the park is a pilgrimage site. They come to the *Klinik* every year with no apparent illness, as the park – once a royal folly – is the main draw: a sacred and hallowed ground where they commune with nature, the spirits, and themselves, and perhaps re-experience, every year, an epiphanous moment at the place where they were once healed.

The park, from the little we have said so far, evidently functions as a recreational, therapeutic and para-therapeutic site; and for some, as a place of pilgrimage. The therapies range from physical and natural ones, such as walking or treading cold water, to divinatory techniques such as using dowsing sticks to find energy spots, or spiritual scoping for trees and flowers to commune with. What kind of *Klinik* houses patients who talk to flowers and trees, or who see the surface of the earth as a series of way stations that can re-fuel them when they are low on energy? And why is the *Klinik* happy to have patients return as "guests" every year to occupy a room, with all three meals, for just €65 a night (2010),[6] along with a host of para-therapeutic activities such as yoga, tai chi, pottery, silk-painting, teddy bear making, and meditating thrown in, and the unlimited use of the *Therme* to boot? And what are we to make of the panoply of therapies on offer? What do they set out to accomplish, and for whom? And, finally, who pays for such a broad therapeutic palette?

If the park is uphill from the *Klinik*, then downhill is the *Therme*. It too is a recreational, therapeutic and para-therapeutic site. The recreational and public entrance, with a mock British phone booth at its entrance, repeats and elaborates the Anglo-oriental theme in the park with a Chinese-style pagoda in red. The Far Eastern theme is given further rein in the internal

---

6   As "guests" they are not entitled to any of the "formal or official" therapies, or nursing care, by the hospital during their stay. But they are entitled to all the para-therapeutic activities as indicated in the text.

architecture of the warm mineral water swimming pool, which is ringed by Jacuzzis, fitness rooms, massage parlours, water slides, and the like. One floor up is an elaborate set of themed and aromatic European and Japanese saunas, including an enormous salt sauna resembling a dinosaur's foot as the centrepiece, ringed on the outside by an assortment of *Kneippkur* douches, a fresh water swimming pool, an electric fireplace with a Greco-Roman facade, and a café that serves up hot and cold beverages along with sausages and pretzels.

The *Therme* is connected by an underground walkway to the *Klinik*. Every morning patients use it to reach the *Therme*, some of them in wheelchairs, for a supervised session of aqua gymnastics in an extra-warm water pool. While this is part of the formal therapeutic timetable, its para-formal part sees patients come in the mornings and evenings, either alone or with members of their cohort, to use the *Therme*, or to congregate after dinner in the larger café on the ground floor for a para-therapeutic session of bonding with their cohort of eleven, who for six to twelve weeks are their substitute family and whose members do not merely bond but often fall in love, and are even tacitly encouraged to do so as part of the therapy.

The private walkway from the *Therme* to the *Klinik* opens out into a labyrinthine maze of several floors with several hundred rooms. Depending on the time of the day and the season, one may see patients actively treading water in *a Kneippkur*, or passively taking a warm *Dauerdusche* (prolonged and continuous shower from head to toe that one self-oscillates by a pulley from the shower bed). Or one might see patients painting and dancing, or doing body work and power breathing, or practicing yoga and tai chi, or chanting mantras in the chapel and meditating in themed meditating rooms and, on a Good Friday, listening to Bach's aria, *Erbarme dich, mein Gott*, from *Matthäuspassion*, in the auditorium. The aria that reflects Peter's lament and solitary heartache in the garden after having denied knowing Jesus three times.[7]

---

7   This theme of betrayal, I soon realised, was a recurring motif for some German patients. Peter denied Jesus; and Germans (though not all) denied Jews during the holocaust. One telling example of this – and there were variants on this theme – was of a 70-year-old patient who has a recurring dream of a Jewish woman knocking on her door. She tosses and turns in her dream. And before she can resolve her quandary, of whether to admit or deny the woman entry into her house in the dead of night, she wakes up in a cold sweat. And then she comforts herself by saying that she was born after the war – albeit on the cusp – and this is a decision that is not hers to make. But this act of self-cajoling brings her little comfort. She belongs, according to Bilger (2016), to a generation of Germans, for some of whom "historical guilt" reappears, night after night, as the "Jewess" at the door. Hence, we can only imagine the kind of resonance that the aria – a litany of lament – sets up in such patients' soul.

One might also witness patients sitting upright on large plastic balls and attending a class on the spine and on posture, or making ghee (clarified butter) as part of their Ayurveda cooking class, or listening to a lecture in the lecture hall on a range of topics from Ayurvedic diet, multivitamin therapy, and macrobiotics, to talks on burn-out, diabetes, cancer and psycho-oncology. And elsewhere, patients may be quietly working their way toward a room labelled *Seelsorge*: which in this *Klinik* functioned as a non-denominational "secular" chaplaincy, in keeping with the increasing rechristening of the hospital chaplaincy in the Anglophone world from one meant for pastoral care to spiritual care (Thierfelder 2017), with some hospital chaplaincies in Scotland and England (based on my fieldwork) having special "secular chaplains" on the roster, who *only* offer non-religious "spiritual" care to patients, though they may be Presbyterians or Anglicans fully trained in Protestant theology.

The *Klinik*, built around a handsome pre-war *Kurklinik* (rehabilitation hospital)[8] belonging to the Deutsche Bahn (German Railway Corporation), was designed around a courtyard that more than mimicked a cloister garth. According to the apocryphal story of the building of the *Klinik* (and earlier the *Therme*), the owner told the contractor to lay the foundation stone a second time because the latter had not taken seriously his injunction to do so at the precise time determined by his astrologer. When we asked Max (pseudonym), the owner, about this, he just smiled mysteriously. Ostensibly designed to resemble a cloister, the chapel occupied one point of the compass, and the buildings appeared to be oriented towards the seasonal declination of the Sun, like much of pre-modern European architecture. The *Klinik* was built before *Vastushastra* (the Indian equivalent of feng shui) arrived on the global architecture-scape. But Max had its layout confirmed later by the appropriate experts, and was pleased to find that it accorded well with it.

The water source for the *Therme*, developed a few years earlier by Max,[9] was located by a water diviner, who evidently appeared on the scene when the engineers were scouting around with their equipment for a precise

---

8   Before the building became a *Kurklinik* of the German railway, it was a *Wasserheilanstalt* (i.e. a clinical institution for hydrotherapy) built in 1883 by a medical doctor. Such institutes mushroomed in the late nineteenth century in Germany, inspired by the movement for *Natur-heilkunde* (nature cure). And both hydrotherapy (the German version is called *Kneippkur* after its inventor, Fr. Kneipp) and *Naturheilkunde* are central parts of the current *Klinik*, and of this narrative. As for the meaning of *Kur* in the German context, see Naraindas (2011).

9   He first built the *Therme* in 1982, and later (in 1986) bought the *Klinik* from the German Railway and started renovating and enlarging it.

spot to drill the well. He accosted Max soon after the boring had begun and told him that the engineers had got it wrong. He indicated a spot that he said was better on two counts: The water would be found a couple of hundred metres higher, and it would be the right temperature. He invited Max to go into town and double-check with an astrologer, which Max did. But much to their horror and indignation, he first asked the engineers to halt the drilling. He then had them drill at the diviner's spot, and when they expressed dismay at their science being trumped, Max, much to their chagrin, said that it was his money and he would rather bet on the diviner than their science. He apparently backed the right horse as the water was indeed found at a lesser depth, thus saving him a small fortune, and it was the right temperature as promised, thus saving him the additional cost of heating it, in perpetuity, to the temperature required for the *Therme*.

Max, who owned nearly two-dozen similar *Klinik*s in the same state, was formerly a devotee of Sai Baba (an Indian Guru) and said he was an Ayurvedic physician in his previous life. This particular *Klinik* was rather special, as it had a full-fledged Ayurveda department, and was situated in the city of his birth. He had personally designed much of it, and had a cardinal role to play in the colour scheme of the curtains, the furniture and the upholstery, with a preponderance of yellow, gold, and burnished gold symbolising the Sun and good health. The *Klinik*'s foyer in particular was decorated with large mandala paintings made by a well-known local artist; and next to the *Klinik*'s café was a Mandala Studio, where patients could learn mandala colouring for a nominal fee. The acme of the architectural design was to crown the Ayurveda department with an octagonal belvedere overlooking the cloister garth, and with a nice view of the *Bergpark* beyond the *Klinik*. Christened the *akasha* ("sky" or "ether") room, it was once a regular prayer house presided over by Max. It now functioned as the weekly meeting room for the Ayurvedic physician Dr. Kapoor (pseudonym) and his team, and also as an occasional prayer house where Dr. Kapoor, a German of Indian descent, who trained initially as a paediatrician and later as a *Vaidya*, conducted *puja* (worship) according to a nominal Hindu liturgical calendar. Apart from being a Hindu by birth and upbringing, and the son of a Sanskrit/Hindi professor, Kapoor had graduated in Indology from the University of Heidelberg and was also an accomplished Indian musician. He was also a historian of medicine (with a PhD) and straddled the Indo-European scholarly world, being conversant in Latin, Sanskrit, Pali, and Bengali, and fluent in German (including several local dialects), Punjabi, French, Hindi, and English.

The other three departments were Internal Medicine, Oncology, and Psychosomatic medicine, the last of which was the largest of all. In fact, the

Klinik was well known to schoolteachers in the city as the "loony-bin",[10] since nearly half the patients were indeed schoolteachers in the decade (2008-2017) I spent at the *Klinik*. All three departments, unlike the Ayurveda department, which was reached by a separate entrance, were eligible for the mandatory German health insurance that roughly covered 85 per cent of the German population (the other 15 per cent subscribed to private health insurance), and most of the patients who came to these three departments appeared to be covered by medical insurance of various kinds. Ayurveda was not covered by any of the insurance schemes, since it was not (yet) recognised as a medically reimbursable expense by the insurance companies.

Against this backdrop we will, for the purposes of this chapter on global mental health, enter the central panel of the triptych – the *Klinik* – and see what transpired in the Psychosomatic department (Scheidt 2017; Zipfel et. al 2016) in the decade that I spent there.

II   The Psychosomatic Department and Its Regimen

The formal regimen of the *Klinik* was like a school timetable. It ran from 7:30 a.m. to 4:30 p.m. In the Psychosomatic department, the therapies seemed to be roughly organised according to three bipolar distinctions between mind and body therapies, active and passive therapies, group and individual therapies. Each group of eleven participants was led by a psychotherapist.

One of the groups that I observed and followed for around six weeks was led by a 6-foot 5-inch therapist called John (pseudonym). The son of a pastor, he had a PhD from a German University in Protestant theology and a degree in psychotherapy. He had spent a part of his adolescence and youth – given his height and reach – in California playing professional basketball and hence spoke excellent English. A part of his time each year was spent interning with shamans in Brazil, another part was spent learning the flute with a Manipuri guru in Bombay, and the rest of the time was devoted to treating patients in the *Klinik*, and some privately at home, where he brought his shamanic training to bear upon his treatment.

John's group of eleven patients also had an art therapist, a body therapist, a nurse, and a "body" doctor, that is, a non-psychiatric doctor. It was overseen by an *Oberarzt* (senior doctor), responsible for several such groups, who was a psychiatrist cum psychotherapist. John led his patients in forms of active

---

10   I am quoting a schoolteacher patient who said this in a gathering of other patients, all of who agreed with her depiction.

and passive group therapies, and also had one on one sessions with each of them. The group therapies consisted of passive imaginative journeys followed by a public verbalisation of what these journeys had produced, or other forms of active therapies where patients were expected to publicly talk about their problem, or even more actively to be part of a group therapy where they arranged their substitute family of eleven at particular angles in particular parts of the room and got them to play their mother, father, boss, spouse, or other interlocutor. Called *Familienaufstellung*, this form of group psychotherapy (more on it further in the essay) invariably produced uncanny results as persons chosen to play these roles, who knew nothing about the persons they were playing, seemed able to impersonate their emotions, sensibilities, and sometimes even tone and cadence, leading to the possibility of self-discovery not only for the patient but also for the "impersonators". The body therapist had her patients work with their bodies, often accompanied by music, in various group formations. The cardinal theoretical assumption being that psychotherapeutic work was best addressed if various non-verbal body work was used to get patients, many of who could no longer "feel their bodies", to feel and express through such work where their pain and trauma were localised. Hence, body work was always followed by trying to verbalise what emotions and thoughts the body work had summoned from the depths of their being. But this was easier said than done. Many patients were initially unable to move their bodies, let alone dance to music. They often broke down and began to cry or left the room, and were invariably attended to by a co-therapist, usually the nurse, who was present. The same thing happened when patients were asked to draw or colour a piece of paper with a crayon in the art class. Art therapy, seen as another mode of addressing emotions, and again as a non-verbal way of working out distress through a continuous and evolving series of paintings over the weeks, often proved initially to be traumatic for some patients. Some of them simply could not put brush or crayon to paper and broke down at the prospect.

The third kind of therapy, not part of every "normal group" – there were special geriatric and adolescent groups, and specific disease groups, with a roughly similar format but with special variations – was called "breathwork" (German *Atemtherapie*) in the psychotherapeutic literature. The variant practiced here, modelled after Grof and Grof's Holotropic breathwork (2010), was to get the patient to lie down and hyperventilate to loud and rhythmic music. Theoretically the music should have no cultural resonance with the patients and hence it was sourced from non-Euro-American sources. But the therapist made an informed choice and the selection played in my honour was

first the Hanuman Chalisa and then a Sufi Dhikr,[11] neither of which (much to
the dismay of the therapist) I recognised. The hyperventilation was meant to
send the patient into a trance and transport them to a preverbal or perinatal
phase and, in rare cases, to their past lives. If body therapy was partly based
on notions such as body-memory and the "body knows better", variants of the
breathwork seemed to be partly based on the treacherousness of the word
and the supposed irreconcilable differences in the various psychoanalytical
traditions, based as they were in giving primacy to the word. One facet of
this discomfort was to lead the patient into the womb, and if possible beyond
into their previous lives, thus drawing upon Buddhist and Hindu theories
of past lives. But, more importantly, all these therapies were meant to make
the patient partly her own therapist and to empower her to undertake the
journey to recovery. The verbal and non-verbal, group and solo, active and
passive methods were all used in tandem, with this objective in mind.

Apart from these core psychotherapeutic gestures in the timetable, the body
doctor also prescribed a host of treatments depending on the condition and
somatic complaints of each individual patient. These again were divided into
active and passive, with the passive including massage, sitz bath, foot bath,
Dauerdusche, foot reflexology, and so on. The active therapies could be aqua
gymnastics in the warm water pool in the *Therme*, a swim in the mineral water
pool, Nordic walking in the *Kurpark*, brisk walking in the *Kurpark*, tai chi, the
fitness parlour (gym), power breathing, a *Kneippkur* in the form of walking in
circles in a cold-water pool, or attending classes on posture, which was both
a theory and practice of how to stand, sit, bend, pick up heavy objects, and so
on. All the activities in the timetable were performed under supervision. They
were reviewed once a week in a meeting led by John, in which each therapist,
including the body doctor and the nurse, recounted the patients' progress.
Every patient's artwork was put up on the wall and was collectively analysed
by John and the rest of the team, and overseen by the *Oberarzt*. The timetable,
as is by now evident, put patients on a treadmill. They often got lost running
from one therapy session to the next and felt as if they were back in school.

---

11   The Hanuman Chalisa is a popular Hindu devotional hymn in North India. It comprises 40
verses and acts, among other things, as a kind of sonic armour against adversity. The Dhikr is an
analogous repetitive utterance of short phrases or prayers, either from the Quran or the Hadith,
in Sufi practice. The Dhikr is now a popular tourist attraction where "Sufi dervishes" perform
it in public: for example, in a hall near the main railway station in Istanbul. The Hanuman
Chalisa recording played in the *Klinik* was sung by an American. The therapist said so when
I told him that the accent and cadence were strange – at least to my ears. Hence, we have an
American singing a Hindu devotional, consciously chosen by a German therapist to have no
cultural resonance for his German clientele.

Parts of the formal timetable were replicated in the informal therapies on offer, either early in the morning or after 4:30 in the afternoon. This was purely voluntary and virtually all of it was free of cost. Participants had to pay for the silk in the silk painting, or the wool in teddy bear making. But the silk scarves or stoles they created, or the teddy bears they made with one eye shut, were theirs to take away. And catatonic patients sometimes benefitted from this informal programme, especially the evening dance, led (as they said in their written testimonies placed in a folder in one of the several foyers) by a "young and angelic 79-year-old", who also read them stories during the Christmas season, led them in carol singing, and virtually put them to bed. Her greatest achievement was to have led scores of patients, year after year for the last twenty-odd years, to rediscover and recover their bodies through movement and dance. It was here that body work actually began for many, and then worked its way into the formal body work in the timetable. Both therapists and patients were acutely aware of how *the formal and the informal bled into each other.* But on the face of it the informal appeared to be, at first sight, an even more superfluous panoply than the formal timetable, with no more use than as recreational devices to pass the evening away. In fact, one could argue that the entire therapeutic palette on offer may have seemed to an uninformed outsider (in this case, me) like a lark, and the panoply of activities like singing, dancing, painting, meditating, walking, swimming, showering, going into a trance, or being endlessly massaged, as something ludicrous bordering on the outrageous, since the insurance – just €156 per day per patient for the entire array – paid for what may have appeared to be patients having a good time. From the Anglophone point of view, it could have looked like *Germans* – and elderly ones – simply enjoying themselves at the expense of a mandatory socialised insurance and pension scheme.[12]

But it was a form of *therapy* that evidently worked as there were several such *Klinik*s – both public and private – throughout Germany, where the *Reha* (rehabilitation) industry was worth €6 billion in 2010 (Wirth et al. 2010). And many of the therapies – or variations of them – were not only offered privately as stand-alone therapies but also practiced in public and university hospitals. This was because the therapies were largely determined by various

12 John, who continued to have one foot in California, where many of these therapies were invented by German and East European expatriates, says his US colleagues, who offer a similar palette, but for private patients in the American "rehab system", and as stand-alone offers, are green with envy that John is able to practice his craft in a mandatory insurance-scape for "common" patients who would never be able to afford this out of pocket, or through a private insurance (the premium would be too high) in the US.

umbrella organisations, with the insurance companies, pension organisations, and the ministry of work on the one side, and doctors' associations on the other, deciding on the gamut of therapies. The price per patient per day was determined by the setting, the selection on offer, and whether the patient was privately insured or was coming through the mandatory insurance scheme. Hence, in the private *Klinik* under study, the "common patients" admitted under the mandatory insurance were charged €156 euros, while privately insured patients were charged more for the same therapies,[13] with cosmetic differences like a slightly larger room with a small private TV, and some seemingly real differences such as the privilege of more private meetings with the *Chefarzt*[14] (the chief physician) on their weekly timetable, though the standing joke among both physicians and well-informed patients was that in most cases the Chief was best not met, as his methods were probably dated and he had become more of a manager of operations than a practicing doctor, and was hence of no real help – though this was not always the case.[15] In effect, this meant that the two types of patients were administratively and cosmetically separated but received roughly the same kind of therapies, except perhaps for the opportunity of seeing the *Chefarzt* more often. They were part of the same cohort of eleven, and thus could even fall in love.

13   Dr. Kapoor explained it thus: "Technically speaking it is not that privately insured patients are charged more; the difference is the way the reimbursement works: the mandatory/public insurance negotiates a lump-sum for all necessary therapy (in this case e.g. €156) and pays that sum per day, no matter what is actually done. The privately insured patient is charged separately for each "therapeutic service" so to say, but on the other hand he/she is charged only for the therapies he/she has actually used. In effect, private patients may land up paying about €176. And if they do not exercise their privilege to see the *Chefarzt* – and they are often encouraged through financial incentives not to do so – they may end up paying the same amount." This kind of financial arrangement also allows the therapists to offer therapies that they deem fit, that is, therapies – such as *Atemtherapie* or *Familienaufstellung* – over and above, or other than those routinely mandated by the insurance companies, the ministry of work, and doctors' associations. And these therapies – both the formal and the informal – then determine in part why and how patients, and their referring physicians (*Hausarzt*/GP), may exercise their choice to go to a particular *Klinik* where a particular panoply is on offer. For example, there are *Klinik*s for the wealthy where a similar bouquet could cost as much €400-600 a day.
14   In Germany, to quote Dr. Kapoor again: "The *Chefarzt* occupies a unique position in the medical hierarchy. In a hospital/department he/she is the lone medical head and normally the only person granted the right to charge patients for personal services separately. This is very different from, for example, the American system, where usually all attending physicians have similar rights and the medical head/chairman is a *primus inter pares*, and often by rotation."
15   This is particularly true of medical disciplines that require technical or even manual expertise (like surgery or paediatrics). But for a discipline like psychosomatics, or even oncology as was the case in this *Klinik*, where diagnostic acumen and therapeutic common sense is often arrived at only over time, seeing a *Chefarzt* may be far more useful.

III Cosmopolitics: Reflections on Formal/Informal, Recreation/ Therapy, Spiritual/Medical

How are we to make sense of the *Klinik* and its two associated institutions? And what bearing, if any, does this have on Global Mental Health? It is evident, from what we have said so far, that the triptych of the *Bergpark*, the *Klinik* and the *Therme* constitute – to borrow lightly and tangentially from Stengers (2004) – a kind of *Cosmopolitics*. They are, singly and together, *queer* spaces where the distinction between recreation and therapy, the material and the ineffable, the formal and the informal, the living and the dead, or between magic, science, and religion is, at the least, held together in some kind of articulated tension, and at best blurred if not altogether effaced. In this Cosmopolitics, queer, rather than being a homophobic epithet through which the binaries of sex are ushered in, now heralds the interrogation of all binaries (Butler 1990) and makes possible several forms of orientations to the world at once. Both Stengerian Cosmopolitics, and Povinelli's *Geontologies* (2016), show us, each in their own way, Western social theory's long and continuing preoccupation with accounting for the distinction between Life and Non-life (Povinelli 2019), or the distinction between an inert world that is the provenance of Science, and an animate world which, rather than being metamorphic, is reduced to the metaphoric and the symbolic under the epithets of "belief" and "culture" and thus becomes the provenance of all the non-scientific disciplines including anthropology (Stengers 2012). Under the banner of anthropology and its colonising impetus, "animism" supposedly sets the ball rolling as the quintessential mark of non-European others and their "cultural beliefs". For Povinelli, this distinction is fundamentally one of governance through classification which, as we will presently see, is central to the argument of this paper. It sets up an us-them distinction that plays out in interesting ways. She says that "the attribution of an inability of various colonised people to identify the kind of things that have agency, subjectivity, and intentionality of the sort that emerges with life has been the grounds of casting them into a premodern mentality and postrecognition difference" (Povinelli 2019).

But what do we find in our ethnography of such a queer space at the edge of an industrial European city – a city bombed to smithereens since it produced armoured tanks for the Wehrmacht? We have a transubstantiation: the *Bergpark*, an eighteenth- century folly probably born of royal conceit and for royal pleasure, *metamorphoses* into a pilgrimage site where "common" patients commune with nature. Not, as Stengers puts it, the "sad nature devoid of life" and the provenance of science, but an animate/d one that she wishes to recover – as do several centuries of European philosophy ever since Enlightenment, if not since the Reformation.

It appears that this animate/d nature is not only being recovered but is in full play in the hands of the largely geriatric, female, and German patients. And we have a *Therme* whose source is divined by a dowsing stick, confirmed by an astrologer, and dug by engineers. And finally, we have a *Klinik* whose foundation stone is laid by astrological dictum, is designed by ostensibly secular architects in a monastic idiom, and built by engineers to resemble a cloister garth in tune with the seasonal declination of the sun, with a chapel at its cardinal end. Into this European setting that is astronomical, astrological, monastic, and religious, we not only have Eastern forms of askesis like yoga and tai chi, but also an entire wing dedicated to an Eastern medical therapy called Ayurveda, with frescos and statues of Dhanvantri (the god of Ayurveda) in different parts of the *Klinik*. The crowning architectural glory is the octagonal belvedere with an altar at its centre where a *puja* could be performed, and is indeed performed according to a liturgical calendar by a German Hindu who, like John the psychotherapist, straddles at least two therapeutic and scholarly worlds at once. This ensemble is assembled by a German (Max), who claims to be a reincarnated Ayurvedic physician, and whose preceptor was a Hindu guru to whom Max donated a large sum of money (as did scores of his other devotees) to build a state of the art "modern" allopathic (biomedical) hospital in Puttaparthi – the Guru's abode in India: a not-so-ironic exchange of faces to which we will presently return.

In his "Politics of Nature", Latour writes that Stengers' idea of Cosmopolitics may be seen as a "progressive composition of the common world". A "common world is not established at the outset (unlike nature and society) but must be collected little by little through diplomatic work" (2004, 247). It appears that in the assemblage above, what we are witness to is the "progressive composition of [a] common world", of the human and the non-human. It seems that this conscious, careful and diplomatic composition is not merely built into the very architectural sinew of the *Klinik*, nor merely sourced from the mineral water for the *Therme*, but also embedded in the therapeutic modalities of each of the departments, especially the Psychosomatic department.[16] *Atemtherapie* (breathwork) – a version of

---

16   This was equally true, if not more so, in the oncology department. The *Chefarzt*, when I first arrived, had won a state award for his work as an oncologist and another from patient support groups. He was on the verge of retirement and had already treated 120,000 patients. His room was like that of a Chinese herbalist with scores of jars that housed substances that he had *collected* from all over the world. He practiced what he called "multi-modal" therapy, and one of his main

Grof and Grof's *Holotropic Breathwork* (2010) – is a case in point, where the patients are regressed not only to their perinatal stage but to their past lives. If Grof and Grof's *Breathwork* collects and composes Buddhist and Hindu ideas of past lives and Western psychological theory, John the psychotherapist personally collects and composes Brazilian shamanism and Western psychological theory.

Atemtherapie is also predicated on the principle that the music col-lected by the therapist should have no cultural resonance to the German/European patients and hence it is sourced from non-Western cultures. But the therapist, as collector and composer, makes an informed choice and often collects music that has a religious (rechristened as "spiritual" as in the case of *Seelsorge*) significance in their native settings.[17] Finally, the patients themselves go a step further (and are not discouraged from doing so by the therapists) by *transubstantiating* the *Bergpark* – a *straight* recreational site for tourists – into a *queer* space for patients: a place where they hug trees, talk to flowers, and use their dowsing stick to find energy spots – and not just water sources – to recharge their bodies. By doing so, these post-industrial German patients – who are hardly Australian aboriginals – raise visions of hylozoism, panpsychism and animism of the so-called "primitive man". Such a panpsychism, hylozoism or animism could be the point of departure for a philosophical excursus, as it is for Hans Jonas (1982), the stock-in-trade of anthropology, or a historical narration. In fact, in Jonas' excursus, it is all three at once, and implicitly functions as the quintessential perigee to the apogee that is Western civilisation.

The invoking, however, of this ostensibly annulled animism by these elderly German women seems to call into question, if not altogether ab-rogates, not only the distinction of life/non-life (Povinelli 2019)[18] on which all of the above are predicated, but the very "evolutionary history" of the planet where the so-called "primitive man" is the originary, simple, and animistic moment in an evolutionary ladder – bequeathed by Darwin – that

---

ways of prescribing drugs was through Kinesis (cf. Naraindas 2011). He warrants a paper in his own right.

17   As Dr. Kapoor perceptively put it: "the rechristening of the religious as the spiritual marks a characteristic of contemporary German/European society. Educated people and intellectuals here are extremely uneasy with all forms of denominational religion but apparently still feel a need for the religious to give meaning to their life. Calling your religious practices spiritual practices then is a way of avoiding this dilemma."

18   By life/non-life I don't mean things – or only *things* like photons and viruses – that can, like Schrodinger's cat, be dead and alive at the same time. We are talking of living and dead ancestors, and of the ensoulment and consciousness of inanimate matter, including trees, stones, and flowers.

Jonas (1982), as mentioned above, persuasively charts in *The Phenomenon of Life* (1982).

But these patients are able to go that crucial step further, since all these techniques – dowsing, hypnosis, meditation, breathwork, *Familienaufstellung*, and many more – are assiduously and formally taught throughout Germany (and perhaps Europe), and widely practiced as stand-alone therapies.[19] As an example, a 33-year-old Swiss-Tunisian therapist in Lausanne, whose biography I hope to write, treated me with a host of therapies ranging from a photon emitting gadget, to colour emitting laser rays, to incense, to African percussion music, and all in tandem, before ending with an intense deep tissue massage in the attic of a Zwinglian Church. She had already travelled to 37 countries collecting therapies. When I last met her in Lugano, she was headed to Jerusalem for a formal Shamanic training of solitary fasting and meditating in the Sinai desert for 40 days with a cohort of fellow seekers – the same number of days that Jesus spent in the desert. She collects, composes, and houses the therapies in her being. And she treats a range of patients with her panoply in the attic of an old Zwinglian Church, which is her abode – patients for whom conventional psychotherapy has not worked; or patients who come to her for self-improvement or self-enhancement, or for an altered state of consciousness and a journey of self-discovery. Her own therapeutic work is a journey of self-enhancement and self-discovery, including the discovery that her healing art is a gift that she has inherited from her Tunisian grandmother. Perhaps one day, like Bert Hellinger and his

---

19   This is especially the case with *Familienaufstellung* (family constellation therapy), which seems to be tailor-made for that lost generation of children born just before and during the war (*Kriegskinder*), and looking for ways to heal not only the trauma of the holocaust but the trauma of 14 million post-war refugees. These were German refugees who largely came from Eastern and Central Europe, as they were no longer welcome there. They continuously streamed into an already devastated German landscape, ravaged by war (Bilger 2016). But according to Bilger (2016), this streaming facilitated the healing of the wounds of war. Bilger's own journey in search of his Nazi grandfather, who turned out to be *a fanatical Nazi and a very good man*, is a beautiful rendering of how the *Familienaufstellung* works, its genesis as a healing technique in Germany, and how it is cardinally interwoven with a traumatised post-war German psyche. It apparently got an enormous fillip in the 1990s with the emergence of the *Kriegskinder*, who needed to know the past and talk to their dead – and possibly Nazi – ancestors. But now this therapy has travelled worldwide, is used for purposes other than an intergenerational conversation, and has also, as Bilger alludes, its share of critics, especially of its putative founder Bert Hellinger, who is seen by many persons practicing this therapy as a cultist, including William (Bo) Sax (personal communication). In fact, Sax insists in his communication with me that the therapy originated in the US with Virginia Satir, and it was taken up in Germany by some therapists, while at the same time acknowledging that Hellinger is by far "the best known *Famillienaufstellung* guy" (ibid.).

version of *Familienaufstellung*, which appears to be, among other things, a collection of Christian belief, Zulu techniques and Viennese psychoanalytical theory (Bilger; Sax et al. 2010),[20] her composition too, collected through assiduous diplomatic work, may be practiced widely and globally.

Several such therapies, composed by therapeutic entrepreneurs or by gifted individuals called to the healing art, or by formally trained psycho-therapists, have been "scientifically discredited" (this is the case, for example, with past life regression). Or they are not "fully accredited", as is the case of *Familienaufstellung*, which is premised on the notion of "disembodied memories" and "morphogenetic fields" – as explained to me by a de-baptised Sardinian therapist who had assumed the Hindu name Anandam (Bliss), in whose weekend therapeutic session in Geneva I did participant observa-tion. But they nevertheless find their way into German and Swiss *Reha Klinik*s. And some of these not "fully accredited" therapies (again, like the *Familienaufstellung*) are so respectable that they are not only practiced in the psychosomatic department of university teaching hospitals, but are the subject of randomised clinical trials – perhaps with a view to accredit them fully – with surprisingly positive outcomes, as was the case recently at the University of Heidelberg (Zipfel et al. 2016). Further, a professor from the Institute of Medical Psychology at the same University of Heidelberg has co-authored a paper with William Sax – the co-editor of this volume – in which *Familienaufstellung* is fruitfully compared with forms of "possession" and ritual healing in the Himalayas, which, like *Familienaufstellung*, evidently repairs and reconciles broken family relationships within and across genera-tions by invoking the dead and their spirits (Sax et al. 2010; Sax 2009).

I can personally testify to this as I spent a substantial part of that week-end in Geneva first resurrecting miscarried and aborted foetuses, then

20   Note how, nominally, the heart (Christian belief) and the mind (Viennese psychoanalytical theory) are vouchsafed to the West, while the hand/body (Zulu techniques) is the provenance of Black bodies. This is a standard narrative. Both the hand (technique) and the heart (lament, and paroxysms of ataxia, but not "true" faith) may have Black provenance, but not the mind (reason, theory). Acupuncture, till recently, was a "technique" that was wedded to and *explained* by modern physiology (it works because it releases serotonin and not because of Chinese "theory"), and was used as therapeutic mode to address not a Chinese but a biomedical nosology (Naraindas 2006). If this is the case with so-called "codified systems" like Ayurveda (ibid.; Naraindas 2014a, 2014b) and Chinese medicine (Adams 2002; Adams and Fei-Fei 2008), systems without an ostensible codex (or codices that went up in flames in the Latin American autos-da-fé) have little chance of being acknowledged to possess a theory. And even if they are granted one, the fact that these therapeutic modes are used to address a biomedical nosology, based tacitly on a biomedical physiology and anatomy, means that non-European theories have to be jettisoned and supplanted, as in the above case, by "Viennese psychoanalytical theory".

acknowledging and naming them, and then saying tearful goodbyes before finally burying them again on behalf of and with my cohort of eleven. This seemed to result in "closure and healing" by recognising unknown ancestors, like one's mother's miscarried or aborted foetus, and thus one's unknown brother or sister; and on other occasions acknowledging and then reconciling with one's own miscarriage or abortion. In the former case, some women, startled by the discovery that they had a dead sibling, called their mothers soon after the séance, only to be told that it was indeed true.

While my weekend therapy was paid for privately from my research grant, if the same thing is done in Germany in a hospital setting *as part of a suite of therapies*, it may be paid for by the mandatory health insurance, or by the pension scheme, or by the Ministry of Labour, or by the insurance provided for German civil servants like school teachers and university professors, including William Sax. Hence, Sax the anthropologist, who unlike John the psychotherapist, unwittingly straddles two worlds (one as a vocation and one as a potential patient), can either have his broken family relationships (if any) with his ancestors, including unknown siblings that will be revealed during the séance, repaired and restored by *Familienaufstellung* at a *Klinik* near Heidelberg, or he can have it done through the "rituals" associated with the Hindu god Bhairav in the Himalayas and pay for it with his research grant. But the latter is unlikely as Sax, according to my reading of his work, is deeply apprehensive of Bhairav and his cult and, if one reads him right, it also may not "work" as it is not *his* local and lived context (cf. Sax 2009; Naraindas 2017). But this is the least of it. What is far more interesting and germane to this paper and this volume on Global Mental Health, is that when healing involves possession, as it often does in the Himalayas for Sax (Sax 2009), or for example in the Chota Nikara shrine in Kerala (Padmanabhan 2017), it is seen by the current Diagnostic and Statistical Manual (DSM-V) of the American Psychiatric Association as a Dissociative Identity Disorder (Padmanabhan 2017). In other words, a séance that is referred to as *possession* – which according to Sax (2009) is often quite violent and scary with a lot of screaming and bodily contortions, but fully effective in its *local* context – if done in the Global South is a pathology according to psychiatry.[21] And a

---

21   The DSM-V purportedly makes a distinction between voluntary and involuntary possession and makes only the latter a pathology. But this is, says Padmanabhan (2017) through her
ethnography, an untenable distinction on the ground and has all sorts of consequences for
the phenomenon of possession in a shrine. For a similar critique from a Brazilian context, see
Delmonte et al. (2016), who say that the DSM-V is ambiguous and unhelpful when it comes to
differentiating "between non-pathological forms of possession and dissociative identity disorder
(DID)". And as practitioners from India point out: "Dissociative disorders can be called as the

séance that is referred to as *Familienaufstellung*, which can also be quite dramatic, with wailing and crying, if done in the Global North in a medical setting may, for Sax, not only be called a variation of either psychodrama, group psychotherapy, or systemic therapy, but may also be studied by an RCT and paid for by government insurance. How have we come to such a pass? And what does it mean for that movement called Global Mental Health?

IV Epistemic Impasse: The Therapeutic Need for Re-composing a Common World

What travels, and what does not? Or, in other words, we now need to ask, perhaps *contra* Latour, who is empowered to compose, through careful diplomatic work, the common and composite world of humans and non-humans that we have alluded to above? And why would anyone even want to compose such a common world? It appears that rituals of possession, or variants thereof, may not travel well outside of their local contexts, unless they are collected and composed by persons such as Bert Hellinger the ex-priest, Bliss the de-baptised Sardinian, or John the psychotherapist, or unless the *ojha* who does the divination in Sax's Himalayas, or the guru who summons the spirits and ancestors, is invited to a special event by either the likes of Bert, John, or Bliss. Bliss, in fact, does invite Brazilian shamans and African percussion healers to his annual retreat in Southern Italy. Thus, rather than travelling, collecting and composing, he gets the therapies to travel to him and his European clientele, so that they can be experienced in the *now*, and perhaps collected and composed for the future.

The other way in which possession, either by Bhairav or by the Jinn, could travel is through and for the Southern diaspora. Hence, we could have Islamic Jinn catchers in Leamington, and perhaps some version of the Bhairav cult on 74th Street in Jackson Heights in Queens. It is extremely unlikely for either Bhairav or the Jinn to travel on their own, *exclusively* through their *ojhas*,

---

controversial child of Psychiatry" (Malhotra and Gupta 2018). That apart, seeing "healing shrines" as native versions of "mental hospitals", and subsuming them under such a rubric is problematic to say the least. While we too have *partly* resorted to such a gloss for heuristic purposes in this article, we have elsewhere (Naraindas 2017) squarely addressed it, as do Padmanabhan (2017) and Basu (2014), albeit in different ways, in their ethnographies. For a study that grapples with the possible distinction between mental illness and possession in a Catholic context in the Global North, see Emily Dowdell's (2018) work on a psychiatrist who is a consultant to exorcists in the United States; and for a distinction in general between mental illness and spiritual affliction, again in the United States, see Verschaet (2018).

gurus, and *hakims*, to Tory Row (the chimneys of the old "Anglican worthies" here are painted differently) in Cambridge, Massachusetts. In the unlikely event that they did, they would certainly not be likely to enter the portals of a hospital in Massachusetts and be fused with Christian belief and Viennese psychoanalytical theory and be offered as psychotherapy for hospital patients. In fact, Bhairav may not even travel from the Himalayas to a Delhi hospital, let alone one near Tory Row, or *formally* even from the streets of Delhi to the portals of a hospital, unless Bhairav is collected by the native version of John, or more precisely, by the native version of the *Oberarzt* who, unlike John, is not *merely* a psychotherapist but a psychiatrist (that is, the person who has a licence to prescribe psychopharmaceuticals and is, in professional parlance, a medical doctor). But this is unlikely for *psychiatry as a discipline*, although some individual psychiatrists may be warm to the idea, perhaps to the extent that they may work with *ojha*s and *hakim*s in the interest of their patients (Chakravarthy 2014). Hence, Bhairav can only travel from the Himalayas or a Delhi street to a Delhi hospital through an *ojha*, *guru*, or *hakim* surreptitiously or informally, but not formally and institutionally as of now.

In other words, Bhairavs, Jinns, the Buddhist past life, Zulu techniques, and so on, ideally travel from the Global South to the Global North (these need not necessarily and always map on to the literal North and South) under medical or para-medical expertise, in quite the same way these objects, by and large, travel as ethnographic objects from the South to the North, with all our Anglo-European contributors to this volume being good examples. When they so travel, they are likely to be collected and composed into a common world of humans and non-humans and offered as therapy within a hospital or medical setting. Next, they may travel under lay Anglo-European aegis, as it is Anglo-Europeans who, by and large, have the wherewithal to traverse the world and, more importantly, *do* traverse the world carrying these quiddities from the South to the North. For, if Latour (1993) is to be believed, they are the ones who ostensibly inhabit an inanimate world of Nature and the symbolic world of Culture, while the "rest" are all "mixed up", or presumed to be mixed up (Povinelli 2019); and the "mixed up" rest have evidently no need to either collect or compose!

Thus, while Latour, Stengers, and Povinelli profess the need for and the possibility of a common world, the licenced and lay healers of Anglo-European provenance actually set out to collect and compose this common world, born no doubt out of pressing therapeutic need. And what might this pressing therapeutic need be? It is a need that is evidently born of the same dualism of nature and culture and its homologues of body and mind, or the real and the symbolic, or inanimate and animate, where, when all is said and done, the animate is sought to be reduced to the inanimate. Such a reduction results in that "sad nature" from which life is extruded (Stengers 2012), and whose metaphysical premise is a "materialistic monism" based on an "ontology of death" (Jonas 1982, 12, 15): all life in terms of non-life, or the irony called a *science of life* based on an *ontology of death*. In the case of psychiatry, this is tantamount to reducing the mind and consciousness to the organic substratum called the brain, with its neurons, synapses, and so on, in an attempt to ground a collocation of external symptoms to an invisible and material substratum called the *lesion*, which from 1800, with the advent of histology, has been the *sine qua non* of modern medicine (Foucault 1973). Its therapeutic corollary now[22] is the psychopharmaceutical drug that will presumably act on this substratum, implicitly and ideally based on a notion of "causal specificity" (Carter 2003), thus completing the triad of cause-lesion-drug, and its homologue of aetiology-disease-cure. While this normative triad is seemingly successful with somatic diseases (though decreasingly so, if it ever was the case other than as a normative ideal), this is evidently not the case for the most part with mental diseases, which as early as the mid-nineteenth century, and soon after the advent of the lesion and histology, were classed (along with the epidemic fevers) as diseases with no organic (lesion) correlates (Stokes 1874; Naraindas 1996). We can therefore speculatively surmise, if we read backwards from the present, that this probably led to three principal trajectories. Firstly, given the shaky foundation vis-a-vis other branches of medicine with the advent of histology, it is none too surprising that one part of psychiatry has always longingly looked, and continues to look, for an organic and material substratum to anchor its mobile and mutable nosology: *the recurring dream of the apodictic in the aberrant tissue*. Hence, it comes as no surprise, as the editors point out in the introduction, that the latest DSM has been rejected by one constituency as it is seen to be lacking such a material basis. The second trajectory is to propose an entirely different way to approach the psyche. One symptom of this in its chequered history, especially in psychoanalysis, was to eschew names for diseases, as such a naming and its possible fixity (so important to insurance reimbursements that, among other things, presumably waylaid it)[23] was considered anathema to the

---

22   I say now, as in 1831 the mainstay may have been the lancet and the leech (bloodletting). This is borne out by the fact that "the number of leeches imported into France grew from 300,000 in 1824 to 33 million in 1837" (Longmate 1966, 19, quoted in Naraindas, 1996, 7).

23   But post war insurance requirements and the US Veteran Health Administration (VHA), among other things, seem to have led the condition to be pinned down as part of the paperwork needed for reimbursements and so forth.

psychoanalytical encounter. The final trajectory is the attempt to stitch psyche and soma together, and to situate both in a social field leading to a broader psycho-bio-social (and "spiritual") model.[24]

If we marry this to current notions of plasticity and the contemporary recovery of a porous and impressionable body (Meloni 2019), as opposed to a closed and impermeable one that the lesion, and its subsequent avatars in the form of the cell and the gene, had ushered in (e.g. genetic destiny), what we have in the making is an epigenetic body rather than a genetic one, where mind, body, biography, milieu, environment,[25] and soul are all mutually and reciprocally implicated in both falling ill and becoming well. Or, to put it differently, it is as if the six Galenic non-naturals – the causes that vitiate the four naturals/humours – are now back as the "epigenetic triggers" of diseases: not by acting on the four humours but on gene expression.[26] And once again the dynamic play between the naturals/genome and the non-naturals/epigenome is staging a comeback – and we can only hope it is not as a farce, though there is a real risk of it turning farcical[27].

24   Kurt Goldstein's *The Organism* (1939), with his emphasis on wholeness and Holism, is perhaps the urtext that offers and keeps alive the possibility of this other trajectory. Hence it is none too surprising that both Hans Jonas and Georges Canguilhem draw on his work. And Canguilhem's idea that disease isolates, and establishes a diminished but new norm, a norm to which the patient needs to be rehabilitated, is uncannily and tellingly echoed by Jonas (1965) in his short memoriam, which he delivered in 1959 on Goldstein's 60th birthday. And again, it is wholly unsurprising that contemporary psychosomatic and rehabilitative medicine trace their genealogy, in part, to Goldstein.

25   This has led Niewohner to propose a "somatic sociality" (Niewohner 2011, 14) and a "customary biology" (ibid., 15) rather than a universal one. While he sees Margaret's Lock's work on menstruation as heralding this through the notion of a "local biology", the first salvo, and perhaps a more radical one, comes from Canguilhem in 1943, when he says that all physiology should be comparative physiology like comparative literature. And any notion of a universal one, based on universal norms is both untenable and misplaced. For it is not possible, if one reads him right, to say what is normal and what is pathological *a priori*.

26   The six Galenic non-naturals are: (1) ambient air, (2) food and drink, (3) exercise and rest, (4) sleep and wakefulness, (5) retention and evacuation of wastes, and (6) the perturbations of the mind and the soul. The derangement of the four humours (naturals) of bile, black bile, phlegm, and blood are *caused* by not being *mindful* of the six non-naturals. The notion of the mindful body, mind-body medicine, and so on, are all echoes of Galenic medicine, which as I have argued elsewhere, never exits the European imagination. The advent of "biomedicine" simply pushes it to the margins, and it becomes the secret and not-so-secret wellspring of large swathes of European alternative medicine, including spa (Kur) medicine (cf. Naraindas 2011).

27   Epigenetics, rather than "freeing" one from fixity and "genetic destiny", may enfold the environmental and the social into the somatic. For example, childhood nutrition or trauma may "imprint" itself, ostensibly through DNA methylation, in the gut or the brain and thus become biomarkers for the advent of either colon cancer or mental illness, respectively. In other words, we may be saddled with an "epigenetic destiny" through a somatisation of the social, thus

In any case, this mutual and reciprocal movement, as it unsurprisingly turns out, is the avowed aim of the *Klinik* under study. The *Klinik*'s brochure proclaims as much, and every department except Ayurveda (where everything is ostensibly mixed up!) attempts to stitch together body, mind, soul, society, and nature, which the oncologist calls *multi-modal* therapy. In fact, multi-modal therapy is the leitmotif of German psychosomatic medicine (Zipfel et al. 2016). A medicine that largely deals with neurotic conditions rather than psychotic ones, and one that attempts to eschew the use of psychopharmaceuticals and supplants it with the panoply on offer. The fact that it deals largely with neuroses rather than psychoses is attested by the fact that the *Klinik*, like all psychosomatic *Klinik*s (ibid.), follows an open-door policy where in-house patients are free to come and go. The psychiatric departments on the contrary deal primarily with psychoses and do use psychopharmaceuticals. This means, rather than being "open door", patients' movements are closely monitored, they are often confined during certain phases of their treatment, and sometimes even shackled. In effect, as the Chair of Psychiatry at the University of Heidelberg told me when I interviewed him, "We are left holding the difficult cases."

Interestingly, and perhaps not so surprisingly, this rough nosological distinction between psychoses and neuroses, between "difficult" and "less difficult" cases, was overlaid, according to the Chair, by a class distinction. He told me, and quite bitterly, when I interviewed him, that they are not only left holding the difficult cases but also persons from the lower end of the social order. He said, quite categorically, that this is likely to be denied by the psychosomatic department, which was indeed the case when I interviewed them – professor, nurse, therapist – soon after. Unfortunately, it is difficult for me to disprove either of these claims as I did not pursue this line of enquiry by looking at the demographics and social class of both these disciplines across the whole of Germany. But what I did discover over time was that the Germans have a not-so-secret caste-like system that is worked out through their extremely well-oiled three-tier school system, which triages students at the age of ten, often (not always) determining their class, work, and life trajectory. Roughly speaking, the blue-collar workers are perpetuated by doing only ten years of schooling at a *Hauptschule*. The lower-end of white-collar workers do eleven years schooling at a *Realschule*. And the daughters and sons of the upper echelons of white-collar workers like university professors, doctors, lawyers, architects, and the like – what

---

making it the latest instance of a trajectory that begins in 1800 with the advent of the lesion and histology.

Bourdieu would call the *petit bourgeoisie* – do twelve or thirteen years of schooling in a *Gymnasium* and pass an exam called the *Abitur*, without which one cannot go to university. This system has been repeatedly critiqued and, starting in the 1970s, the Germans have addressed it by enabling persons without an *Abitur* to get to university via other routes – such as the extended *Realschulabschluss, Fachabitur*, and *Fachgymnasium* – and thereby enable social mobility by making the tiers more permeable. Finally, alongside this three-tier system, "regular" or "mixed" schools called *Gesamtschulen* have been set up, where there is no "triage at ten". But despite these measures, the three-tier system with its "triage at ten" continues to hold considerable sway, and seemed particularly true for the generation of quasi-geriatric women who, between 2008 and 2017, were the subjects of my study.

If this educational structure is sutured to the health insurance-scape, then things become a bit clearer. Eighty-five per cent of Germans come under a mandatory social insurance scheme. The other fifteen per cent are on private insurance. One has to earn €50,000 for three successive years to be able opt out of the mandatory social insurance. Most of the school teachers and several others who came to my *Klinik* would not have qualified for private insurance as, even with ten years of experience, they would have fallen short or hovered around the risky €50,000 barrier – "risky" because once you opt out of the mandatory scheme, coming back is frightfully difficult. In fact, many of them earned – when I categorically asked them – no more than €20,000 to €30,000 per annum as part-time teachers. But they had all been to the *Gymnasium* and had passed the *Abitur* so that they could be trained to be school teachers at the university in their *Pedagogische Hochschule*. Hence, though they were not wealthy by any stretch of imagination, they were well educated.

If the above two scenarios are viewed together, it is possible that both the *Chefs* – of psychiatry and psychosomatic medicine – may have been right in their own ways. At least half the patients in my *Klinik* may not have earned above the €50,000 mark and hence were not wealthy; however, they were well educated. In fact, as Dr. Kapoor pointed out to me, psychosomatic medicine requires verbal skills that go well with a certain level and kind of education. This did not mean that persons who had only been to either a *Realschule* or *Hauptschule* were not present, but they were fewer. And among the latter, they were usually "civil servants" like policemen or soldiers, who had a privileged insurance fully paid by the state. One suspects that in psychiatry this pyramid would be partly inverted. In other words, there were probably more "well-educated" but not necessarily "well-paid" persons in psychosomatic medicine; while in psychiatry the proportion of less educated patients may have been greater, without necessarily presuming that they were *all* also less well-paid because a lot of blue-collar work could be far better paid. In fact, Germany may have a "wealthy blue-collar strata", as it is the home of the small family-owned business that is often seen to be the backbone of the German economy, with many of these "blue-collar persons" going on to become millionaires, including the owner of our *Klinik*, who began life as a mason and a builder! Finally, according to Dr. Kapoor (who reads everything I write), these "class distinctions", which as one can see play out in interestingly different ways in Germany, is likely to be flattened out in city-run public hospitals, unlike either private ones, or tertiary university hospitals.[28]

But irrespective of this nosological and "class" distinction – not necessarily by income but by education – what is nevertheless common to both psychiatry and psychosomatic medicine is the therapeutic palette, including in public institutions like the university hospital in Heidelberg. Here too, the therapies in both departments are multi-modal: the music, dance, art, and body work are all available. But the mix and extent to which they are made available, and when, could vary. And this variation is a matter of both theoretical and clinical judgement, as the patients in psychiatry are seen to be more fragile.

It is thus evident that German psychiatry, and especially psychosomatic medicine, is busy collecting and composing a common world through assiduous diplomatic work to address a therapeutic impasse at the heart of its craft, a craft where one could have *diseases with no patients* (e.g. kidney stones with no symptoms, or the asymptomatic Coronavirus carrier),[29] or

28 If we compare this with the Anglophone world – the NHS in particular, as I have already done elsewhere (Naraindas 2011) – such a therapeutic palette may not be available. One may need to step outside the NHS to avail oneself of it. And in the case of the US, given its different healthcare system, such a palette may be available only to a far smaller segment the population, if it is available at all, unless one is willing to pay for it out of pocket; meanwhile, in the third world, no such palette is available in an institutional setting, either public or private. Hence, it is none too surprising, as we pointed out earlier, that John's Californian psychotherapeutic colleagues are green with envy, because John, unlike them, can offer this for a larger segment of the German population. And he is sitting pretty because he knows that it is an all-inclusive package – one that could include sending patients into a trance and regressing them to their past lives. Moreover, the package varies between €156 and roughly €176 per day per patient, irrespective of the type of insurance. By contrast, this is clearly not the case in the Ayurveda department in the same *Klinik*. There, patients roughly pay €250 per day (2010) out of their own pockets, depending on what therapies they are availing themselves of. And the majority of the patients in the Ayurveda department are above the €50,000 mark, and have been to the *Gymnasium*.

29 This is the leitmotif through which Georges Canguilhem (1978) constructs his oeuvre and argues that the diseases of the pathologist (kidney stones) need not be the disease of the sick

patients with no disease, such as lower back pain without a lesion, or, in the context of this paper, mental illness with no lesion. Given the primacy of the lesion (Foucault 1973), when symptoms present without a lesion, doctors are seemingly lost. This may result, if there is no resolution through symptomatic treatment, in the patient being referred to a "shrink" on the presumption that it is a "mental" rather than a physical condition. But the psychiatric encounter between doctor and patient can only proceed if the patient accepts the narrative that the psychiatrist constructs of the patient's physical symptoms. If she does not, it leads to a "broken narrative" (Kirmayer 2000) with the patient abandoning the psychiatrist.

But this "broken narrative", as I have argued elsewhere (Naraindas 2006, 2011), is merely the beginning of other trajectories germane to this paper. Patients, often belittled by the fact that their physical symptoms are now seen as mental ones (with its attendant stigma), turn to either alternative systems like Ayurveda in India (Naraindas 2006), or to chiropractic treatment in the United States (Rhodes et al. 1999), both of which may take pain as a *sui generis* category rather than as a symptom of an underlying organic cause.

In Germany, they may go to a *Heilpraktiker* (a lay and legally licenced practitioner). The *Heilpraktiker* are often poly-therapists and may offer an amazingly rich therapeutic palette that addresses mind, body, emotion, soul, past lives and astral planes, among other things, through the use of

---

man. He invokes Rene Leriche to argue that if the person exhibits no symptoms, it should give us pause and we should not immediately presume that the local lesion is the disease and this disease is identical with the experiential reality of the sick person, thus annulling the sick person's speech and her testimony (Canguilhem 1978; cf. Jewson 1976, Fissell 1991). Rather than seeing sickness as a form of pathology that is identical to the normal, except for being a quantitative deviation from the former, we may want to see it, he says, as a novelty and hence a new way of being in the world, with its own norms – for "life is polarity" (Canguilhem 1978), with a capacity to be normative and establish new norms, rather than being judged with reference to a norm. If I extend this line of argument and extrapolate, I could say that disease as a new norm is an invitation to all and sundry to step up and be accepting of the new norm and the new world that the diseased person now begins to inhabit. Therapy then becomes a mode of rehabilitation: that is, rehabilitating the patient to this new world. This is the theme, I believe, that Mol takes up in *The Body Multiple* (2003), where she makes a plea for the equal importance of a *clinical* understanding of atherosclerosis and the possibility of *rehabilitation*, rather than mere amputation due to a pronouncement by the pathologist, who historically has been the kingpin and "legislates" the business of diagnosis as shown wonderfully well by Atkinson in is *Medical Talk and Medical Work* (Atkinson 1995). But Mol's work notwithstanding, living up to the dictums that ensue from Canguilhem's critique is easier said than done, especially in large swathes of clinical practice, as the local lesion (and its latter-day avatars, the cell and the gene) soon becomes, with advent of Xavier Bichat and histology, the *causal* site of modern clinical medicine (Foucault 1973), and thus the cornerstone of the epistemic impasse and its fallout.

photons, body massages, laser beams, flower essences, Ayurveda and so on, given the fact that patients are often at the end of their tether, having tried both conventional therapy (biomedicine) and a host of other therapies en route to the *Heilpraktiker* (Naraindas 2011).

It is thus evident that the *Heilpraktiker*'s poly-therapy, or the Swiss-Tunisian's global composition, is like the "multi-modal" therapy in the psychosomatic department, and the *Klinik* as a whole. The difference being that the multi-modal offer by the oncologist, for example, is within a formal medical setting (with its own informal twin – all that happens after 4:30 pm, as we pointed out); while the poly-therapy of the *Heilpraktiker* is within a legal but para-medical setting; and finally, the Swiss-Tunisian's composition is within a non-medical and, from a legal point of view, perhaps in an "illicit" setting. But many of the therapies and techniques, with *Familienaufstellung* being a prime example, are found in all three settings. In fact, Familienaufstellung begins life in a non-medical setting and crosses over to a medical setting.

They all appear to be symptoms of an underlying cause: the epistemic impasse at the heart of biomedicine and its resultant inability to treat a whole class of diseases that propel patients to look for what in popular parlance is called Holistic Medicine – a form that is invariably seen as a sign of the New Age movement, and often explained without recourse to the paradoxes of the biomedical episteme. It is this same impasse, and its resulting limitations, that also propels biomedical practitioners – including the oncologist in the *Klinik* – to look for alternatives in an attempt to expand their armoury. In other words, such patients and practitioners are obverse sides of the same coin.

While this epistemic impasse in the Global North leads to a multi-modal poly-therapy in an assiduous attempt to "mix things" that have been separated, it appears that in the Global South, where things are presumably "mixed up", or where the "non-naturals" effects on the "naturals" are presumably in full swing, what modern medicine traditionally advocates, and the Movement for Global Mental Health seems to reiterate, are "purified wholes" (Latour, 1993): that is, the clear and hierarchical separation of science and religion. In India, this takes the form of a clear hierarchy as far as formal statecraft is concerned (not necessarily in lived practice), with psychiatry as a medical degree at the top, followed by forms of clinical psychotherapy (under the appellation of counselling), practiced by persons usually trained in university psychology departments. The great number of vernacular forms of healing that are largely practiced by healers under the sign of "religion", and institutionally housed in religious shrines, whether they be

Christian (Sébastia 2007), Muslim (Basu 2014), or Hindu (Sax 2009; Quack 2014; Padmanabhan 2017; Ranganathan 2015a, 2015b), come last of all.[30]

But the last is first in terms of both sheer reach and quantum. For example, the religious shrine of Balaji near Agra, widely studied by anthropologists, or the Badaun shrine about 230 kilometres east of Delhi in Uttar Pradesh, each draw more pilgrims than the entire psychiatric establishment throughout India would be able to house as in-patients. In Badaun, the three saints (two brothers and a sister) with the appellations of Bade Sarkar, Chhote Sarkar, and Banno Bi, are visited by all faiths: "They [come] to ask for settlement of land disputes, forgiveness for robberies committed, punishment for errant lovers, sanity for the insane, health for the sick, vindication for crimes" (Badhwar 1986). And they may do this by shaking their fists at the saints and saying: "Haramzadi Banno toone mujhe maar diya. Aa jaa mere saath pun[g]a le! (You bitch Banno, you have done me to death. I dare you to come and [f]ight with me)" (ibid.). Despite their quantum and reach, and despite the great range of problems they address, and despite often being the first resort for the disenfranchised, these "vernacular" (a misnomer?) forms of healing can never be global. *Or to put it more precisely: they may not be "universal" even if they are global.* And the shrines themselves are seen as places meant largely for the poor (though this may not be empirically true): paroxysmal spaces that are aesthetically displeasing and hence fearful for the urbane. But most of all, they labour under the designation of *religion* and hence are classed as "faith healing", purportedly tied to a "local" context, although this "local" may have a wide regional (and increasingly global, through the diaspora), and multi-faith spread. Finally, they are stigmatised by two cognate constituencies. The paroxysms of ataxia and shaking, under the appellation *possession,* is pathologised by the current DSM as Dissociative Identity Disorder (Padmanabhan 2017) and, in earlier editions of the DSM and the ICD (International Classification of Diseases), as Tourette's syndrome, hysteria, mania, psychosis, epilepsy, and schizophrenia

---

30   Before the ostensibly non-codified vernacular forms come the so-called codified systems. While codified/non-codified is a problematic distinction, remnant of "the great" and "little" traditions of erstwhile anthropology, we are, through a self-fulfilling prophecy, saddled with them because they have been institutionalised in the form of modern medical colleges for Ayurveda, Unani and Siddha. These institutionalised forms, although they have an alternative nosology, invariably use the biomedical nosology and, in the bargain, they produce, through translational work, a creole that is neither fully Ayurvedic nor biomedical. This creolisation leads to a radical transmutation of these systems (cf. Naraindas 2006, 2014a 2014b) in ways that are cognate to the so-called non-codified forms that are practiced in the "healing shrines". See footnote 35 for a further elucidation.

(Naraindas 2017).[31] And as disenfranchised spaces seemingly meant for the poor, with presumably no codex to back their claim, they are, along with a large class of other faith-based behaviours practised by the poor, classed as superstition by the Rationalists, in whose view they are based on "blind faith" (*andha vishwas*) and exploitative of the disenfranchised, and should therefore be banned under the law and actively stamped out (Quack 2011).

In other words, Global Mental Health (like Global Reproductive Health?) runs the risk of epistemically disregarding, if not actively pathologising, vernacular forms of healing, especially those that labour under the epithets of faith and religion, and especially those modes where humans invoke, converse, beseech, and abuse non-humans (saints, ancestors, ghosts, spirits, gods) through paroxysms of ataxia. In its stead, MGMH appears to privilege Western psychiatry and psychotherapy, with its arsenal of psychopharmaceuticals and modes of counselling, along with its hospitals and out-patient clinics, as the principal and "correct" form of cure for a large number of presumably misdiagnosed and non-diagnosed patients under the notion of a "treatment gap".

In doing so, the MGMH runs the risk of extirpating the vernacular, the non-human, and the East from the East; and, like species-death in that "sad Nature devoid of life", it intentionally or unintentionally contributes to the marginalisation and radical transformation, if not the demise, of other cognitive and epistemic modes with their attendant ontologies. Ironically, while this trajectory – a trajectory of ontological genocide that eviscerates other ways of being in the world – is likely to unfold under the banner of MGMH in the Global South, the Global North appears to be importing, through assiduous "diplomatic work", the past and the East into the West, melding them with Western psychological and psychoanalytical theory,

---

31 Possession appears to be a stigmatised term native to Catholic theology. It primarily indexes possession by the Devil. Hence, it is none too surprising, as Smith (2007) points out, that it can only be sinister and evil in the West, while this is evidently, as Smith (2007) also compellingly shows, not the case elsewhere, especially in South Asia. But both psychiatry and Anglo-European anthropology, without let or irony, take what appears to be a stigmatised Catholic term and use it as a descriptive and analytical tool to understand a large class of phenomena worldwide, under the sign of another problematic word called "ritual" (cf. Davis-Floyd 1990), through this single epithet. While Western psychiatry seems to follow its religious roots, and unsurprisingly pathologises and thus stigmatises such phenomena, anthropology struggles (and often fails given the sheer weight of the term) to demonstrate why it may be neither sinister nor evil but ostensibly "functional" and hence useful. But its *explanations*, as I have pointed out (Naraindas 2017), often belie these unenviable intentions. And the surprising thing is it continues to use words like possession and ritual, despite their pejorative weight. And the rest of the world follows suit, including me, as it is, by sheer inertia, the lingua franca of the discipline.

and offering them in medical, para-medical, and non-medical settings to address a large class of mental problems in the West. It is as if under the pressure of religion and superstition – lenses through which India and the Global South are often seen – both doctors and rationalists should aim to prevent disciplinary contamination and ensure that the world of science and the world of religion are kept apart. Meanwhile, the "sterile West", with its ostensibly sad and dead Nature, seems to necessitate the "composing of a common world of humans and non-humans", and of the living and the dead.

V   Coda: Whither Cosmopolitics and Global Mental Health?

Is this something that is true only of mental health? I suspect not. Would it be fruitful to pause and compare it to the cognate practice of reproductive health, which we believe has been there and done what the MGMH is likely to do? It may be instructive to do so as it could allow us to (a) legitimately extrapolate, (b) see the MGMH as part of a larger historical trajectory, and (c) offer it is as a cautionary critique of the MGMH. But once again, it is pointless if we were to dwell on reproductive health only in the Global South, as is invariably the case with most studies, especially those on South Asia. We need to once again constitute an ethnographic object where the North and South are in a relational play. If we do, we may see startling similarities to the arguments we have been advancing.

Home births, largely of rural provenance in India, are also seen, like religious shrines and their misdiagnosed patients/pilgrims, as being both backward and the principal cause of maternal and infant mortality in India. Like *andha vihswaas* (Quack 2011), they have a long history that goes back to the late nineteenth century and the institution of the Lady Dufferin Fund (Pinto 2006; Ram and Jolly 2001; Van Hollen 2003). The contemporary mode of addressing home births – both by the Indian State and international NGOs (the Movement for Global Reproductive Health, like the Movement for Global Mental Health) – is to extirpate them via inducement (money) and threat (targets, failing which health providers may lose their jobs). This is done by offering both pregnant women and the auxiliary nurse-midwives (ANMs) a sum of money to ensure that women have a "medical" rather than a home-based delivery.[32] In an exact parallel, what we are witness to in the

---

32 In rural Tamil Nadu, which prides itself on achieving the target of medicalised deliveries (98 per cent), many rural women first give birth at home and then go to the primary health centre to illegally claim the money: but the money – both for the women and the ANM – is handed over

West is the turn away from hospital births to home births under the banner of the "natural birth" movement, spearheaded by highly educated women like gynaecologists and certain kinds of feminists, along with hippies, anthropologists, and the Christian far right (in the US). While the actual number of home births in both the US and Germany is not more than two to four per cent (Naraindas 2014a; Loytved 2012) – which is a testimony to the hegemonic nature of hospital births – nevertheless, it has led to the "natural birth" movement in the US and elsewhere.

Quite like *Familienaufstellung*, which begins life outside a medical setting but then works its way into formal psychosomatics, contemporary home births in the US were initially nurtured by the lay midwifery movement, which is still illegal in 22 states in the US (Butter and Bonnie 1988; Naraindas 2014a). It first gave rise to the institution of nurse-midwife within the hospital, and subsequently transformed the very nature of the birthing experience for American women. It is now possible for American women to be seen almost exclusively by a nurse-midwife instead of a gynaecologist in the case of "normal" pregnancies. In other words, the hospital, stung by the critique, and sensing competition from lay midwifery, begins to incorporate several elements from lay midwifery. But it retains the power of the physician by designing a new birthing table to address the disempowering lithotomy position of birthing women: a table that twists, turns, and even decomposes, but is always at a certain height, thus allowing the physician to stand upright rather than get on the floor (as may be the case with lay midwives) to "catch the baby". And the final icing on this "natural birth cake" is to offer prospective mothers an underwater birth with neither epidurals nor episiotomies and, if need be, in a Jacuzzi.[33]

In India, on the contrary, home births and religious shrines are not only assiduously kept apart from hospital births and psychiatry, but are to be actively stamped out or ignored, as they are perceived as dangerous or unhelpful for

---

only after the state leaves its imprimatur in the form of a needless post-birth episiotomy on the bodies of such women. It is as if the episiotomy, like childhood vaccination, is a rite of passage that sets apart citizens from others (Naraindas 1998): the latter to prevent children from dreaded infections, and the former to prevent "baby death" (as the head might get stuck), and to prevent natural third degree vaginal tears that may lead to lifelong incontinence. For the problematic and at times dubious nature of these claims, see Woolley (1995) and Naraindas (2014a, 2008). In any case, the born-again fervour with which these are followed in the Global South makes episiotomy a *sine qua non* for hospital births (Selvaraj et.al. 2007; Otoide et.al. 2000).

33 A nurse-midwife, who had spent 40 years on the job at the University of Iowa Hospital, said as much to my students when I invited her to address my class: "We'll do whatever it takes to keep the competition at bay; and if they want an underwater birth, and in a Jacuzzi, we'll give them one".

mothers and the mentally ill, respectively. While the WHO mandates a 10 per cent rate for episiotomies, the rate of episiotomies among first-time mothers in public tertiary hospitals (with the most qualified doctors) in South India is 98 per cent, and in private ones 100 per cent (Selvaraj et al. 2007).

Hence, it would not be surprising if we soon read a news item in the Times of India that the State of Tamil Nadu has successfully closed the "treatment gap" for the mentally ill, in quite the same way it has achieved a 98 per cent success rate for institutional as opposed to home-based deliveries (Padmanabhan 2008). The sure sign of this success, the article may proclaim, is that psychopharmaceuticals are now prescribed at a rate three to five times more (as with the prescription of antibiotics, or the "super success" of episiotomies) than in countries like the US or Germany. A decade later, we may have a new research programme to address the fallout of this "success" in exactly the same way that the Global South's "super success" with antibiotics has led to the global epidemic called anti-microbial resistance (AMR) – though the cognate and more pronounced reason, in terms of sheer scale and metabolic intensity, may well be the extensive use of antibiotics in the global practice of industrial poultry and pig farming.[34]

One could easily multiply the above scenarios ad nauseam: for example, the "prophylactic" use of oxytocin during non-high-risk deliveries in the Third World (Mukherjee, Forthcoming) – rather than administering it in either high-risk ones, or post-partum to stop the haemorrhage, as is the case in the Global North – has resulted in the widespread and tragic practice of rural patients *routinely* demanding it even during deliveries at home, and paying handsomely for the illegal service. In the same vein, we may soon see, with the advent of the Movement for Global Mental Health, patients (or their families) demanding drugs "over the counter" (without a prescription) for "depression", so that they can "treat", or "chemically castrate", ill/troublesome members of their family. And the first responders for this latent sensibility, say in a city like Delhi, may well be the 40,000 non-qualified practitioners (often called quacks) in the slums of Delhi (Barua 2014): the perfect handmaidens (though not the cause) waiting to detonate a "depression epidemic" among the poor, whose implications for the pharmaceutical industry can well be imagined.

34 70,000 lives are presumably lost to AMR every year. It is estimated that by 2050, 10 million people may die from AMR alone, which is more than cancer and road traffic accidents combined. The Centre for Disease Dynamics, Economics & Policy says in its report (2015) that Indians consumed more antibiotics than any other country. In 2010, it was 12.9 billion units. But such figures are to be partly expected given India's population.

While the above prophecy – based on cognate and tragic examples we have alluded to above – may come true across all social classes, it would be particularly true for the poor (India has more of them than sub-Saharan Africa), since rank poverty, in search of declining wages and spiralling aspirations, may mean a desperate clamour for quick solutions with quick and cheap drugs. If a large number of poor rural women in Maharashtra can practice "elective hysterectomies", in a desperate attempt to work uninterrupted by menstrual cycles in sugar cane plantations during the high harvest season in search of lucrative seasonal wages (Shelar 2019), we can only imagine what new forms of "industrial agriculture" may bring in its wake for families of the poor with persons who have been diagnosed as "mentally ill". And once statecraft, prompted by the Movement for Global Mental Health, puts in place ready and easy diagnostic templates for diagnosing mental illness in primary health centres (this is already afoot), and sets targets to boot, there is likely to be a veritable epidemic of mental illness, in quite the same way that a revised Body Mass Index (BMI) led to an epidemic of obesity in India amidst a sea of malnutrition, leading to that peculiar metabolic disorder called the thin-fat syndrome (Solomon 2016).

This is likely to see the demise of other ontologies, through their sanitation and creolisation (Naraindas 2014a, 2014b) at best, or evisceration at worst, indexed by the incipient transmutation of places like Badaun and Balaji, quite like the radical transformation of rural home births. We may not be too far from a scenario where a new class of compounders – like the ones administering oxytocin for rural home births – set up shop in Badaun and Balaji with their disposable syringes to administer psychopharmaceuticals on demand to the "mentally ill", especially the poor. These "prophecies" or extrapolations are based on the fact that the Indian state, and a "well-meaning" NGO, recently inserted psychiatrists into the Mira Datar sufi shrine in Gujarat to re-diagnose "pilgrims" as "misdiagnosed patients" and offer them psychopharmaceuticals alongside their "religious ritu-als" (Basu 2014). This is likely to have a trickle-down effect and "religious functionaries" could easily rename and rebrand their "jinn catching" as "Islamic psychotherapy", as is evidently already the case in North Africa (Sax, this volume; Sax 2017).[35] But since possession by the jinn is marked by paroxysms of ataxia, the North African jinn exorcist has hired a professional

---

35   The best example of such rebranding is yoga for fitness, health etc. It is now claimed that "modern Hatha Yoga" was, from its very inception, an amalgam of Western and Eastern forms of body work rather than a "purely" Indian technique.

"jinn catcher" to be possessed on behalf of his middle-class clientele (ibid.), for whom public paroxysms are unseemly and beyond their ken.

Nothing prevents this newly arrived Islamic psychotherapist from taking the next step and administering intravenous psychopharmaceuticals to middle-class bodies, politely segregated behind translucent muslin curtains, from where they can silently watch their paid doubles vicariously and publicly enact, through wailing and contortions, *their* possession. And, as perhaps a final step, the psychopharmaceutical could be mixed with distilled water infused with incanted verses from the Quran, rebranded as *jinee dava* (jinn medicine), and administered by our neophyte to his well-heeled clientele.[36]

But home births, hospital based "natural births", and versions of *Familenauf-stellung* are now possible in India. All three, however, are meant for a sliver of the urban elite. A private hospital in South Delhi began to offer natural births about five years ago. We now have women in Bombay writing blogs of their home births in a bathtub, attended by an American or American trained midwife – not a native one of rural provenance. In the same vein, there are the bare beginnings of both doctors and lay persons offering a suite of therapies (like past life regression) that are found in the psychosomatic department of the *Klinik* in Germany. And like the American or European trained midwife, these doctors/healers have been trained in the US or Europe, or trained by Indians in Bombay or Delhi who were trained in Europe.

---

36 He could then become a "global entrepreneur" and teach his new Islamic psychotherapy through online courses, and then mass produce his *jinee dava* and sell it, as a one-size-fits-all-substitute to "jinn catching", to his students and imitators *globally* – the only caveat with the last step may be him running afoul of the local drug controller, and then the FDA, if the *jinee dava* contains prescription drugs that he is not licenced to administer. While all this is pure speculation, intended as a futuristic fable, such fables are firmly based on extant forms, such as the periodic accusations of Ayurvedic doctors administering steroids in the guise of Ayurvedic drugs, or Ayurvedic drugs mixed with steroids – and on occasion this may well be true. And, just so as to not be misunderstood, Hindu and Buddhist religious functionaries, or Shinto and Amazonian "shamans", may do similar things. Such speculation is further buttressed by the fact that most of contemporary Ayurveda (or TCM, or Siddha), even when it is legitimately and ethically practised, especially its arsenal of "proprietary" drugs, as I have argued elsewhere (Naraindas 2014b, 2014c), is a creole: that is, rather than addressing an Ayurvedic nosology, they primarily address a biomedical nosology – a good example in the current context may be "depression", which is not native to their nosology. The Ayurvedic "appropriation" of depression (as it is with so many other disease categories) leads to a creolised diagnosis through a kind of translational work (Naraindas 2014a), and then it results in a creolised "Ayurvedic formulary" for these alien diseases categories (Naraindas 2014b). A formulary that is neither Ayurvedic, nor herbal, nor biomedical but a full-fledged creole that runs the risk of radically transmuting, if not altogether eviscerating, its extant ontology.

I studied two such practitioners recently – a doctor and an ex-diplomat's wife – with a view to ascertain the theoretical premises of their clinical craft and discovered that their past-life models, originally of Buddhist or Hindu provenance, have all come to them through an Anglo-European prism after it had been wedded to Western psychological theory. Their models and theories have nothing to do with Badaun or Balaji *directly*. And the doctor charges 4000 rupees an hour (in 2016) for a psychotherapeutic encounter – which is likewise a panoply of options, with past-life regression being one of the several therapies offered. But this therapeutic encounter is more expensive than the most expensive super-specialised private doctor (like an endocrinologist) that I have ever seen. As a university professor at the top end of the Indian civil service pay scale, I can ill afford him. Nor will my university medical insurance pay for it. But if the new age Indian doctor is to be believed, he has no dearth of patients and is booked for several weeks by patients belonging to a gilt-edged sliver,[37] who go in search of something other than the quotidian – or the "unknown" made up of multiple and divergent worlds. And perhaps for perfectly understandable reasons, since the known and the familiar were unable to cater to their needs, in quite the same way that the discipline of psychiatry was unable to address his needs. He said he had quit his psychiatric training in South India halfway through because not only did psychiatry, as it was then taught in his medical college, *not* speak to him, but as a budding gay person trying to come out of the closet, he was deeply troubled by the way its nosology saw homosexuality as pathological. And part of its therapeutic arsenal to cure it (and by implication him of his "disease") was to get prospective patients to read pornography and subject them to "electric shocks" (ECT). He told me that he, quite like his future patients (with their "broken narratives"), went in search of something divergent and unknown and thus came to inhabit a cosmos – not a discipline – that was seemingly more open, at times contradictory, but certainly more meaningful, fulfilling *and* lucrative.

For Stengers, "in the term cosmopolitical, cosmos refers to the unknown constituted by [...] multiple, divergent worlds, and to the articulations of which they could eventually be capable, as opposed to the temptation of a peace intended to be final, ecumenical" (Stengers 2004, 3). If a "common world" (Latour 2004), made up of the multiple and the diverse, is to be

---

37   These patients, like the ones in the psychosomatic department in Germany, are likely to be not merely educated but, in the Indian context, anglicised; unlike the German patients covered by the mandatory insurance scheme, they are likely to be, in current banking parlance, either "high income" or "high net worth" individuals.

diplomatically composed/recomposed, in an attempt to "return us" to an animistic and "panpsychic" world (Goff 2019), by blurring the distinction between human and non-human, life and non-life, and thus of "us and them" (Povinelli 2016, 2019), the question we need to pose once more is: who has the power and/or authority to diplomatically re-compose such a world? It appears that if such re-compositions are not to be final and ecumenical in the service of a lasting peace, then they must be kaleidoscopic: an endless, never settled, shifting pattern. But again, who gets to compose them? And where? For what ends? And for whom? It appears that they are, at the moment, largely the prerogative – *a prerogative evidently necessitated by an epistemic impasse* – of John, Bert, and Bliss, and their Southern understudies like my gay doctor in Delhi. Such re-compositions, especially where the living and the dead are brought together, are always to be wedded, in the context of this paper, to psychological and psychoanalytical models and theories, whether they happen in the North or the South, *in quite the same way the "codified medical systems" of the Global South, even when they are practiced by Southerners, are invariably wedded to a biomedical anatomy, physiology, nosology, and pharmacology*. It is within the ambit of such Northern theories and models that they can and do function as legitimate or quasi-legitimate forms of therapy, especially if they are to be reimbursed by health insurance and are to travel worldwide not merely as *global* but as *universal* forms of therapy. And by doing so, the distinction between us (those who inhabit the "sad Nature devoid of life") and them (those who inhabit the strange world teeming with life, and whose anthropological and philosophical epithet is animism) is not only *not* bridged but perhaps intensified.

Acknowledgements

This paper owes its existence to all the doctors, therapists (especially John), administrative and support staff, and most of all to the patients at the *Klinik* and *Therme*, all of whom gave of themselves so generously. None of it would have been possible without Herr Max graciously agreeing to have me at the *Klinik* year after year as a guest. And the person who made it all happen and ensured that all went well for three months every year for a decade was Dr. Kapoor. I can't thank him enough for his time, warmth, and generosity. I would not have met Dr. Kapoor if not for William (Bo) Sax, who I can't thank enough either for all that he has done, but most of all for his intellectual companionship. This paper has benefited from the perceptive and thoughtful comments of Ananda Samir Chopra, Claudia Lang, Sinjini

Mukherjee, Tanmoy Sharma, Purbasha Mazumdar, Subhashim Goswami, Tuhina Ganguly, Arnav Sethi and, most of all, Bo Sax. I have been generously supported over the years by the following agencies and institutions: A joint-appointment professorship (2008-2012), and projects C3 and MC11.1 (2008-2016), of the Cluster of Excellence, Asia and Europe in Global Context, at the University of Heidelberg; a DAAD visiting professorship at the SAI, University of Heidelberg in 2017; sabbatical leave from JNU in 2013-2014 that allowed me to spend eight months at the *Klinik*; the Indo-Swiss Joint Research Programme in the Social Sciences, jointly funded by the Indian Council for Social Science Research (ICSSR) and the Swiss State Secretariat for Education, Research and Innovation (SERI), for my work in Switzerland, which was housed in the Institute for Ethnologie at the University of Zurich; and the Jawaharlal Nehru University's UPOE-II grant (Project No. 242) on well-being. I would also like to thank Sylvia Sax for being a wonderful and gracious host; Johannes Quack and Ananda Samir Chopra, who have, among other things, been my fellow-travellers on several projects during the decade; and Annette Hornbacher for her sparkling conversations and being such a welcoming host. And last but not least, Gabi Alex and Karin Polit for their warmth, friendship, and collaborative work over these years.

References

Adams, Vincanne. 2002. "Randomised Controlled Crime: Postcolonial Sciences in Alternative Medicine Research." *Social Studies of Science* 32 (5-6): 659-90.

Adams, Vincanne, and Fei-Fei Li. 2008. "Integration or Erasure? Modernising Medicine at Lhasa's Mentsikhang." in *Tibetan Medicine in the Contemporary World: Global Politics of Medical Knowledge and Practice*, edited by Laurent Pordie, 105-31. London: Routledge.

Atkinson, Paul. 1995. *Medical Talk and Medical Work. The Liturgy of the Clinic.* London: Sage Publications.

Badhwar, Inderjit. 1986. "Miracles in Ziyarat of Badaun in Uttar Pradesh Rain down in Benevolent Abundance." *India Today*, 15 February 1986. Accessed 29 August 2019, https://www.indiatoday.in/magazine/living/story/19860215-miracles-at-ziyarats-of-badaun-in-uttar-pradesh-rain-down-in-benevolent-abundance-800575-1986-02-15.

Barua, Napur. 2014. "Medical Pluralism in a Slum in Delhi: Global Medicine in a Local Garb?" in *Medical Pluralism and Homeopathy in India and Germany (1810-2010). A Comparison of Practices*, edited by Martin Dinges, 203-16. Stuttgart: Franz Steiner Verlag.

Basu, Helene. 2014. "Dava and Dua: Negotiating Psychiatry and Ritual Healing of Madness." in *Asymmetrical Conversations: Contestations, Circumventions, and the Blurring of Therapeutic Boundaries*, edited by Harish Naraindas, Johannes Quack, and William Sax, 162-99. New York, Oxford: Berghahn Books.

Bilger, Burkhard. 2016. "Where Germans Make Peace with Their Dead." *New Yorker*, 5 September 2016. https://www.newyorker.com/magazine/2016/09/12/familienaufstellung-germanys-group-therapy.

Bracken, Patrick, Joan E. Giller, and Derek Summerfield. 2016. "Primum Non Nocere. The Case for a Critical Approach to Global Mental Health." *Epidemiology and Psychiatric Sciences* 25 (6): 506-10. doi:10.1017/S2045796016000494.

Butter, Irene H., and Bonnie J. Kay. 1988. "State Laws and the Practice of Lay Midwifery." *American Journal of Public* Health 78 (9): 1161-69.

Canguilhem, Georges. 1978. *On the Normal and the Pathological*. Boston: D. Reidel Publishing Company.

Carter, K. Codell. 2003. *The Rise of Causal Concepts of Disease: Case Histories*. Aldershot, UK: Ashgate Publishing.

Chakravarthy, Tina. 2014. "Interface in Approaches to Mental Disorder: A Study in Psychiatric Sociology." Unpublished PhD diss. Mumbai: Tata Institute of Social Sciences.

Center for Disease Dynamics, Economics & Policy. 2015. *State of the World's Antibiotics, 2015*. Washington, D.C.: CDDEP.

Davis-Floyd, Robbie E. 1990. "The Role of Obstetrical Rituals in the Resolution of Cultural Anomaly." *Social Science & Medicine* 31 (2): 175-89.

Delmonte, Romara, Giancarlo Lucchetti, Alexander Moreira-Almeida, and Miguel Farias. 2016. "Can the DSM-5 Differentiate between Nonpathological Possession and Dissociative Identity Disorder? A Case Study from an Afro-Brazilian Religion." *Journal of Trauma & Dissociation* 17 (3): 322-37. http://dx.doi.org/10.1080/15299732.2015.1103351.

Dowdell, Emily. 2018. "Evaluating an Experienced Psychiatrist's Assessment of Possession from a Catholic Perspective." Doctoral diss., Institute of Psychological Sciences. Divine Mercy University.

Fissell, Mary E. 1991. "The Disappearance of the Patient's Narrative and the Invention of Hospital Medicine." In *British Medicine in an Age of Reform*, edited by Roger French and Andrew Wear, 92-109. New York: Routledge.

Foucault, Michel. 1973. *The Birth of the Clinic*. Translated by Alan Sheridan. London: Tavistock.

Freeman, Melvyn C. 2016. "Global Mental Health in Low and Middle Income, Especially African Countries." *Epidemiology and Psychiatric Sciences* 25 (6): 503-05. doi:10.1017/S2045796016000482.

Goff, Philip. 2019. *Galileo's Error. Foundations for a New Science of Consciousness.* New York: Pantheon Books.

Goldstein, Kurt. 1939. *The Organism: A Holistic Approach to Biology Derived from Pathological Data in Man.* New York: American Book Company.

Grof, Stanislav, and Christiana Grof. 2010. *Holotropic Breathwork.* Albany: State University of New York Press.

Jonas, Hans. 1965. "In Memoriam: Kurt Goldstein, 1878-1965." *Social Research* 32 (4): 351-56.

—. 1982. *The Phenomenon of Life: Toward a Philosophical Biology.* Chicago: University of Chicago Press.

Jewson, Nicholas D. 1976. "The disappearance of sick man from medical cosmology, 1770-1870." *Sociology* 10 (2): 225-44.

Jolly, Margaret, and Kalpana Ram. 2001. *Borders of Being: Citizenship, Fertility, and Sexuality in Asia and the Pacific.* Ann Arbor: University of Michigan Press.

Kirmayer, Lawrence J. 2000. "Broken Narratives: Clinical Encounters and the Poetics of Illness." In *Narrative and the Cultural Construction of Illness and Healing,* edited by Cheryl Mattingly and Linda C. Garro, 153-80. Berkeley and Los Angeles: University of California Press.

Latour, Bruno. 1993. *We Have Never Been Modern.* Translated by Catherine Porter. Cambridge, MA: Harvard University Press.

—. 2004. *The Politics of Nature: How to Bring the Sciences into Democracy.* Translated by Catherine Porter. Cambridge, MA: Harvard University Press.

Longmate, Norman. 1966. *King Cholera: The Biography of a Disease.* London: Hamish Hamilton.

Loytved, Christine. 2012. "Qualitätsbericht 2010. Außerklinische Geburtshilfe in Deutschland." Edited by Gesellschaft für Qualität in der außerklinischen Geburtshilfe e.V. (QUAG e.V.). Auerbach/V.: Verlag Wissenschaftliche Skripten.

Malhotra, Nidhi, and Nitin Gupta. 2018. "Dissociative Disorders: Reinvention or Reconceptualization of the Concept?" *Indian Journal of Social Psychiatry* 34 (5): 44.

Meloni, Maurizio. 2019. *Impressionable Biologies: From the Archaeology of Plasticity to the Sociology of Epigenetics.* New York: Routledge.

Misra, Supriya, Anne Stevenson, Emily E. Haroz, Victoria de Menil, and Karestan C. Koenen. 2019. "'Global Mental Health': Systematic Review of the Term and Its Implicit Priorities." *BJPsych Open* 5 (3): 1-8. doi:10.1192/bjo.2019.39.

Mol, Annemarie. 2003. *The Body Multiple: Ontology in Medical Practice.* Durham, NC: Duke University Press.

Mukherjee, Sinjini. (Forthcoming). "Vital Flows: A Comparative History of Umbilical Cord Blood and Obstetric Practice in Europe and India", in Gerritsen, A. &

Cleetus, B. ed. Health and Materiality in the Indian Ocean World 1600-2000: Medicine, Material Culture and Trade. London: Bloomsbury Press.

Naraindas, Harish. 1996. "Poisons, Putrescence and the Weather: A Genealogy of the Advent of Tropical Medicine." *Contributions to Indian Sociology* 30 (1): 1-35.

—. 1998. "Care, Welfare and Treason: The Advent of Vaccination in the 19th Century." *Contributions to Indian Sociology* 32 (1): 67-96.

—. 2006. "Of Spineless Babies and Folic Acid: Evidence and Efficacy in Biomedicine and Ayurvedic Medicine." *Social Science & Medicine*, 62 (11): 2658-69.

—. 2008. "Mainstreaming AYUSH and Ayushing Obstetrics." *Health for the Millions* 34 (2&3): 33-37.

—. 2011. "Of Relics, Body Parts and Laser Beams: The German Heilpraktiker and His Ayurvedic Spa." *Anthropology and Medicine* 18 (1): 67-68.

—. 2014a. "Nosopolitics. Epistemic Mangling and the Creolization of Contemporary Ayurveda." in *Medical Pluralism and Homeopathy in India and Germany (1810-2010). A Comparison of Practices*, edited by Martin Dinges, 105-36. Stuttgart: Franz Steiner Verlag.

—. 2014b. "My Vaidya and my Gynecologist: Agency, Authority, and Risk in Quest of a Child." In *Asymmetrical Conversations: Contestations, Circumventions and the Blurring of Therapeutic Boundaries*, edited by Harish Naraindas, Johannes Quack, and William S. Sax, 118-161. New York, Oxford: Berghahn Press.

—. 2014c. "Of Shastric Yogams and Poly Herbals: Exogenous Logics and the Creolisation of the Contemporary Ayurvedic Formulary." *Asian Medicine* 9 (1-2): 12-48.

—. 2017. "Of Sacraments, Sacramentals and Anthropology: Is Anthropological Explanation Sacramental?" *Anthropology & Medicine* 24 (3): 276-300.

Niewöhner, Jörg. 2011. "Epigenetics: Embedded Bodies and the Molecularisation of Biography and Milieu." *Biosocietes* 6 (3): 279-98.

Otoide, Valentine O., Sunday M. Ogbonmwan, and Friday E. Okonofua. 2000. "Episiotomy in Nigeria." *International Journal of Gynecology and Obstetrics* 68 (1): 13-17.

Padmanabhan, Divya. 2017. "From Distress to Disease: A Critique of the Medicalisation of Possession in DSM-5." *Anthropology and Medicine* 24 (3): 261-75.

Padmanabhan, P. 2008. "Integrated Service Delivery in Primary Health Care. The Tamil Nadu Experience." Paper presented at Jawaharlal Nehru University, September 2008.

Patel, Vikram, Ricardo Araya, Sudipto Chatterjee, Dan Chisholm, Alex Cohen, Mary De Silva, Clemens Hosman, Hugh McGurie, et al. 2007. "Treatment and Prevention of Mental Disorders in Low-Income and Middle-Income Countries." *Lancet* 370 (9591): 991-1005. doi: org/10.1016/S0140-6736(07)61240-9.

Patel, Vikram, Pamela Y. Collins, John Copeland, Ritsuko Kakuma, Sylvester Katontoka, Jagannath Lamichhane, Smita Naik, and Sarak Skeen. 2011. "The

Movement for Global Mental Health." *British Journal of Psychiatry* 198 (2): 88-90. doi:10.1192/bjp.bp.109.074518.

Patel, Vikram. 2012. "Global Mental Health: From Science to Action." *Harvard Review of Psychiatry* 20 (1): 6-12. doi: 10.3109/10673229.2012.649108.

Patel, Vikram, Mario Maj, Alan J. Flisher, Mary J. De Silva, Mirja Koschorke, Martin Prince, Raymond Tempier, Michelle Riba, et al. 2013. "Reducing the Treatment Gap for Mental Disorders: A WPA Survey." *World Psychiatry* 9 (3): 169-76. doi:10.1002/j.2051-5545.2010.tb00305.x.

Pinto, Sarah. 2006. "Divisions of Labour: Rethinking the 'Midwife' in Rural Uttar Pradesh." In *Birth and Birthgivers: The Power Behind the Shame*, edited by Janet Chawla, 203-38. New Delhi: Shakti Books.

Povinelli, Elizabeth A. 2016. *Geontologies: A Requiem to Late Liberalism.* London: Duke University Press.

—. 2019. "Life/Nonlife: A Response." Accessed 10 August 2019. http://somatosphere. net/forumpost/life-nonlife-a-response/.

Quack, Johannes. 2011. *Disenchanting India: Organised Rationalism and Criticism of Religion in India.* New York: Oxford University Press.

Ranganathan, Shubha. 2015a. "A Space to 'Eat, Trance, and Sleep': The Healing Power of Mahanubhav Temples in Maharashtra (India)." *Mental Health, Religion & Culture* 18 (3): 185-95.

—. 2015b. "Rethinking 'Efficacy': Ritual Healing and Trance in the Mahanubhav Shrines in India." *Culture, Medicine, and Psychiatry* 39 (3): 361-79.

Rhodes, Lorna A., Carol A. McPhillips-Tangum, Christine Markham, and Rebecca Klenk. 1999. "The power of the visible: The meaning of diagnostic tests in chronic back pain." *Social Science and Medicine* 48 (9): 1189-03.

Sax, William S. 2009. *God of Justice: Ritual Healing and Social Justice in the Central Himalayas.* New York: Oxford University Press.

—. 2017. "The Birth of the (Exorcism) Clinic: Media, Modernity and the Jinn." Paper presented at the Medical Anthropology Forum, South Asia Institute, University of Heidelberg, 2 May 2017.

Sax, William S., Jan Weinhold, and Jochen Schweitzer. 2010. "Ritual Healing East and West: A Comparison of Ritual Healing in the Garhwal Himalayas and 'Family Constellation' in Germany." *Journal of Ritual Studies* 24 (1): 61-78.

Scheidt, Carl Eduard. 2017. "Psychosomatic Medicine in Germany." *International Journal of Body Mind Culture* 4 (2): 78-86.

Sebastia, Brigitte. 2007. *Les Rondes de Saint Antoine. Culte, Affliction et Possession en Inde du Sud.* Paris: Aux Lieux d'Etre.

Selvaraj, Alphonse, A. Chitra, and S. Parvathy. 2007. *Episiotomy: Real Need or Ritual?* Poonamalee, Chennai: Institute of Public Health.

Shelar, Jyoti. 2019. "A harvest of crushed hopes: Why number of hysterectomies are high in Maharashtra's Beed district" https://www.thehindu.com/news/national/other-states/in-beed-a-harvest-of-crushed-hopes/article28969404.ece.

Smith, Frederick M. 2007. *The Self Possessed: Deity and Spirit Possession in South Asian Literature and Civilization.* New York: Columbia University Press.

Solomon, Harris. 2016. *Metabolic Living: Food, Fat, and the Absorption of Illness in India.* Durham, NC: Duke University Press.

Stengers, Isabelle. 2004. "The Cosmopolitical Proposal." Accessed 10 October 2019. https://balkanexpresss.files.wordpress.com/2013/09/stengersthe-cosmopolitcal-proposal.pdf.

Stengers, Isabelle. 2012. "Reclaiming animism." *e-flux* Journal 36, July 2012. Accessed 6 October 2019. http://www.e-flux.com/journal/reclaiming-animism/.

Stokes, William. 1874. *Lectures on Fever. Delivered in the Theatre Hospital and County of Dublin Infirmary*, edited by John William Moore. London: Longmans, Green and Co.

Summerfield, Derek. 2008. "How Scientifically Valid Is the Knowledge Base of Global Mental Health?" *BMJ* 2013 (336): 992-94.

—. 2013 "'Global Mental Health' Is an Oxymoron and Medical Imperialism." *BMJ* 2013 (346): f3509.

Thierfelder, Constanze. 2017. "Pastoral Care (Seelsorge) and Spiritual Care in Germany." *HTS Theological Studies* 73 (4): 1-6.

Van Hollen, Cecilia. 2003. *Birth on the Threshold: Childbirth and Modernity in South India.* New Delhi: Zubaan.

Verschaet, Nathan P. 2018. "Differentiating Spiritual Affliction from Mental Disorders: Reports of Experienced Practitioners." Doctoral diss., Institute of Psychological Sciences. Divine Mercy University

Wirth, Alfred, Gernot Klein, and Hans-Joachim Lepthin. 2010. "Medizinische Rehabilitation: Bessere Vernetzung notwendig." *Deutsches Ärzteblatt* 107 (25): 1253-6.

Whitley, Rob. 2015. "Global Mental Health: Concepts, Conflicts and Controversies." *Epidemiology and Psychiatric Sciences* 24 (4): 285-91. doi:10.1017/S2045796015000451.

Woolley, Robert J. 1995. "Benefits and Risks of Episiotomy: A Review of the English-Language Literature Since 1980. Part I." *Obstetrical & Gynaecological Survey* 50 (11): 806-20.

Zipfel, Stephan, Wolfgang Herzog, Johannes Kruse and Peter Henningsen. 2016. "Psychosomatic Medicine in Germany: More Timely than Ever." *Psychotherapy Psychosomatics*, 85 (5): 262-69.

About the Author

Harish Naraindas is currently professor of sociology at Jawaharlal Nehru University, and honorary professor at the Alfred Deakin Institute, Faculty of Arts and Education, Deakin University. He works on the history and sociology of science and medicine and has published on a range of topics, including an epistemological history of tropical medicine, a comparative history of smallpox from the eighteenth to the twentieth century, and work on the creolisation of contemporary Ayurveda, spa medicine in Germany, pregnancy and childbirth within the context of competing medical epistemes, and recently, how anthropology attempts to explain the non-human. He is currently working on AyurGenomics and P4 medicine, past-life aetiologies and therapeutic trance in German psychosomatic medicine, and a multi-sited study of perinatal loss and bereavement in the Anglophone world. His most recent publication was a co-edited special issue of *Anthropology and Medicine* called "The Fragile Medical: The Slippery Terrain between Medicine, Anthropology and Societies" (2017).

Alternatives

7 The House of Love and the Mental Hospital

Zones of Care and Recovery in South India

Murphy Halliburton

Abstract

The Movement for Global Mental Health has defined the person suffering psychopathology in low-income countries as an abused and suffering subject in need of saving by biomedical psychiatry. Based on fieldwork in Kerala, South India, carried out at psychiatric clinics and a psychosocial rehabilitation centre, this paper examines patients' experiences of illness, the degree and quality of family support, and attributions made to the role of 'sneham', or love, in recovery. The role of love and family involvement may help explain the provocative finding by WHO epidemiological studies that 'developing' countries – and India in particular – showed better rates of recovery from severe mental illness when compared to developed countries.

Keywords: love, schizophrenia, social support, Kerala, Movement for Global Mental Health

In recent years, prominent articles in the *New York Times*, with titles like "A Mission to Heal Minds" and "A Call to Foster Mental Health Across the Globe," reported on psychiatrists and mental health workers who have been addressing the supposedly underserved mental health needs of people in developing countries.[1] These individuals, many of whom are part of the Movement for Global Mental Health (MGMH), have led efforts to scale up psychiatric interventions, counter abuse of the mentally ill, and close what

---

1   Carey 2015a, 2015b, 2016a, 2016b.

Sax, William, and Claudia Lang (eds), *The Movement for Global Mental Health: Critical Views from South and Southeast Asia*. Taylor & Francis Group, 2021

DOI: 10.5117/9789463721622_CH07

they claim is a "gap" between the needs of the mentally ill in these countries and the mental health services that are available to them.[2] Such media coverage sometimes includes a photo of the legs of an African or Asian man or woman with a chain around one ankle, iconically representing abusive treatment of the mentally ill that is supposedly the result of ignorance about mental illness and traditional methods of healing employed in these settings.[3] These stories are compelling, but what this media coverage does not tell the reader is that according to the WHO, people with schizophrenia and related diagnoses in these countries are actually doing better in terms of improvement and recovery than the mentally ill in developed countries where psychiatric services are more widely available and the mentally ill are supposedly better treated. Also, such forms of restraint through an ankle chain are infrequently used in sites I have visited in India and are arguably no worse than methods of incarceration and physical restraint used in biomedical mental hospitals (Mills 2014) – though both forms are problematic.

Since the 1960s, the World Health Organization (WHO) has examined the course and outcome of schizophrenia and related diagnoses at "developed" and "developing" country sites across the globe, and determined in multiple follow-up studies one of the most striking and robust findings in epidemiology, which is that people with these disorders in "developing country" sites showed greater degrees of improvement than subjects at "developed country" sites (WHO 1973, 1979; Sartorius et al. 1986, 1996; Hopper et al. 2007). The data from the WHO studies has been further parsed to reveal that among all sites, India shows the best prognosis for these illnesses (Hopper 2004; Cohen et al. 2008).[4] But instead of trying to assess what India and the other developing countries are doing right and applying it to places like the US and Europe that have a poorer outcome, the MGMH, as well as the WHO itself, have created programmes to "save" the mentally ill in India and other developing countries through interventions based on western models of mental health care.

In the last decade or so, anthropologists too have focused on "suffering subjects" (Robbins 2013), including cases of people suffering mental illness, and like the MGMH and WHO, this had led researchers to overlook more

2   Patel et al. 2007, Patel et al. 2011, Patel et al. 2016.
3   Such a photo is featured in Carey (2015a), and was the lead photo on the front page of the *New York Times* that day. See also Dey (2016) and Soudi and Patel (2016)
4   Despite the title of their article, Cohen et al. do not so much "question an axiom" of better results for developing countries as demonstrate that not all developing countries did well in the WHO studies, at the same time highlighting that India showed the best results.

fortuitous, caring encounters with the destitute and those suffering serious pathologies.[5] From December 2013 to August 2014, I conducted fieldwork at mental health centres in the state of Kerala in south India to help explain why people in India fare better in recovery from schizophrenia and related disorders. While recognising the contribution of studies that examine cases of abandonment or apply Agamben's (1998) perspective on thanatopolitics (power that operates by the threat of repression and death) to contemporary ethnographic settings and the need to remain vigilant about cases of abuse of the mentally ill in all settings, this paper answers Robbins' (2013) call to go beyond our focus on the "suffering subject" and build what he calls an "anthropology of the good". Robbins' purpose is not to ignore suffering and oppression, but to also attend to and learn from what goes right and what people strive for. Thus one aim of this paper is to inform medical anthropologists, advocates of the MGMH, and mental health policy professionals about what India may be doing right, in the hope of improving the lives of people suffering psychopathology in low- *and* high-income countries and to rethink current efforts to make India's mental health system over through interventions developed, mostly, in the West. I do so by examining cases of success in treating mental illness in Kerala, paying special attention to the role of the family and caring relations between healers and patients, who are not abandoned or reduced to "bare life"[6] but are treated as qualified life, with dignity and also, often, with *sneham* or love. These caring relations, aside from affirming the humanity of the person suffering distress, also appear to contribute to improved functionality and recovery from psychopathology.

After a discussion of the anthropology of abandonment and care and a sketch of the variety of meanings of "love" in South Asia, this article will consider caring and loving relations in the lives of patients I spoke to at a mental hospital and community health centres. This will be followed by a more explicit consideration of *sneham* at a psychosocial rehabilitation centre known as Snehaveedu or "House of Love".[7]

---

5   Examples include Biehl (2013 [2005]), Cohen (2005), Marrow and Luhrmann (2012), Povinelli (2011), and Goldstein (2013 [2003]).
6   This term comes from Agamben (1998) for persons also referred to as "zoë", or those who are alive but abandoned rather than living the qualified, social life of the citizen.
7   More literal translations would be "home of love" or "love home" because of the notion of belonging in the term "home", but these translations are more awkward. Another rehabilitation centre in another district of Kerala that is operated by the same church organisation that runs Snehaveedu is known by the English name "Love Home".

Anthropologies of Abandonment and Care

In his influential ethnography *Vita: Life in a Zone of Social Abandonment* (2013 [2005]), João Biehl depicts Vita, a psychosocial rehabilitation centre in southern Brazil, as a place of abandonment where the poor are left to live and die as non-, or formerly, social beings, and he makes his case primarily through his examination of the life of Vita resident Catarina who is abandoned by her family and by the state and apparently left alone with no meaningful social relations. Catarina's case is disturbing and Biehl's presentation is compelling, but I am concerned about how much Biehl's explanation of social abandonment hangs on the experience of this one individual and how we have seen a proliferation of other ethnographic studies of abandonment and examples that speak to Agamben's theory of sovereign power in the neoliberal world, several directly influenced by Biehl's analysis.[8] I am not suggesting that Biehl or those who called our attention to cases of abandonment have nothing important to say about social relations in our neoliberal word or that Agamben's argument is not compelling. However, as with Rabinow and Rose's (2006) critique of Agamben's (1998) and Hardt and Negri's (2000) focus on thanatopolitics (where Rabinow and Rose remind us that biopower works not only by threatening death or abandonment but also by making live, such as through programmes of public health, which also create and discipline subjects), we need to be sure we are capturing the larger panoply of power relations and experiences operative among the abandoned and those who are attended to.

Critiques of the rubric of abandonment are raised in ethnographies by Clara Han (2012) and Anita Hannig (2017) who speak of an anthropology of care that considers how people attend to and care for others who are suffering structural violence or stigmatising illness and how those others can have vital lives despite the challenges with which they struggle.[9] Additionally, Ma (2012) critiques studies that depict pharmaceuticals as simply reducing valued, social lives (*bios*) to bare life (*zoē*). She also highlights the centrality of love in the case of Mei, who is given a psychotic diagnosis, but "complained to me [Ma] that what drove her crazy was a lack of love" (53).

---

8   See Povinelli (2011) and note 5 above.

9   Hannig (2017) shows that despite great suffering and stigma, women with obstetric fistulas in Ethiopia maintain social relations and engage in other vital parts of their lives, such as their religiosity. She explains that "most women with fistula remain entangled in intimate networks of kin and community obligations that defy their supposed relegation to the margins of society. And while some of their relations might be changed by fistula, they are rarely dismantled by it" (8).

But this is a case of unrequited romantic love, from a significant other who constantly defers plans to marry while Mei is under psychiatric treatment, while the present article focuses on the caring love of *sneham* (although one can receive caring and romantic love from the same person and unrequited romantic love is a source of mental distress for many in India as well).

I did meet people in Kerala whose situation resembled that of Catarina from Biehl's *Vita*. They had been rejected by family and in some ways were abandoned although they were attended to in rehabilitation centres I visited in a way that took their humanity seriously. I could have focused on one of these individuals and depicted a case of abandonment similar to the case of Catarina. But most of the destitute mentally ill I met in Kerala were cared for or, in significant ways, developed a social connectedness that is highly valued by people in Kerala, which they refer to as *bandangal* in Malayalam. *Bandangal* refers to valued and loving or caring social connections. A literal translation would be "relations", but *bandangal* refers specifically to concerned and supportive social relations which can come from family and friends or a romantic partner and which are seen as necessary for a healthy and complete life.

Snehaveedu and Biehl's Vita are both psychosocial rehabilitation centres, though they are in very different parts of the world. Conditions in Kerala, with its communist social interventions and relatively robust social safety net, may be quite different from the context where Biehl worked in Brazil or from Chennai in South India where Cohen (2005) examined the abandoned and the "bioavailable" who were victims of the organ trade. This article does not so much challenge the claims of these studies as show other things that are also going on, although I would like to know how representative Catarina's experience is compared to others in rehabilitation centres in southern Brazil or other parts of the world.

There is a danger in promoting an anthropology of the good and of critiquing the Movement for Global Mental Health by pointing out what works well in mental health care in low-income countries. Following Robbins' suggestion risks romanticising human interaction and obscuring suffering, and, for this reason, I struggle with the terms I use to describe the encounters considered here.[10] It is difficult to name a situation where the individuals I describe in some cases recover or create something like a normal or satisfying life while others who have seen improvement – and are attended to and cared

10 Leo Coleman (2016) discusses the limitations of what he calls "vitalist" ethnographies that, in line with Robbins' proposal, follow stories of hope and caring while he also claims that Biehl does point out moments of hope and agency in Catarina's life.

for – are still abject and living in problematic relationships. These cared for individuals are not necessarily living a "good" or "happy" life. They may be struggling with adversity, but what is significant is that they are living a valued or vital life that includes *sneham* and *bandangal*. Because of the role I believe family involvement and care play in recovery, my analysis also risks romanticising the Indian family as an inherently nurturing institution when in fact, as elsewhere, abuse and abandonment occur in families of the mentally ill in India and family relations can contribute to the onset of psychopathology.[11] Still, I would argue that the taking in of and the interacting with mentally ill members by families in India has significant merits over the frequent lack of involvement in other localities, such as the United States, as we see in Tanya Luhrmann's (2007) work on "social defeat" among the mentally ill in Chicago who have lost connections to family and friends. While both situations merit improvement, this analysis of the role of family and loving relationships helps explain recovery from psychopathology and counters simple caricatures of the treatment of the mentally ill in low-income countries as abusive. Indeed, this work builds on other research that claims a significant role for family attitudes and involvement in explaining the favourable outcome in the WHO studies for people diagnosed with schizophrenia. Such research has considered family "support" and "expressed emotion" (which refers to the *lack* of expression of *negative* emotions toward the ill family members) but not love per se (Leff et al. 1990; Thara 2004; Warner 1994).

Benefitting from the serendipity that often accompanies fieldwork, I was led to consider caring love, or *sneham*, as a salient quality of family and other social relations by Father George Joshua Kanneeleth, who runs Snehaveedu, and by staff and residents at the centre. *Sneham* in Malayalam refers to the love between parent and child, husband and wife, friends, and other relations. Another term for love in Malayalam, *premam*, refers to romantic love, the passionate love of two individuals for each other – although some who share *sneham* also share *premam* for one another. Father George Joshua explained that what people like the residents of Snehaveedu were lacking most in their lives was love: that is, someone who is devoted or loving toward them, which could be but was not necessarily a spouse or romantic partner.

Scholars have examined the various meanings of love in South Asia, including, perhaps most prominently, work on the religious idiom of *bhakti*, which refers to devotional love for a/the deity. David Haberman (1988) considers *bhakti* in the context of a Hindu religious sect known as Gaudiya

---

11   See, for example, Marrow and Luhrmann (2012) and Kottai (2020).

Vaishnavism. "[L]ove itself" he says, "is identified as an aspect of the essential nature of God", and "[t]he desired aim of Gaudiya Vaishnavism is to
participate (*bhakti*) in this aspect of God, defined as love or infinite bliss"
(32).[12] *Bhakti* is thus often seen as a form of ecstatic devotion to the deity.
This is different from romantic love and from sneham, mainly in the sense
that the object of love is divine in one case and human in the others, but
there are degrees of overlap including styles of romantic and parent-child
love in expressions of bhakti. Love as *bhakti* is also transcendent, implying
not just an exalted emotion but, in Haberman's terms, "infinite bliss". Love
(*anpu* in Tamil) within the family has been considered as profound affective
ties that emerge from slow habituation and are marked by ambiguity and
paradox (Trawick 1990).

In her work with women in mental hospitals in northern India, Pinto (2011)
depicts love and marital relations as central concerns for women diagnosed
with serious psychiatric disorders and to the psychiatrists who treat them.
"[P]ractitioners – doctors, residents, social workers, psychologists – read
patients' lives for signs of illness by evaluating emotions related to marriage"
(378), we are told, and they develop their treatment recommendations based
on this. Although Pinto doesn't explicitly reflect on the differences between
caring love and romantic love, these cases tend to focus on romantic love,
the kind of love that can make one crazy, especially when gone awry, when
it remains unrequited or when it results in divorce, as is the case for many
of the women Pinto met. This kind of "crazy love" is commonly depicted
in South Asian expressive genres: "in Hindu devotional, Sufi, and Urdu
poetry, it allegorizes the lover to the devotee, while in Hindu mythology
gods go crazy with love, just as people do" (386). Affective relations toward
family other than the spouse is also important in the realm of psychiatric
scrutiny and for the women themselves. This kind of love along with the
love of parents for children is what is referred to as *sneham* in Kerala.[13] In
Claudia Lang's work (2019) on surveillance and care in Kerala community
mental health work, we see an emphasis on family care and *sneham* in
the discourse of patients and healthcare workers. In fact, for junior health
inspector Sanjeev who visited patients in their homes, "it was the disruption

---

12   See also Haberman 2003 and 2006 on *bhakti* and love.
13   In Sanskrit and North Indian languages, *sneham* or "oily love" is the love of the superior for
the inferior: paradigmatically of parent for child, although also of guru for disciple and other
relations (William Sax, personal communication). This may be the case in Malayalam as well
though the hierarchy is less manifest. As in the North Indian context, parent-child relations
are the epitome of *sneham*, but in Kerala, friends who are social equals speak of their relations
in terms of *sneham* as well.

of caring family relations much more than the neurochemical imbalance in a patient's brain that was key to the etiology of depression, and therefore to its treatment" (600). Patients used Sanjeev's home visits to complain about and mobilise family care and attention. In one case, Sanjeev admonished a patient's daughter-in-law to treat her mother-in-law with "*sneham* and consideration" adding "[w]e can change a person only through *sneham*" (606).

Additionally, *sneham* has physiological connotations in the context of Ayurveda, South Asia's largest formalised, indigenous medical system. *Sneham*, or the prefix *sneha-* in this context, refers to an oily, lubricating substance such as that used in *snehapana*, a treatment where the patient drinks ghee in an effort to lubricate the body as part of the multi-phase *panchakarma* treatment used in ayurvedic treatments of psychopathology. Later, we will see this form of *sneham* also described as "lubricated affection" in the comments of an ayurvedic doctor who attends to patients at Snehaveedu.

It should be added briefly that it is not my claim that it is only in India that love is considered important to psychic healing. Luhrmann (2016) observed that Massachusetts Mental Health Center psychiatrist Elvin Semrad "took seriously Freud's dictum that psychoanalysis was a cure through love, and he taught that a doctor's ability to cure came from his ability to care". He also spoke of "'loving the patient as he is'" (12).[14] Chloe Silverman's study of autism in the US focuses on love as central to treating and caring for autistic children. She explained "I use 'love' because it is the term used by the people and found in the texts that I have studied" (2011, 3). Thus, like me, she was led by her informants to take love seriously in her analysis. But while the importance of love in healing is not confined to India, there is evidence, as will be discussed later, that people with whom those suffering psychopathology have affective ties are present more often at treatment centres and in the lives of the afflicted in India than they are in Europe and North America.

While the role of love is occasionally cited by researchers, this concept   •
is usually left out of scholarship on mental health, according to Tjeltveit (2006), possibly because it appears unscientific and difficult to quantify. While psychological research points to "social" or "family" "relations", I would add that such generic labels elide the caring love, or *sneham*, that is key to the therapeutic power of those relations. In discussing psychological research, Tjeltveit says "love is too bound up with emotions, is too closely linked with religion, and slips too easily into sentimentality. Love, that

14   See also Good (2009) on Semrad.

is, is a topic that is not well-suited for a discipline that is, and should be, striving mightily and manfully to be a 'hard' science" (13).[15] The role of family involvement and love – often but not necessarily from family – is central to the following analysis of the experience of patients at a psychiatric hospital and community health centres. In this analysis, "love" is not always the explicit label for what is experienced, but love and caring interactions that recognise the ill individual as valued life (something more enhanced than Agamben's "qualified life") are arguably what makes family relations and support empowering or, to borrow an ayurvedic concept, "lubricating", and thus aiding in recovery.

Research Methods

As an anthropologist who focuses on cross-cultural approaches to mental health, I utilised methods that are typical of research in medical anthro-pology and ethnographic research in general. Thus, I undertook largely qualitative interviews with patients and with their family members who accompany them to clinics, and employed participant observation which involved observing everyday routines at healing centres. Research for this chapter was conducted in Thiruvananthapuram District in Kerala, India over nine months in 2013 and 2014. Fieldwork I undertook on treatments for mental illness and related problems in Kerala in the 1990s (Halliburton 2009) also informs the analysis. In Kerala in 2014, I conducted interviews and participant observation at an urban government hospital, neighbourhood state-run primary health clinics, and charitable psychosocial rehabilitation centres, all of which primarily use biomedical psychiatric interventions. I interviewed 43 patients with diagnoses of serious mental disorder, mostly schizophrenia, and I engaged in other forms of observation and interaction at these centres and other locales including interviews with healers. I attempted

---

15   Psychological research on "social" and "family" relations is so vast that it is not easy to quantify. Psychologists occasionally study love or loving relations, though this, as Tjeltveit (2006) says, is quite rare. He claims this is because of psychologists' ambivalent feelings about love as an analytic tool for research. There is a mystical sense associated with love that makes it appear less scientific, and it is difficult to measure objectively. One of Tjeltveit's concerns is Christian notions of love (rather than romantic/erotic love), which is fitting for this article since it is a Christian organisation, Snehaveedu, that invokes the importance of love more explicitly than the mental hospital. It is Jesus's mandate to love your neighbour and be self-sacrificing or altruistic that is reflected in Tjeltveit's analysis and in Snehaveedu director Father George Joshua's attitude toward the destitute mentally ill, as will be seen a little later.

to assess the degree and quality of family involvement in the lives of those being treated for major psychopathology by obtaining illness histories and inquiring into perspectives on recovery from patient-informants as well as from family members who accompanied patients.

My assistants, T. R. Bijumohan and Tintu James, and I interviewed in-patients at the Thiruvananthapuram Mental Health Centre, a large government mental hospital, and out-patients at this hospital and neighbourhood primary health clinics in order to speak to patients who were ill and individuals who were recovered or recovering. Informants whom we considered to be "ill" were those who were admitted to the hospital while those we considered recovered or recovering were out-patients at the hospital and community centres that psychiatrists identified as being recovered or much improved, and all of these informants were diagnosed with schizophrenia or bipolar mood disorder. I used the English term "recovered" with psychiatrists who used the same term to indicate patients they thought were doing well and were significantly functional. In some cases, as with Sreedevi presented below, patients appeared completely normal and signs of pathology were undetectable, but this was unusual. More commonly, "recovered" patients were able to live with family and work and have some quality to their life even if they did not feel fully normal or were not thriving. The out-patient health centres where we interviewed recovered individuals are known as "primary health centres" and "community health centres" and are part of a state-run network of community-based centres that dispense medicines and offer consultations for people with all kinds of illnesses.[16] Individuals with mental illness diagnoses who were living at home went to these centres to get their medications refilled and occasionally for follow-up consultations with psychiatrists, which were usually brief encounters oriented toward medication management. In addition, we visited three charitable, church-affiliated psychosocial rehabilitation centres which care for people who do not have family to whom they can return after hospitalisation.

Interviews were either semi-structured, enquiring about informants' illness histories and therapy-seeking experiences, or unstructured, addressing the same topics but allowing for more diversions into other areas of interest to the interviewee. Altogether 45 people with schizophrenia and related diagnoses (such as paranoid schizophrenia or schizoaffective disorder) and

---

16 For more on the network of health centres in Kerala and how their mental health workers constitute a network of care and surveillance of Kerala communities, see Lang (2019). This network can, and to some degree already does, operate as a conduit through which MGMH ideologies and practices are disseminated.

bipolar mood disorder were interviewed. I also spoke to doctors and other staff at the various centres about their experiences working with these patients and observed daily routines and intake sessions at the research sites. Interviews with patients were conducted mostly in Malayalam, the official language of Kerala, while interviews with staff were conducted in English.

Family, Care and Recovery in Kerala

One feature of the hospital where I conducted research that is striking compared to hospitals in the West and to the rehabilitation centre in Brazil studied by Biehl, is the presence of family members on the hospital grounds. Patients are usually accompanied by family members when they go for out-patient treatment, and in-patients are often visited by family or have family members staying with them at the hospital. The women's section of the hospital featured a "family ward" where, usually, mothers would stay with daughters who are patients or daughters would stay with mothers. In other words, a family member lives in this section of the hospital, in the same space as their in-patient relative and helps take care of them. Addlakha describes the same situation at a psychiatric hospital in Delhi, and for her it is not just the care and support of family that is important: "The presence of the family and the relative permeability between the ward and the outside world help in sustaining the social persona of the patient during hospitalisation, and consequently play a positive role in therapy as well" (2008, 110). This, she claims, helps patients in India avoid the "role dispossession" of Goffman's (1961) total institutions. Nunley (1998) examines the heavy involvement of families in in-patient and out-patient psychiatric care in hospitals in northern India in relation to the low level of family involvement in the US, and argues that this high level of involvement benefits patients. He also observes that family attendants in in-patient facilities in India provide assistance that is often provided by auxiliary staff in the US, such as feeding, bathing and maintaining medical records (by keeping prescriptions from previous treatments) for the patient. Nunley says that at the hospitals where he worked in Uttar Pradesh, each in-patient is required to have an attendant stay with him or her at the hospital, explaining that this arrangement "is a case of cultural expectations making permissible what the economics of health care makes necessary" (332). The economic pragmatism aspect is less present in out-patient care where Nunley and my research show that close to 90 per cent of patients are accompanied by family members. In this setting, they do not replace staff functions except for maintaining records, and their attendance costs the family financially as transportation to health centres is the main economic burden on low income families seeking care. In the hospital where I conducted research in Thiruvananthapuram, there is no requirement for in-patients to be accompanied by an attendant, and the hospital appears to have the staff necessary for the auxiliary functions that are addressed by family members where Nunley worked. However, there are some wards at the Thiruvananthapuram hospital where families are allowed to stay with relatives – suggesting that family presence is due more to cultural expectations than economic expediency in this case.

In examining patient interviews, I found that the quality of a person's family life and family members' involvement in their relatives' care consistently relate to their degree of illness or recovery (as measured by the Global Assessment of Functioning, an instrument used by mental health professionals – see below). I propose that love and caring social relations are at the core of what is beneficial about family involvement in the lives of those diagnosed with serious mental disorder, and illustrate this with the following three sketches of patients, all diagnosed as schizophrenic, which represent a sample of the variety of family relations.

Hari

Hari was a 39-year-old Hindu man and a former teacher whom we interviewed while he was undergoing in-patient treatment at the Mental Health Centre in Thiruvananthapuram. Hari had a degree in electrical engineering, and said he was diagnosed with a mood disorder, a problem that, he explained, has been with him since childhood (though he was diagnosed as schizophrenic according to the staff and his chart). My assistant Biju and I interviewed Hari on the grounds outside the concrete cell block where he and several other male in-patients were staying during their hospitalisation. This was not a family ward like the one described earlier in a women's section of the hospital, but family often visited patients in this ward. When we asked Hari what bothered him most about his problem, he pointed to a lack of home and family life:

> Biju: What problem is bothering you most now?
> Hari: The problem that bothers me is that I have no home. That's my biggest problem: at home, in the home, there is no one. That I am living alone at home is my biggest problem.
> Biju: Are your father and mother still alive?

Hari: Not father, mother passed away. Father is alive. But it has been six years since I have seen my father.
Biju: What is the reason for being separated from your father like this?
Hari: With my father... I fought with my father.

Hari says he fought with his father about money and about his inability to work due to his *"vata* illness" – using a diagnosis from ayurvedic medicine, related to an excess of *vata*, one of the three *dosha*s or embodied essences of physiology. This seems to be a reference to his current problems, but it was not clear whether it may have been a separate health issue or something he had suffered from in the past.

Biju asked whether previously "You and your father had good relations [*snehabandham*]?", and Hari responded, "We did have good relations [*snehabandham*]." The term *snehabandham* in Malayalam translates as "good relations", but literally it means "loving relation/connection". Hari explained that he had two younger brothers who support him to some degree, but "they are staying aloof, saying that I have been coming and just lying around here, without trying to get work." The brothers brought him to the hospital, but now they are aloof, seemingly annoyed and dismissive of Hari, accusing him of being lazy.

Hari was experiencing changing moods, depression, and burning sensations in his body, and he heard voices, though he said the voices had recently receded. He explained that he has no future plans, and that it is hard for him to work because labour is painful for him and he doesn't have the mood for it. Hari was not doing well in terms of his functioning. Earlier he explained that he left teaching to work in security, "because of decreasing memory power and being unable to take any mental strain," since he felt security work was less demanding. He was hospitalised with incapacitating symptoms, and the quality of his family relations seemed to correspond to his moderate- to low-functioning state. His primary complaint about his current condition is what I am claiming is a major cause of the persistence of his affliction: his lack of a good relationship with his family. This was indicated by his estrangement from his father, the loss of *snehabandham*, and the lukewarm support of his brothers.

Satheesh

When we met Satheesh, a 47-year-old Hindu male, he was visiting Malayin-keezhu Primary Health Centre for follow up care. This centre was in a quiet,

tree-canopied neighbourhood away from the bustle of central Thiruvananthapuram in area well off the main road to the city. Just a handful of patients
and staff are around at any time at the Malayinkeezhu Centre which is in
striking juxtaposition to the out-patient clinic in the city's mental hospital
that is regularly crowded with patients and their families.[17] Satheesh's life
too seemed calm now, but he was diagnosed as schizophrenic and was
hospitalised twelve years earlier at the Mental Health Centre where Hari
was a patient. According to his chart, he was talking and laughing to himself
at the time, he had little sleep or appetite, and he suffered from persecutory
delusions. Satheesh seemed to us to be doing well, though, when we met
him. He was very articulate, and it was hard to perceive anything wrong
with him. He was doing "coolie work" he said, which refers to the occasional,
general manual labour in which many working class and poor people in India
engage, and he claimed he was doing okay economically. When we spoke to
him, he also claimed he was not having any mental problems, either. "I am
not as I was earlier. Now I am married. I have two children," he declared,
emphasising that these were the main reasons for his improvement. He had
a large, supportive family, but, according to the notes in his chart, this was
also the case during his hospitalisation several years before his marriage.

As always, we asked if there were currently any issues at home with
the family. With a nurse from the health centre joining our conversation,
Satheesh responded by saying that all was well with his family. In response,
Biju referred to sneham in his interpretation of how Satheesh explained
his family relations:

Satheesh: No such difficulties in home, no problem at all.
Biju: Everyone is loving [ellarumaittu snehamaittu].
Nurse: Did your relatives or someone inhibit you in some way or
something?
Satheesh: No, nothing like that. There are no such problems in the family.
Nurse: Nothing like that.
Biju: Who among the family is helping you more in connection with this
problem?

---

17   Despite the quite different feel of the place, this primary health centre is connected to the
Mental Health Centre hospital due to the outreach programme of the District Mental Health
Programme (DMHP) which is based at the hospital and visits the primary health centres. In
addition, the DMHP has placed a poster at the Malayinkeezhu centre informing the public how
to identify and seek help for mental health problems. According to some in Kerala, such efforts
reflect the effect of the MGMH although a direct connection between the Kerala DMHP and
the MGMH is hard to establish. Certainly, their methods and ideology are similar.

Satheesh: Well, I have a mother, a sister, an elder brother is there, then my wife, and his wife. Then I have my children. That's who is helping me. They are helping.

The nurse continued this line of inquiry:

Nurse: When the problem started, who was the first person to come forward to take you to the hospital?
Satheesh: That was my father and mother.
Nurse: After that...
Biju: Who is caring (*paricharikkunnathu*) for you the most? Caring for you the most?
Satheesh: It is my wife who is doing the most caring.
Biju: Because of your problem...
Satheesh: Then, my sister, mother and elder brother are looking after me well.

Satheesh was dismissive about his problem, claiming he did not have an illness at present, not as if he were in denial about his diagnosis, but casually, as if he no longer had concerns about his state of mind, that he felt stable and content. He was not accompanied to the health centre by a family member. This may have been because he was in a good state of mind and this was a routine follow up visit, with him no longer needing family support to stop into the health centre for this purpose which usually amounted to just picking up a prescription renewal. He said that he had "kutumbatthil santhosham" or happiness in the family, and Satheesh was one of the most completely recovered interviewees we spoke with. It was hard to detect anything unusual about his affect or demeanour, and Biju told him he didn't seem to have any illness at all. He had come a long way from in-patient care with a diagnosis of schizophrenia. Satheesh also reported one of the most supportive families of any person we met, where a great variety of relatives were involved in his care, and it is caring family relations that Satheesh, Biju and the nurse mobilised as an explanation to account for Satheesh's recovery.

Sreedevi

Sreedevi, a 44 year-old Hindu woman we met at the Mental Health Centre's out-patient unit, also seemed completely recovered from schizophrenia. She and Satheesh may represent the kind of patient that make the WHO studies of schizophrenia intriguing. Complete recovery, in the sense of being not just merely functional and staying out of the hospital but highly functional, symptom free and even thriving, is usually considered outside of the realm of possibility in North American medical and popular discourse on schizophrenia, but both individuals were highly functional and it was not possible to detect any sign of pathology.[18]

Sreedevi was hospitalised in 2002 in the Mental Health Centre, and at the time she was running about, screaming, exhibiting *bahalam* (boisterous behaviour), and hearing voices. Her husband's family beat her for acting this way, she recalled. While she said her problem was exacerbated by her husband's family beating her, she didn't explain what she thought was the cause of the original onset of symptoms. Both her father and mother helped a lot with her struggles with her illness, and, she claimed, did everything for her, but her husband did not help at first. She said she has been working in a variety of manual labour positions for the last ten years, including working as a maid for other families and as a day labourer for a community programme. When we enquired into her views about her future and her prospects for her work life going forward, she explained that she is a workaholic who works hard out of fear of becoming "sad" – a reference to a possible return of her mental troubles – if she doesn't.

Sreedevi's demeanour seemed completely normal to Biju and me when we spoke to her, and she was hospitalised only once, for a week, fourteen years ago. With all other patients we spoke to who had schizophrenia diagnoses, even if they were significantly recovered, we could detect some atypical affect or interaction in our conversations, but with Sreedevi, as with Satheesh, there was no hint of a past episode of psychosis. She has been coming to the Mental Health Centre outpatient unit every couple of months for follow up treatment since her hospitalisation and is still taking medications. She recounted as well that she helped others in her community with similar problems by talking to them about her experience and guiding them to the Mental Health Centre when necessary. When I asked specifically what helped

---

18   The Mayo Clinic website, for example, describes schizophrenia as a chronic condition requiring "lifelong treatment" (2018) and does not discuss the possibility of recovery. Yet Hopper, Harrison, and Wanderling (2007) say that over half of the subjects followed up in the ISoS, the latest follow up to the WHO studies, at all of the research centres were "rated as 'recovered'" (27) suggesting a general course of improvement in this diagnosis in most settings over the long run. When I report to people in the US that I interviewed patients in India who had recovered from schizophrenia, their most frequent response is that they thought one could not recover from this illness. However, the "recovery movement" in the US claims a greater potential for change for people with serious mental illness (Arenella 2015).

her recover, she said it was because of "my husband's *sneham*". Her husband eventually came around to her side, and he was able to cut off ties with his family because of their abuse of Sreedevi. Her supportive parents and the caring love[19] of her husband who dissembled at first, perhaps because of not wanting to be in dispute with his natal family, seemed to have aided her recovery. Sreedevi's case is intriguing given Kottai's (2020) observation in his work in Kolkata that mistreatment by in-laws was a common cause of women becoming homeless and being deemed mentally ill.

These sketches illustrate the role of family support in general as well as specific claims regarding the role of love/*sneham*. These two factors are hard to isolate from one another, and I am assuming that love, or the caring love that is *sneham*, is a key element of family support. Certainly, pragmatic, financial and other aspects of family support are also crucial to maintaining stability or achieving recovery, and these can be part of *sneham* as well. These sketches represent points on a continuum of family involvement and degrees of illness and recovery I observed in my interviews with patients at the Mental Health Centre and the community health centres. I also used the Global Assessment of Functioning (GAF – from *Diagnostic and Statistical Manual of Mental Disorders IV-TR*) to score those patients with schizophrenia diagnoses for whom there was sufficient data to do so: there were nineteen such patients in all. I also evaluated the quality and degree of involvement of family in patient care on a scale from 1 (lowest) to 5 (highest). Quality of family involvement scores strongly correlated with GAF scores of patients ($r=0.8687$) such that the higher the degree and quality of family involvement the higher functioning the informants were, and these results were statistically significant ($p<0.001$).[20]

While there is a correlation between the quality of family involvement and the level of functioning of people diagnosed with schizophrenia in at least one niche of southern India, this does not tell us whether there is more family involvement in India than in Western/Northern countries, which might help explain the differences in the WHO studies on the course of schizophrenia mentioned earlier. There are, however, many indications along these lines in the research literature. Kallivayalil et al. report that an "important difference in which India differs from the West is that [in India] more than 90% of the patients of schizophrenia stay with their families" (2010, 39), by which they mean patients live with their families. In the US, by contrast, people with

---

19   This illustrates how *sneham*, caring love for the other, more than *premam*, romantic love, is operative in recovery, though both may be present in this relationship.
20   More details about these results and how work lives correspond to functionality and recovery will be published in a separate article addressing a clinical audience.

schizophrenia diagnoses often live alone and, increasingly, in prison (Prins 2014). Sartorius et al. mention that in the WHO studies, the Aarhus, Denmark site had one of the highest percentages of people with schizophrenia living alone, with 35 per cent, while the percentage of people with schizophrenia living alone in the India sites, Agra and Chandigarh, was "virtually nil" (1986, 916). My research assistant Tintu James, in her Master's thesis on mental illness in Thiruvananthapuram, shows that among out-patients at community clinics and psychiatric hospitals doing follow-up outpatient care, 93 per cent were living with family and 87 per cent were living in joint, as opposed to nuclear, families (2013, 33-34). The majority of these patients were diagnosed with severe mental illness (schizophrenia, bipolar mood disorder, or psychosis) (ibid., 37). Reviewing the Indian psychiatric literature, Addlakha says that several studies claim "to show the lower prevalence of all types of mental disorders in the joint family, accounting for it in terms of the greater social, economic and moral support provided by this type of household to its vulnerable members" (2008, 101). Ethnographic work by Luhrmann (2007), Brodwin (2013), and Myers (2015), meanwhile, indicate that people with serious psychopathology in the United States have little connection to family. Additionally, providing a comparison between India and the US, Nunley says that the problem of where the patient will go after hospitalisation which is "so critical in the practice of acute psychiatry in the United States, essentially vanishes in India, where it is taken for granted that the patient's family will continue to care for the patient" (1998, 334). In a study of a mental health clinic in the US, Myers says that "most members [referring to patients] had lost touch with their families after various kinds of problems – arguments over alcohol and drug habits, legal problems, homelessness, and so forth" (20). This is rare among patients in India. Hari was estranged from his father, but had not lost touch with his family and had some involvement with his brothers. Health centre staff regularly showed me patients' charts when I was conducting interviews, and of all the patients my assistants and I spoke with, there was only one whose chart listed no family contacts, a woman who had the lowest level of functionality of all of the patients we met. Normally patient charts report mobile contact numbers for several family members, even among those who have strained relations with their families.

Snehaveedu: The House of Love

Snehaveedu is one of many psychosocial rehabilitation centres established in Kerala in recent years, partly in response to a Supreme Court mandate to increase the availability of resources for the mentally ill. These centres are mostly Church-run, charitable organisations that are licensed and monitored by the state government and care for the few individuals who are not able to return to family after leaving in-patient mental health treatment. I visited two other centres, Menni Family Home and Divy Shanti Ashram, but spent far more time at Snehveedu, which means "House of Love" or "Love Home". While "sneha" refers to love, "veedu" means house or home, and this "veedu" provides an illustrative counterexample to João Biehl's "Vita" (which means "life", 2013[2005]) in terms of the quality of relations between people with mental illness diagnoses, their caregivers, their families, and their social context.

Snehaveedu is a project of the Malankara Syrian Catholic church, one of the many constituents of Kerala's large Christian community which dates back two thousand years. Christianity is not a colonial import here, although European colonisers did bring their own styles of Christianity to India starting in the 1500s, and the Syrian Catholic church, as the name implies, is a hybrid of a sect that dates to the first century and a European liturgy brought by the Portuguese in the sixteenth century. Snehaveedu takes in the destitute mentally ill who have no homes to go to or whose families are unable to care for them. Since, as reported earlier, 80 to 90 per cent of people in India with serious psychopathology live with family, institutions such as Snehaveedu are not a primary recourse for the mentally ill but a refuge for those few who have no other place to go.

As a form of psychological and work rehabilitation, residents of Snehaveedu partake in animal husbandry, gardening, and the maintenance of a self-sustaining, ecological system that provides food, water, and fuel for the institution. Residents also pray and eat together, and they are taken to the Mental Health Centre once a month for follow-up assessments; but Father George Joshua Kanneeleth, who runs Snehaveedu, and a college student I will call Suresh who volunteers and lives with the residents, emphasised to me that the key thing that is missing in the lives of their residents that their institution offers is love. "For this rehabilitation process," Father George Joshua explained, "love is the best quality", and he added "quality is better than qualification", explaining that the capacity to be loving and compassionate is more important for rehabilitation than professional expertise. Father George Joshua referred to Snehaveedu residents as his "mukkal", his children, and spoke of his "affection" for them. One does not generally hear this kind of language from psychiatric staff about their patients, even though some hospital staff have been described by patients as caring or loving. One exception comes from a hospital social worker who explained that when she has success with a patient, it's because of "the love I have for the person across the table." Father George Joshua added that "[t]hose who are working here, my staff, they should have affection as a mother or a father with these people. He [a patient] may be [like] my brother or my father or my sister. Likewise, such kind of family affection we should have".

As per government regulations, the staff at Snehaveedu brings the residents to the Mental Health Centre hospital once a month for evaluations. While psychiatric follow-up is done at the hospital OP by a biomedical practitioner, weekly general health check-ups at Snehaveedu are provided by doctors of Ayurvedic medicine, since state regulations allow psychosocial rehabilitation centres to utilise Indian systems of medicines for regular health maintenance. Father George Joshua is a supporter of Ayurveda and its supposedly gentler methods of treatment, and while I was doing fieldwork at Snehaveedu, he organised a seminar to train rehabilitation workers from all over Kerala in Ayurvedic methods of mental health care.

Father George Joshua explained that Snehaveedu was established after a cardinal from his church saw a mentally ill man wandering in the streets, and decided the church should open a home for the destitute mentally ill. Father George Joshua took on this project, and in addition to receiving patients who are discharged from the mental hospital who do not have family they can return to, Father George Joshua brings in mentally ill individuals he finds wandering in the streets. Father George Joshua explained that when they bring someone in this way:

> After bath and cleaning, after cleansing, we give food and an embrace, and immediately half of the problem is gone away. We just take the patient from the road and within hours, without medicine, half of the problem is [...] It is because of the care and protection.

Regarding his approach to the needy and homeless, he added, "I want to see the face of Jesus in that man," and he recalled how he encountered a destitute man on the streets who was angry and aggressive. Father George Joshua kissed him and touched his feet, which, he says, transformed the man. Summing up his attitude, which acknowledges a role for medication, he said "Care and protection is the important thing. We need medication. At the same time, we need care, protection and affection for these people. If we are affectionate, they are very genuine." Care and affection are ways of enacting the kind of love that is referred to as *sneham*. It is these characteristics of emotional and embodied relations, rather than specific therapeutic techniques, that is emphasised here. Caring, affection, and *sneham* are not methods developed by the logic and empiricism of a researcher, but are a calling of this member of the church who follows Jesus's model of caring for the marginalised when he attends to people who experience mental suffering.

Several residents of Snehaveedu whom I spoke to reflected the Father's perspectives on love/sneham. One resident identified a lack of love in his life as his chief concern, using the English term "love" while speaking in Malayalam: "My biggest problem is 'love.' [...] It is 'love' that I'm lacking". Another resident emphasised the curative power of love at Snehaveedu, "Here they are giving food at the right time. Also, sisters [nurses] give medicines at the right time. Also, they love us [avar nammale snehikkunnundu]. Even if we didn't get any food, their love [avarute sneham] is enough for the cure of the disease. [...] This place is called 'Snehaveedu', right? So there is a lot of love here." Timely food and medicine are seen as a critical part of a health regimen in south Indian society. These are stressed here, but love supersedes in this assessment. The psychiatrist who sees the Snehaveedu residents once a month for mental health evaluations, although he did not use the term "love", praised the caring environment at this rehabilitation centre. At a meeting with me at the mental hospital, he explained, "The acceptance by the officials there, by the people who run Snehaveedu, is more than or equal to that of a family member. They actually give them all of the support. They actually treat them with compassion. They never feel ... I have never seen that they are actually looking at them as a patient."

Connections between illness, healing, and love were made in other contexts, outside of Snehaveedu and patient discussions of their families and illness experiences. In 2014, I visited a church in Thiruvananthapuram that, during earlier visits in the 1990s and early 2000s, had served as a place of healing for people with mental afflictions. In 2014, this was no longer the case according to Father Verghese, an official of this church who said that people with mental health problems are now directed to the local mental hospital. This may be the result of efforts by the Kerala or Indian government and the MGMH to direct people suffering psychopathology from religious centres to "proper" treatment at biomedical facilities, efforts that have led to the discontinuation of religious healing practices elsewhere in India (Sood 2016). While Father Verghese felt that sending people to a mental health facility was appropriate, he also thought that the biological model emphasised at such places was limited. He felt that people with mental health problems are reacting to their environment and explained that what they really need is support and love. This shows how MGMH-style changes may be steering patients away from places, such as this church, that emphasise *sneham*. The notion of *sneham* has also been invoked in patients' descriptions of the staff at the Mental Health Centre and of an ayurvedic practitioner who specialises in treating psychopathology. In an interview I conducted in the 1990s, a patient referred to the talk therapy she received from this Ayurvedic psychiatrist as "loving". "[H]e talks a lot," she said and added, "I get relief from his talk itself" and "his talk is very loving."

In addition to the notion of caring love, *sneham* also refers to an embodied, tangible substance. According to Osella and Osella's (1996) work on *sneham* in Kerala, there are two key aspects of the concept of sneham: "*sneham* as love, concrete demonstrations of care which make social relations run smoothly" and "sneham, as a cooling and lubricating fluid within the body, [which] is critical to good health" (38). *Sneham* is thus necessary for good social relations and for general health. *Sneham/sneha-* is also a term in Ayurvedic medicine that has implications similar to the second of these two definitions. Dr. Bindu, an Ayurvedic physician specialising in mental health who sees patients at Snehaveedu, explained, "*Sneham* means, it's not rough. It's a lubricated affection; it's not a rough affection. When we are talking to a patient with *sneham*, communication becomes more lubricated."

Sneha(m) in Ayurveda refers to unctuousness, an oiliness in the body or a lubricating substance used in clinical treatments. One such treatment is *snehapana*, which is administered to patients at Kerala's Government Ayurveda Mental Hospital (GAMH), in Malappuram District. *Snehapana* involves drinking ghee (clarified butter) in increasing quantities over several days in order to lubricate the body. According to Dr. Abdu of the GAMH, this lubrication helps move "impure substances" to the alimentary canal and then to the stomach and intestines during a sweating treatment (*svedana*). Then through *vamana* (drinking a substance to induce vomiting) and *virechana* (taking emetic medicines), two other steps in a regimen that includes *snehapana* and is known as *panchakarma*, these substances are expelled from the body through vomiting and purgation of the bowels. Thus, the lubricating effects of this *sneha-* therapy help remove impurities and detoxify the body. Another step in *panchkarma* used at the GAMH is the administration of *snehavasti*, an unmedicated oily enema which is administered on alternate days, with *kashayavasti*, a medicated enema, administered on the other days.[21]

Perhaps we could say that *sneham* is something like a bio-social lubricant that through affection and caring prepares the body and mind for recovery

---

21   For more on Ayurvedic treatments for mental illness in Kerala, see Halliburton (2009) and Lang (2018).

among those diagnosed with serious mental illness. That is, *sneham* as caring love may activate *sneham* as tangible substance in the body, although no one I spoke to made this explicit connection – and I did not ask about it at the time. In her fieldwork with a mental health outreach worker in Kerala, Lang (2019) interprets references to *sneham* among patients as lubricated affection, and considers the potential connections between Ayurvedic treatments that lubricate the body and love as *sneham*: "Although Ayurvedic psychiatrists did not talk explicitly about snehapana in relation to the physio-social notion of sneham as love, these concepts might be related and further studies are needed to explore the relationship of snehapana to Malayali concepts of bodies, morals, care and well-being" (607).

While this idea of *sneham* as lubrication may help explain how, along with care and affection, it enables recovery, what is equally significant is that these cases of love and caring show how people in this low-income setting treat vulnerable people as qualified, even valued, life and have seen success in recovery from diagnoses thought to be intractable. Individuals diagnosed with severe mental illness that my assistants and I met in Kerala have regular, significant social interactions with family, other patients, mental health workers, and volunteers, some or much of which is marked by *sneham*. For those who are abandoned by family (or whose families cannot take care of them), the slack is often taken up, at least in Kerala, by others such as the staff and the community of residents at Snehaveedu and other similar institutions.[22]

Concluding Remarks

The Movement for Global Mental Health – like the WHO mhGAP programme and, to some degree, the Government of India – has declared India a place of deficiency and abuse in terms of its mental health care and vowed to "save" it from these problems. The findings of the WHO studies of schizophrenia should however make us ask what places like India, with its especially high recovery rate, are doing right, and apply whatever that is in places that are not doing as well, such as the United States. The involvement of family and of caring love/*sneham* are areas to investigate further about what is going right and should give pause to claims that mark India more as a place that

---

22 This may be less common in other states. Davar (2012) claims that Kerala has more psycho-social rehabilitation centres than any other Indian state, even though it has a lower population than most states.

is abusive or neglectful toward the mentally ill than as a model for caring relations toward those suffering mental distress. Similarly, Nunley, writing before the advent of the MGMH but concerned about Indian psychiatrists he met trying to emulate psychiatry as it is practiced in the West, asked "whether in this case the emulation ought not to be running in the other direction" (320) – that is, whether the involvement of families in Indian psychiatry ought to be emulated in the US and Europe.

This study also directs anthropological attention to caring relations by foregrounding the role of a certain kind of love among family and non-family members who attended to destitute people with serious psychiatric diagnoses, treating them not as bare life but as qualified, vital life. We should not ignore abuses that occur in the treatment of the mentally ill, whether in India or anywhere else. Nor should we neglect cases of abandonment in developing what Robbins calls an "anthropology of the good." But as Robbins says, we should also find space in our evaluations of human endeavour to attend to "the ways people come to believe that they can successfully create a good beyond what is presently given in their lives" and we should resist the "strong temptation to dismiss people's investments in realizing the good in time as mere utopianism" (458). Both "the abandoned" as ethnographic subjects in anthropology and "the abused mental patients" presented by advocates of the MGMH can be regarded as examples of what Robbins calls the "suffering subject." If we focus primarily on such subjects, we may miss much of what is salutary about human interactions, even if we feel compelled to recognise, in the spirit of the Foucauldian critique (raised earlier in Rabinow and Rose's critique of Agamben) that positive and caring relations can be confining and also create constellations of power. While there is surely some truth to this Foucauldian perspective, it would ultimately reduce love to power relations and overlook its potential as transformative and as aiding recovery. As pointed out earlier in reference to Tjeltveit (2006), it somehow feels "unscientific" to operationalise love as an analytical category or as a variable in studying clinical outcomes. While the present foray into the role of love is somewhat preliminary, it may help us to take more seriously the role of love in the lives of the mentally ill. It seems indeed to be associated with significant improvements in the lives of those suffering from psychopathology, even if many still experience stigma, second-class status within the family, and other kinds of adversity.

Like the MGMH and WHO's attempts to "save" the mentally ill in developing countries, the focus on saving, or lamenting, suffering subjects may preclude an opportunity to learn from others. Indeed, the point of Robbins' provocation was to revive anthropology as cultural critique, in the sense of using other cultural experiences to critique one's own assumptions. The explicit valuation of love in recovery from the perspective of healers as well as people diagnosed with mental disorders in Kerala may contain lessons for improving mental health care elsewhere in a way that goes beyond explicit clinical techniques and interventions.

References

Addlakha, Renu. 2008. *Deconstructing Mental Illness: An Ethnography of Psychiatry, Women and the Family*. New Delhi: Zubaan.

Agamben, Giorgio. 1998. *Homo Sacer: Sovereign Power and Bare Life*. Stanford, CA: Stanford University Press.

Arenella, Jessica. 2015. "Challenges for the Recovery Movement in the US: Will its Light Reach the Darkest Corners?" *Clinical Psychology Forum* 268: 7-9.

Biehl, João. 2013 [2005]. *Vita: Life in a Zone of Social Abandonment*. Updated edition. Berkeley: University of California Press.

Brodwin, Paul. 2013. *Everyday Ethics: Voices from the Front Line of Community Psychiatry*. Berkeley: University of California Press.

Carey, Benedict. 2015a. "The Chains of Mental Illness Across West Africa." *New York Times*, 12 October 2015, A1, A9.

—. 2015b. "A Mission to Heal Minds." *New York Times*, 13 October 2015, Science Times D1, D9.

—. 2016a. "A Call to Foster Mental Health Across the Globe." *New York Times*, 13 April 2016, A4.

—. 2016b. "Mental Illness Left Untreated Burdens China and India." *New York Times*, 19 May 2016, A4.

Cohen, Alex, Vikram Patel, Rangawsamy Thara, and Oye Gureje. 2008. "Questioning an Axiom: Better Prognosis for Schizophrenia in the Developing World?" *Schizophrenia Bulletin* 34 (2): 229-44.

Cohen, Lawrence. 2005. "Operability, Bioavailability and Exception." In *Global Assemblages: Technology, Politics and Ethics*, edited by Aihwa Ong and Stephen Collier, 79-90. Oxford, UK: Blackwell.

Coleman, Leo. 2016. "Inside and Outside the House: A Narrative of Mobility and Becoming in Delhi." *Journal of Contemporary Ethnography* 45 (6): 692-715. https://doi.org/10.1177/0891241616630377.

Davar, Bhargavi. 2012. "Legal Frameworks for and against People with Psychosocial Disabilities." *Economic and Political Weekly* 47 (52): 123-31.

Dey, Sushmi. 2016. "Only 1 in 10 Mentally Ill Gets Aid in India." *Times of India*, 19 May 2016 (electronic edition). Accessed 12 September 2018, http://

www-lexisnexis-com.queens.ezproxy.cuny.edu/lnacui2api/api/version1/
getDocCui?lni=5JTB-C381-JB3N-T18S&csi=8411&hl=t&hv=t&hnsd=f&hns=t&
hgn=t&oc=00240&perma=true.

Goffman, Erving. 1961. *Asylums: Essays on the Social Situation of Mental Patients
and Other Inmates*. New York: Anchor Books.

Goldstein, Donna. 2013 [2003]. *Laughter Out of Place: Race, Class, Violence, and
Sexuality in a Rio Shantytown*. Berkeley: University of California Press.

Good, Michael. 2009. "Elvin V. Semrad (1909-1976): Experiencing the Heart and Core
of Psychotherapy Training." *American Journal of Psychotherapy* 63 (2): 183-205.

Haberman, David. 1988. *Acting as a Way of Salvation: A Study of Raganuga Bhakti
Sadhana*. New York: Oxford University Press.

—. 2003. *The Bhaktirasàmçitasindhu of Rûpa Gosvàmin*. New Delhi: Indira
Gandhi National Centre for the Arts in association with Motilal Banarsidass
Publishers.

—. 2006. *River of Love in an Age of Pollution: The Yamuna River of Northern India*.
Berkeley: University of California Press.

Halliburton, Murphy. 2004. "Finding a Fit: Psychiatric Pluralism in South India and
Its Implications for WHO Studies of Mental Disorder." *Transcultural Psychiatry*
41 (1): 80-98.

—. 2009. *Mudpacks and Prozac: Experiencing Ayurvedic, Biomedical and Religious
Healing*. London and New York: Routledge.

Han, Clara. 2012. *Life in Debt: Times of Care and Violence in Neoliberal Chile*. Berkeley:
University of California Press.

Hannig, Anita. 2017. *Beyond Surgery: Injury, Healing, and Religion at an Ethiopian
Hospital*. Chicago: University of Chicago Press.

Hardt, Michael, and Antonio Negri. 2000. *Empire*. Cambridge, MA: Harvard
University Press.

Hopper, Kim. 2004. "Interrogating the Meaning of 'Culture' in the WHO Interna-
tional Studies of Schizophrenia." In *Schizophrenia, Culture and Subjectivity: The
Edge of Experience*, edited by Janis Jenkins and Robert Barrett, 62-86. Cambridge,
UK: Cambridge University Press.

Hopper, Kim, Glynn Harrison, Aleksandar Janca, and Norman Sartorius, eds. 2007.
*Recovery from Schizophrenia: An International Perspective: A Report from the
WHO Collaborative Project, the International Study of Schizophrenia*. New York:
Oxford University Press.

Hopper, Kim, Glynn Harrison, and Joseph Wanderling. 2007. "An Overview of
Course and Outcome in ISoS." In *Recovery from Schizophrenia: An International
Perspective: A Report from the WHO Collaborative Project, the International Study
of Schizophrenia*, edited by Hopper, Kim, Glynn Harrison, Aleksandar Janca,
and Norman Sartorius, 23-38. New York: Oxford University Press.

James, Tintu. 2013. "Assessment of Internalized Stigma among Patients with Mental Illness in Trivandrum District, Kerala." Masters of Public Health diss., Thiruvananthapuram, India: Achutha Menon Centre for Health Sciences Studies.

Kallivayalil, Roy A., Rakesh K. Chadda, and Juan Mezzich. 2010. "Indian Psychiatry: Research and International Perspectives." *Indian Journal of Psychiatry* 52: 38-41.

Kottai, Sudarshan R. 2020. "An Ethnographic Study of Community Mental Health in Contemporary India: Interrogating 'Care', 'Chronicity' and Expansion of Patienthood." PhD diss., Indian Institute of Technology Hyderabad.

Lang, Claudia. 2018. *Depression in Kerala: Ayurveda and Mental Health Care in 21st Century India*. London and New York: Routledge.

—. 2019. "Inspecting Mental Health: Depression, Surveillance and Care in Kerala, South India." *Culture, Medicine and Psychiatry* 43 (4): 596-612.

Leff, Julian, Narendra N. Wig, Harinder Bedi, David K. Menon, Elizabeth Kuipers, Alisa E. Korten, and Gunilla Ernberg. 1990. "Relatives' Expressed Emotion and the Course of Schizophrenia in Chandigarh: A Two-Year Follow-Up of a First-Contact Sample." *British Journal of Psychiatry* 156: 351-56.

Luhrmann, Tanya. 2007. "Social Defeat and the Culture of Chronicity: Or, Why Schizophrenia Does So Well Over There and So Badly Here." *Culture, Medicine and Psychiatry* 31: 135-72.

—. 2016. Introduction. In *Our Most Troubling Madness: Case Studies in Schizophrenia Across Cultures*, edited by Luhrmann, Tanya and Jocelyn Marrow, 1-26. Berkeley: University of California Press.

Ma, Zhiying. 2012. "When Love Meets Drugs: Pharmaceuticalizing Ambivalence in Post-Socialist China." *Culture, Medicine, and Psychiatry* 39: 51-77.

Marrow, Jocelyn, and Tanya Luhrmann. 2012. "The Zone of Social Abandonment in Cultural Geography: On the Street in the United States, Inside the Family in India." *Culture, Medicine and Psychiatry* 36: 493-513.

Mayo Clinic. 2018. "Schizophrenia – Diagnosis and Treatment." Accessed 16 August 2018. https://www.mayoclinic.org/diseases-conditions/schizophrenia/diagnosis-treatment/drc-20354449.

Mills, China. 2014. *Decolonizing Global Mental Health: The Psychiatrization of the Majority World*. Hove and New York: Routledge.

Myers, Neely. 2015. *Recovery's Edge: An Ethnography of Mental Health Care and Moral Agency*. Nashville, TN: Vanderbilt University Press.

Nunley, Michael. 1998. "The Involvement of Families in Indian Psychiatry." *Culture, Medicine and Psychiatry* 22: 317-53.

Osella, Filippo, and Caroline Osella. 1996. "Articulation of Physical and Social Bodies in Kerala." *Contributions to Indian Sociology* 30 (1): 37-68.

Patel, Vikram, Ricardo Araya, Sudipto Chatterjee, Dan Chisholm, Alex Cohen, Mary De Silva, Clemens Hosman, et al. 2007. "Global Mental Health 3: Treatment and

Prevention of Mental Disorders in Low-Income and Middle-income Countries."
The Lancet 370: 991-1005.

Patel, Vikram, Pamela Y. Collins, John Copeland, Ritsuko Kakuma, Sylvester Katontoka, Jagannath Lamichhane, Smita Naik, and Sarah Skeen. 2011. "The Movement for Global Mental Health." *British Journal of Psychiatry* 198: 88-90.

Patel, Vikram, Shuiyuan Xiao, Hanhui Chen, Fahmy Hanna, A. T. Jotheeswaran, Dan Luo, Rachana Parikh, et al. 2016. "The Magnitude of and Health System Responses to the Mental Health Treatment Gap in Adults in India and China." *Lancet* 388: 3074-84.

Pinto, Sarah. 2011. "Rational Love, Relational Medicine: Psychiatry and the Accumulation of Precarious Kinship." *Culture, Medicine, and Psychiatry* 35: 376-95.

Povinelli, Elizabeth. 2011. *Economies of Abandonment: Social Belonging and Endurance in Late Liberalism*. Durham, NC: Duke University Press.

Prins, Seth J. 2014. "The Prevalence of Mental Illnesses in U.S. State Prisons: A Systematic Review." *Psychiatric Services* 65 (7): 862-72.

Rabinow, Paul, and Nikolas Rose. 2006. "Biopower Today." *BioSocieties* 1: 195-217.

Robbins, Joel. 2013. "Beyond the Suffering Subject: Toward an Anthropology of the Good." *JRAI* 19: 447-62.

Sartorius, Norman, Assen Jablensky, Alisa E. Korten, Gunila Ernberg, Martha Anker, John E. Cooper, and Robert Day. 1986. "Early Manifestations and First-Contact Incidence of Schizophrenia in Different Cultures." *Psychological Medicine* 16: 909-28.

Sartorius, Norman, Walter H. Gulbinat, Glynn Harrison, Eugene M. Laska, and Carole Siegel. 1996. "Long-term Follow-up of Schizophrenia in 16 Countries." *Social Psychiatry and Psychiatric Epidemiology* 31: 249-58.

Silverman, Chloe. 2011. *Understanding Autism: Parents, Doctors, and the History of a Disorder*. Princeton, NJ: Princeton University Press.

Sood, Anubha. 2016. "The Global Mental Health Movement and Its Impact on Traditional Healing in India: A Case Study of the Balaji Temple in Rajasthan." *Transcultural Psychiatry* 53 (6): 766-82.

Soudi, Laila, and Vikram Patel. 2016. "The Global Community Is Failing to Address Mental Health." *The Guardian*, 25 July 2016. Accessed 12 September 2018, http://www-lexisnexis-com.queens.ezproxy.cuny.edu/lnacui2api/api/version1/getDocCui?lni=5K9N-FXB1-JCJY-GoN7&csi=8411&hl=t&hv=t&hnsd=f&hns=t&hgn=t&oc=00240&perma=true.

Thara, Rangawsamy. 2004. "Twenty-Year Course of Schizophrenia: The Madras Longitudinal Study." *Canadian Journal of Psychiatry* 49: 564-69.

Tjeltveit, Alan. 2006. "Psychology's Love-Hate Relationship with Love: Critiques, Affirmations and Christian Responses." *Journal of Psychology and Theology* 34 (1): 8-22.

Trawick, Margaret. 1990. *Notes on Love in a Tamil Family.* Berkeley: University of California Press.

Warner, Richard. 1994. *Recovery from Schizophrenia: Psychiatry and Political Economy – Second Edition.* London and New York: Routledge.

World Health Organization. 1973. *The International Pilot Study of Schizophrenia.* New York: Wiley and Sons.

—. 1979. *Schizophrenia: An International Follow-up Study.* New York: Wiley and Sons.

About the Author

MURPHY HALLIBURTON studied anthropology at Stanford University and the City University of New York (CUNY) Graduate Center, where he earned his PhD in 2000. Currently he is Professor in Anthropology at Queens College and the Graduate Center of CUNY. Since the 1990s, he has been conducting research on mental health and illness in Kerala, India. His first book, *Mudpacks and Prozac* (Routledge, 2009), compared ayurvedic, biomedical, and ritual forms of healing for mental illness and related problems, and he recently completed a Fulbright-Nehru-funded study of recovery from schizophrenia in Kerala. He has also conducted research on the struggle between Indian pharmaceutical companies and global big pharma over patent rights and concerns about biopiracy of ayurvedic knowledge, which is the subject of his book *India and the Patent Wars* (Cornell University Press, 2017). He is currently investigating the history of eugenic research at Stanford University and the role of biological determinism in American culture.

8 Ayurvedic Psychiatry and the Moral Physiology of Depression in Kerala

Claudia Lang

Abstract

The GMH movement has not considered psychiatric traditions outside mainstream psychiatry. By highlighting the existence and significance of Ayurvedic mental health care, I challenge the notion of a "treatment gap" in India. At the same time, focusing on Ayurvedic psychiatry as an alternative to globalised biomedical psychiatry and highly dynamic field, I go beyond the usual dichotomy of global psychiatry and local traditional healing by showing how a (re)invented tradition assembles local bio-moral embodied minds, classic texts, vernacular practices, and globalised psychiatric and psychological knowledge to recognise and treat distressed, embodied minds. Against the narrative of traditional medicine as the epistemic "other" to Western psychiatry, I will describe how Ayurvedic psychiatrists engage elements of globalised psychiatry and psychology while stressing Ayurveda's epistemic difference and embodied alterities.

Keywords: Ayurvedic psychiatry, depression, moral physiology, embodied minds, Kerala

Ayurvedic psychiatry is one of many highly dynamic indigenous medical fields addressing mental health problems. Proponents of global mental health – and most allopathic[1] psychiatrists and health policy makers in India – ignore indigenous medicine when they talk about the "treatment gap" in many lower- and middle-income countries such as India (Chisholm et al. 2016; Patel and Thornicroft 2009): that is, the difference between the

---

1   Allopathy is the most common term used in India for biomedicine.

Sax, William, and Claudia Lang (eds), *The Movement for Global Mental Health: Critical Views from South and Southeast Asia*. Taylor & Francis Group, 2021
DOI: 10.5117/9789463721622_CH08

number of people estimated to need treatment for mental illness and the number actually receiving it. While this ignorance persists amongst many proponents of global mental health, the recently published report of the Lancet Commission on global mental health and sustainable development (2018) provides hope in arguing for "respecting the complementary role of [...] local traditional approaches to treatment" (Patel et al. 2018).

By highlighting the existence and significance of Ayurvedic mental health care, I challenge the notion of a "treatment gap" in India. At the same time, focusing on Ayurvedic psychiatry as an alternative to globalised biomedical psychiatry and highly dynamic field, I go beyond the usual dichotomy of global psychiatry and local traditional healing by showing how a (re)invented tradition assembles local bio-moral embodied minds, classic texts, vernacular practices, and globalised psychiatric and psychological knowledge to know and treat distressed, embodied minds. Against the narrative of traditional medicine as the epistemic "other" to Western psychiatry, I will describe how Ayurvedic psychiatrists engage elements of globalised psychiatry and psychology while stressing Ayurveda's epistemic difference and embodied alterities. Using the case of Ayurvedic psychiatry as a local therapeutic assemblage, I further suggest that indigenous medical knowledge and practices are essential in localising global mental health.

In this chapter, I focus on depression, which is projected by Global Burden of Disease studies to become the leading cause of disability worldwide and a major contributor to the overall global burden of disease Numbers produced by the Global Burden of Disease studies and their DALY metrics (Murray and Lopez 1996).[2] Depression is at the centre of many global mental health initiatives and projects, and has become a major public health concern in India as well (Lang 2018a, 2019). With the focus on depression, I hope to show the complexities and ambiguities of theorising and treating a global mental health priority in a highly dynamic indigenous medical field.

I begin with a brief introduction to the institutional context of Ayurvedic psychiatry in Kerala and to basic notions of Ayurveda that are relevant for mental health problems. Next I elaborate on the notion of "embodied minds," before going on to analyse two different kinds of depression in Ayurveda. In Ayurveda, mental ill health is both a physio-moral problem and a rupture in perception, and I provide an analysis of its theory and its psychotherapeutic and embodied treatment that engage global psy-discourses and local notions of embodied minds and selves.

---

2   For current numbers, see http://www.healthdata.org/gbd.

Institutionalised Ayurvedic Psychiatry

The process of seeking mental health care in Kerala is complex and multifaceted. Patients often visit a variety of specialists, receive care in allopathic mental hospitals, general hospital psychiatric units, or primary health centers in addition to Ayurvedic and Unani define practitioners, homeopaths, psychologists or counsellors, "undisciplined healers", and Catholic priests and retreats. Although Indian allopathic psychiatrists maintained a marginal interest in Ayurvedic notions and treatments of mental illness as part of their interest in an "Indian psychiatry" from the 1960s through the 1980s (Sébastia 2009), this has died away and these days, Ayurveda's role in mental health care in India is rarely acknowledged by Indian allopathic psychiatrists or global mental health actors.

Many Ayurvedic doctors and non-institutionally trained *vaidyas* (traditional Ayurveda practitioners) also treat people with mental health problems such as depression, anxiety, or tension, but institutionalised Ayurvedic psychiatry is mainly practiced at the Government Ayurveda Mental Hospital (GAMH) and the Ayurveda College in Kottakkal in Northern Kerala. This specialty hospital was established in 1974 on the joint initiative of the Arya Vaidya Sala and a member of the Legislative Assembly in Kerala. The first superintendent was both institutionally and traditionally trained; a medical officer hailing from a family of *vaidyas* that had been treating mental illness for generations. Under his management, the hospital joined the state system and came under the direct authority of the Directorate of Indian Systems of Medicine in Tiruvananthapuram and later the AYUSH Department. First housed in a smaller Malabar-style mansion on the premises of Arya Vaidya Sala in Kottakkal, it shifted into a larger, modern facility in the late 1990s. Today, GAMH accommodates up to 50 patients, including (since the 2010 establishment of a child psychiatry unit) children. It boasts free as well as paying wards for inpatients, and a daily out-patient facility that attracts patients from different social and religious backgrounds from nearby villages and towns, other parts of Kerala, and even other states. The in-patient treatment takes around 40 days after which patients return for regular out-patient check-up and treatment. In the same town, the Department of General Medicine (Kaya Chikitsa) of the P.S. Varier Ayurveda College offers outpatient treatment for patients with mental health problems, as well as the Medical Doctor of Ayurveda (M.D.) course *Knowledge of the Mind and Mental Diseases*.[3] This course follows the BAMS (Bachelor of

3   *Mano vigyan avum manas roga.*

Ayurvedic Medicine and Surgery), and is often translated by the students as "psychology and psychiatry," or simply "psychiatry." There are several other Ayurvedic doctors in Kerala who specialise in mental health, some trained at Kottakkal (Lang 2018a), others from a lineage of *vaidyas* (not college-trained Ayurvedic practitioners) specialised in mental health (some integrating religious treatment Sax and Nair (2014)).

Of Doshas, Gunas and Sattvabalam

Scholars of Ayurveda have dealt with Ayurvedic notions and treatment of mental illness and occasionally touched upon depression (Naraindas 2014; Ecks 2013; Giguère 2009; Halliburton 2009; Langford 2002; Obeyesekere 1977; Nichter 2002) but have not described the theorising and treatment of depression in institutionalised Ayurvedic psychiatry (but see Lang 2018a; Lang and Jansen 2013). Ayurvedic practitioners in institutional Ayurvedic psychiatry understand and treat depression as a problem at once physiological, moral, and cognitive. This approach is deeply intertwined with the Ayurvedic concept of mental health as *dosha* (humoral) imbalance and involving mental strength, self-control, equanimity, and clarity. Although in its elaborated form (described below in detail) it is part of an Ayurvedic scholarly discourse, the basic assumptions informing this concept are shared by vernacular physiology, and manifest in embodied experiences of mental health in Kerala. Most Malayalis[4] are not familiar with Ayurvedic psychiatric theory but do have a similar understanding of mental illness as increased heat in the head or other parts of the body, as lack of mental strength, or as weakness. Since medical applications such as oil or medicated mudpacks have long been part of folk medicine for troubled minds and behavioral problems in Kerala, most Malayalis are at least somewhat familiar with many of the Ayurvedic psychiatric procedures. Moreover, many Malayalis share a notion of mental illness as a product of physio-moral imbalance as a result of an "imbalanced lifestyle" or "imbalanced food". The notion of imbalance provides a popular idiom for talking about both physical and mental illness in Kerala. It is, as Rhodes notes for Sri Lanka, "an idiom in which moral and physical balance can be talked of in the same breath, so that excess in the sense of "transgression of moral limits" and excess in the physical sense often go together and provide mutually reinforcing meanings for the events of daily life" (Rhodes 1980, 88).

---

4   People who speak Malayalam, the language spoken in Kerala.

In the "great three" Sankrit texts,[5] that are authoritative for Ayurvedic teaching and practice, and in the clinical practice of Ayurveda, illnesses of the body and of the mind are understood in relation to the *doshas* (humours or principles), *dhatus* (tissues), *agni* (digestive fire), *prakrti* (constitution), and *gunas* (qualities) or mental doshas of the patient. The three doshas – *vata*, *pitta* and *kapha* – may present either in their healthy physiological state according to individual constitution or in their faulty or harmful state. The doshas are both principles and substances governing the physiological functioning of the body and the mind. Health requires their balance while illness is the result of their imbalance.

The idea of *dosha* circumvents the conceptual split between the body and the world (Langford 2002). My Ayurvedic interlocutors translated *vata* as the moving principle, *pitta* as the transforming and *kapha* as the stabilising principle. Additionally, *vata* is dry, *pitta* is hot, and *kapha* is cool. Yet *doshas* are not only an abstract but also a concrete part of the physiology of the body. Many types of pain, emotional upheaval, and distress are related to *vata*. Practitioners speak of *kapha* when referring to mucus or of *pitta* when referring to vomit. Healing consists of pacifying the vitiated *doshas* and bringing them back to their healthy or balanced state. Depression as an illness is, then, a deviation from an individual's normal state of *dosha* balance.[6]

Important for Ayurvedic theorising and clinical practice are the three gunas: *sattva*, *rajas*, and *tamas*. *Sattva* indicates a healthy or pure mind, whereas *rajas* (activity and change) and *tamas* (darkness, heaviness, plumpness, ignorance) are viewed as noxious qualities that can cause mental illness. Persons with a high level of *sattva* have robust mental health and are morally strong while persons with a low level lack these qualities and are therefore more vulnerable to mental illness and more difficult to treat. Enhancing these qualities and increasing the level of *sattva* is thus a key part of rehabilitation or preventive treatment once the acute problem has been addressed through purifying and pacifying therapeutic procedures.

---

5   *Caraka Samhita, Sushruta Samhita,* and *Asthangahrdayam.*
6   Alter (1999) criticises what he calls the "remedial bias" in medical anthropology. Halliburton criticises the "limitation of the ideology of curing" as "the return-to-balance metaphor may involve importing biomedical assumptions about curing as ridding of symptoms and restoring functionality" (ibid., 47). But it was the restoration of functionality that was emphasised to me as the main goal of treatment by the Ayurvedic practitioners in institutional Ayurvedic psychiatry. When I mentioned Alter's argument that the aim of Ayurveda was to make the patient "better than well", most Ayurvedic psychiatrists said that they would be content to see a patient return to normal functioning.

Ayurvedic psychiatrists often psychologise the *gunas* as "mental *doshas*", but according to Samkhya philosophy *gunas* are physio-moral qualities of the material and intangible material world.

The *sattvik* notion of mental health is closely related to *sattvabalam* that many Ayurvedic psychiatrists translated as mental strength or willpower. "If you analyse the depressive patients", Dr. Nayar explained while introducing the concept,

> there will be some weak-mindedness in all these patients. A strong mind means you are equipoise. You are not depressed when you are sad nor are you overthrilled when you have joy. A strong mind means a strong character. But these patients have some type of weak-mindedness, some problems persisting in the back of their mind; subconscious mind is there. Subconscious mind means there will be certain feelings that may have created in you during your childhood, and they may repeat that.[7]

The concept of sattvabalam as it is used by Ayurvedic psychiatrists in Kerala closely resembles the vernacular Malayalam notion of *manobalam* (mental strength, willpower), and many patients and family members perceive a lack of *manobalam* as one cause of mental illness. Both can be seen as a culturally shared notions concerning the foundations of mental health.

How does a *guna*-related predisposition or vulnerability lead to mental illness? To answer this question, Ayurvedic psychiatrists take not only the socialisation of the child into account but also go back to a person's birth, the pregnancy that produced them, and sometimes even to previous lives. The theory of predisposition to mental illness is closely related to other Ayurvedic fields of paediatrics and gynaecology, to the Ayurvedic notion of child development (Halliburton 2009) and to the philosophical notion of karmic traces (*vaasanaa*). "There are several factors that play a role," Dr. Shankaran, a teacher at another Ayurveda college in Kerala, explained. One factor is the *guna* constitution of the parents at the time of conception. "If the *guna* of the father and mother is *rajas* and *tamas* predominant then the child will also be *rajas* and *tamas* predominant. Then the child is a vulnerable person." A second factor is the atmosphere experienced by the

---

7   This last detour into psychoanalysis gives an indication of how the psychoanalytic notion of the subconscious is locally appropriated. In the context of Ayurvedic psychiatry, I occasionally heard the subconscious or subconscious mind constructed not as something deep and essential but rather as an impediment to mental health, an obstacle to be overcome. Religious healers and self-titled counsellors made similar statements.

mother during pregnancy. "If the mother has severe mental stress or tension then that will also affect the progeny; then the progeny will be *rajas* and *tamas* predominant." A final factor in *sattvabalam* is socialisation, including the family atmosphere and child rearing practices. Thus, for Ayurvedic psychiatrists, mental health care and prevention of mental diseases begins not only with the socialisation of the child but already much earlier with the mental health of the parents. A physio-moral notion of mental health is also closely associated and tied up with a normative "traditional" family life involving religious habitual and regular practices.

Embodied Minds

At institutional, educational, and clinical levels, Ayurvedic psychiatry is a new field of specialisation with a focus on mental diseases. But it is not entirely separate from "classical" forms of Ayurveda focusing on the body, and indeed Ayurvedic theory and clinical practice do not, in general, separate mental from physical diseases. Mind and body are seen as closely interrelated. Dr. Ganapati (at another Ayurveda college) explained, "All diseases are both *sharira* (body) and *manasu* (mind)." They are part of what anthropologist Mark Nichter has called a "resonating system":[8] what happens in the body resonates in the mind, and what happens in the mind resonates in the body. "Basically, Ayurveda is a materialistic science and it has got a very materialistic outlook towards the nature, mind, everything," Dr. Praveen, a general practitioner who focused on autism, explained.

   In Ayurveda, the mind cannot be treated directly. So Ayurvedic psychiatrists treat the mind by treating the body. Ayurvedic psychiatrists frequently used the metaphor of water in a vessel to describe the relationship between the mind and the body in Ayurveda. You cannot cool the water in a vessel directly, but by cooling the vessel the water also gets cooled. "By purifying the body," the former superintendent of the Government Ayurveda Mental Hospital Dr. Sundaran explained, "the mind gets clear." On the other hand, Ayurvedic psychiatrists see purity of the mind and an absence of distress and anger as essential for the health of the body. In Ayurvedic theories of the mind and mental illness, physiology, morals, lifestyle, and existential questions are interwoven. *Manas* and mental disorder, for that matter, can

8   Mark Nichter, "Hybrid Medicine for Hybrid People", lecture delivered in Heidelberg, Germany (12 June 2009).

be manipulated and treated in the same way as other bodily and somatic diseases: that is, through purification and diet, but also through cognitive and moral controls (Obeyesekere 1977; Langford 2002) again targeting physiological processes. Consequently, until recently there has not been a separation in Ayurveda between practitioners and disciplines treating the body and those treating the mind. The (re)invention of Ayurvedic psychiatry as a separate theory, practice, and academic discipline in Kerala establishes and institutionalises a Cartesian dualism separating body and mind that did not previously exist in Ayurveda. The permeability and distinctiveness of Ayurveda with respect to allopathic psychiatry are part of the process of producing new institutions, experts, and knowledge regimes in order to enter into the broader glocal network of mental health. As such, Ayurvedic psychiatrists are working to establish the compartmentalisation of body and mind both institutionally *and* pedagogically.

One of the basic characteristics of *manas* is that it is part of matter or the material world that is organised into different levels according to the degree of density. Samkhya philosophy, the school that most closely informs Ayurvedic concepts and practices, does not make a sharp ontological distinction between mental and physical domains. Rather than locating a split between body and mind, Samkhya philosophy distinguishes between consciousness without content or quality (*purusha*) on the one hand and matter (*prakrti*) which is imbued with the three *gunas* (*sattva, rajas*, and *tamas*). The different mental faculties *buddhi* (discriminating intelligence), *ahamkara* (self-identification, ego) and *manas* (mind and emotion – the faculty that comprehends sensory objects) are substances (*dravya*) and part of matter, not opposed to it (Larson 1969; Langford 2002; Halliburton 2002).[9] Ayurvedic psychiatrists treat problems related to manas through the same purification procedures with which they treat other physical diseases: emesis, purgation, vomiting, nasal purification, and diet changes. Purified and balanced bodies and material minds make for purified and balanced thoughts, emotions and behavior (cf. Nichter 2002; Halliburton 2009; Ecks 2013).

9   *Manas* is the densest of these three and thus easiest to therapeutically manipulate. Moreover, the Upanishads and Samkhya, Yoga and Advaita Vedanta philosophies distinguish manas from consciousness (Halliburton 2002; Ecks 2013). While *manas* is subjected to change through sensorial impressions including food, consciousness remains unaffected by them (ibid.). The Sanskrit term *manas* is etymologically related to the Malayalam term *manasa* (Halliburton 2002) and the Bengali term *mon* (Ecks 2013). As *manas* and related terms capture both emotion and mind, scholars have suggested the English translation of "heart-mind" (Desjarlais 1992; Kohrt and Harper 2008; Ecks 2013).

In a healthy person, there is a chain linking sensory objects with the senses, *manas*, and buddhi. To perceive a sensory object, the senses attach to the object and send the information to *manas* that receives and aggregates the sensory information. If the linkage between *manas* and *buddhi* is disrupted or blocked, information cannot be processed or analysed, and it is impossible to construct a rational response. Its emotional and cognitive content can be influenced through the same material means as other physical diseases. Emotions and thoughts thus can be changed and replaced through a process of physio-cognitive self-control. Depression involves the disruption of this connection, which in turn is related to local moral worlds and local ideas of societal functioning. As such, it both results from and leads to *prajnaparadha* (an offence against wisdom or norms).

In the Ayurvedic pedagogic and clinical practice that I observed, *manas* is used interchangeably with "mind". In spite of this apparent synonymy, *manas* does not fully match the psychological aspects of the Euro-American concept "mind". It is understood as somehow more material, epiphenomenal, and inessential than "mind". Both allopathic and Ayurvedic psychiatry have a material approach towards the mind but they differ in fundamental ways: allopathic psychiatry's materialism is the product of a long history of reductionisms. The ancient trialism of soul, mind, and body was reduced to a mind-body dualism, which now is being further reduced to a material-ism that extinguishes the mind by reducing it to a mere epiphenomenon, manifestation, or "function" of the brain. The Ayurvedic concept of *manas*, on the other hand, incorporates mental faculties into the realm of matter and sees the body and the mind as two sides of a resonance system. Other than the biopsychiatric reduction of mind into matter, the Ayurvedic conception of mental health problems is not reductionist. Physiology in Ayurveda, based on *doshas* and *gunas*, diverges from allopathic physiology by including morals and values and differs from it by its strong emphasis on *pathiyam* (diet and daily activities) that are related to South Asian notions of permeable selves.[10] *Manas* includes both mental and emotional processes that affect the humoral balance in the heart, the vessels, and other parts of the body (Zimmermann 1987).

10   In the anthropology of South Asia, significant attention has been accorded to this sociocentric conception of personhood – in particular, the way it differs from the Western, circumscribed construction (Marriott 1976; Marriott and Inden 1977; Dumont 1980). Recent studies transcend this dichotomy and show that both notions of bounded and permeable selves exist and are performed, staged, and evident in different contexts and institutions in South Asia (Mines 1994; Lamb 2000; Sax 2009; Basu 2014).

Two Kinds of "Depression"

The asymmetrical relations between biomedicine and Ayurveda and the prestige of biomedicine leads practitioners and students of Ayurvedic psychiatry to engage and appropriate biomedical psychiatric nosologies, to integrate them into Ayurvedic theories, and translate Ayurvedic knowledge into the language of globalised psychiatry. Although practitioners of Ayurvedic psychiatry emphasise that Ayurvedic terms and concepts cannot be neatly translated into biomedical psychiatric ones, in their interaction with patients, in classroom debates, research, medical charts, and the interviews I conducted, students and practitioners were constantly involved in translation processes.

In the Ayurveda College in Kottakkal, students and teachers of Ayurvedic psychiatry mainly differentiated between two kinds of depression: *vishadam* (sadness, confusion) and *kaphonmada* (a phlegmatic, despondent state, often translated into severe depression). Rather than a categorical distinction, the difference between kaphonmada and *vata* viitation lies on a continuum, similar to the continuum of mild, moderate, and severe depression. They correlated mild depression with *vata* viitation and severe depression with a predominance of *kapha dosha* and a more significant impairment of the mental faculties.[11] They described *vishadam* as a symptom of *vata* viitation, and used *kaphonmada* to refer to a syndrome or illness category. *Vishadam*, they told me, can be translated as the mild or neurotic form of depression or as reactive depression. It manifests mainly as emotional disturbance or tension in reaction to external stressors including depressed mood, crying spells, anxiety, anger, agitation, sleeplessness, and excessive worry. *Vishadam* is further characterised by sleeplessness, physical fatigue, difficulties thinking and speaking, and mild psychomotor retardation or agitation. Some practitioners also translated *vishadam* as "confusion" related to a lack in mental strength and closely associated with Arjuna's *vishada yogam* (yoke of suffering) in the Bhagavad Gita. Ayurvedic practitioners often framed the warrior Arjuna's predicament when he was confronted with his relatives and teachers as adversaries on the battlefield in terms of confusion about which path to take rather than in terms of sadness, hopelessness, or despair. Both framings of *vishada* as sadness, despair, or anxiety on the one hand and as confusion on the other indicate a somatic, cognitive, *and* moral understanding of depression.

---

11   During their academic training, students of Ayurveda are taught the theoretical possibility of diagnosing severe depression and other mental disorder along with certain *graha* diagnoses, but this has little clinical or diagnostic relevance.

Vata vitiation and emotional disturbance are closely interrelated. Grief, anxiety, and confusion can vitiate *vata*, which may then manifest in excessive crying, anxiety, and other signs of emotional disturbance. On the other hand, *vishadam* can "manifest in pure somatic symptoms such as aches and pains only", as Dr. Krishnan explained. By framing depression as an impairment or reduction of *vata*, Ayurvedic doctors elaborated an integrated understanding of "somatisation" that contradicts allopathic psychiatrists' interpretation of somatisation as a process of masking what are assumed to be psychological symptoms behind the expression of somatic symptoms. As *vata* vitiation, depression manifests at both the mental and somatic levels. Depression as *vishadam* is not perceived as a severe condition and does not require purifying inpatient treatment, but can be managed with pacifying and mind-strengthening formulations and applications, counselling or psychotherapy, or yoga. Allopathic psychiatrists in Kerala use the terms *vishadam* and *vishada rogam* are the Malayalam translations of depression and depressive disorder, but for Ayurvedic psychiatrists *vishadam* is not a disease category per se but one of many symptoms of *vata* affliction. However, as many practitioners stressed, if *vishadam* persists it may develop into *kaphonmadam*.

Vishadam is a symptom, or rather a feature or characteristic (*lakshana*), but *kaphonmada* is a syndrome and a specific illness. *Unmada* (madness, mental illness) is characterised, I was taught at the college, by dysfunction of the mind, intellect, orientation of self in time, place and person memory, desire, habits, psychomotor activities, and morals. *Kaphonmada* is one of five forms of *unmada* as described in the classical texts relevant to the teaching and clinical practice of Ayurvedic psychiatry. They describe the features of these forms of *dosha unmada* in physical, cognitive, and emotional terms (Langford 2002, 236). *Vishadam* affects the dysfunction of *manas* (mind and emotions) only but *kaphonmada* additionally includes dysfunction of other mental faculties such as intellect, consciousness, memory, desire, and also manners, behaviour, and conduct. Then, Dr. Krishnan explained, the person becomes "like a chariot without a charioteer", a phrase I often heard in Kerala. In the development of *kaphonmada*, both *kapha* and *vata* are aggravated or vitiated and the accumulated *kapha* spreads to the mind-carrying channels and blocks them. This leads to depression and other mental disorders.[12] For treatment, he continued, *kapha* has to be removed

---

12   I also encountered a few Ayurvedic practitioners (both general and specialised in psychiatry) who differentiated between *vata, pitta,* and *kapha* kinds of depression. Dr Joshua, trained in Ayurvedic psychiatry but working in his own clinic, elaborated: "Those who are daily not able

by *shodana* (purification) treatment and *vata* has to be pacified by *samana* (pacification) treatment. *Vishadam* does not require in-patient treatment and can be managed with Ayurvedic drugs and counselling alone. *Kaphonmada*, however, requires more intensive treatment, through purging and purifying procedures including internal and external oleation of the body, sweating, therapeutic vomiting, and nasal treatment.[13]

Dr. Nayar specified the relationship between *vata* vitiation and *kapha* accumulation, integrating the biopsychiatric concept of depression as the manifestation of neurochemical changes in neurotransmitters. "If *kapha* blocks the *manovahashrotas* [mind-carrying channels]," he explained, "then *vata* cannot pass through. *Vata* is responsible for the regulation of the mind, and stimulates the connection between a sensory object, a sensory organ, the mind, and discriminating intellect." "Modern" (allopathic) doctors, he said, express the carrier function of *vata* in terms of neurotransmitters. Like *vata*, serotonin and noradrenalin carry information from one neuron to another. For allopathic as well as Ayurveda doctors, according to Dr. Nayar, the carrying function of *vata* or serotonin and noradrenalin, is disturbed in depression. In Ayurveda, this disturbance is conceptualised as a blockage caused by aggravated *kapha*. "By reducing the blockage of *kapha*," he concluded, "Ayurvedic practitioners stimulate the neurotransmitters as *vata* and the neurotransmitters are functionally the same." As exemplified by Dr. Nayar's explanation, many Ayurvedic psychiatrists frame the pathogenesis of depression in a hybrid fashion drawing on both Ayurvedic and allopathic knowledge. Ayurvedic pathogenesis, then, becomes just another way to describe biochemical processes in the brain.[14]

Ayurvedic psychiatrists recognise *kaphonmada* when the symptoms correspond with *kapha* vitiation and follow a diurnal course typical for *kapha* afflictions such as aggravation in the morning or immediately after taking food.[15] The symptoms of *kaphonmada* largely correspond to the symptoms of

to sleep, they will get the *vata* type of depression. Those who are taking greater amounts of meat or alcohol or spicy food, they will get the *pitta* type of depression. Those who take more sleep and *kapha* food items, they will get the *kapha* type of depression. If a person has been psychologically weak from the childhood onwards, then according to their lifestyle and diet she will get the *kapha, vata, pitta* type of depression.

13 Purification in which drops of medicinal oil are administered through the nose.

14 This is an example where Ayurvedic knowledge is seen to both anticipate "modern" discoveries and to be confirmed by modern neuroscientific research.

15 If the mental illness does not follow the path of any of the *doshas, graha unmada* [madness of the *graha* kind] is – theoretically – suspected.

what psychiatrists call "severe depressive disorder".[16] Some other symptoms – such as aggravation after taking food or in the night, or increased sexual desire – do not. However, most Ayurvedic psychiatrists agreed that mental illness always involves all three *doshas* at the same time, just to different extents. "*Unmada* with a single *dosha* is rare; also pure *kaphonmada* is rare. More often, there is *kapha-vata-paittika* or *kapha-paittika unmada*. If it is *kapha-paittika*, anger is there, the patients are quarrelling with others, and the *kapha* symptoms are also there," explained Dr. Sarasvati. On the other hand, *vata* is involved in other forms of mental illness besides depression, as Dr. Shaila (who also held a PhD in psychology) at the Government Ayurveda Mental Hospital told me:

> *Vata* will definitely be there in all types of mood disorders. Mood, we say, *vega* [emotions]. For the appropriate expression of mood, we need *vata*. *Vata* is the moving force that gives energy. Mood is actually energy or emotion. And that requires *vata*. That is why people say that *vata* is definitely impaired. So there will be *vata* impairment also in *kaphonmada*. Because sometimes this depression is a lack of expression of emotions. Even though they will have sadness, they won't express.

Dr. Sundaran, then the superintendent in charge of GAMH, disclosed the clinical pragmatics of single *dosha* diagnoses. "We don't say it is purely *kaphonmada* because in all the cases of *unmada* it is said it is *sannipad*, three *doshas* are involved. For the convenience of the treatment modality only we differentiate between *vatonmada, pittonmada,* and *kaphonmada*."

Kapha dosha can manifest as many different problems according to where it has localised, but for *kapha dosha* to reach the mind and to develop a *kapha*-related mental illness, specific causative factors and predispositions are required. Ayurvedic psychiatrists take different levels of causation of depression or related Ayurvedic categories like *kaphonmada* into consideration. At the Government Ayurveda Mental Hospital, Dr. Rasheed elaborated on the causal chain of *kaphonmada*: Excessive eating or over-nourishment and a sedentary lifestyle precipitate *kapha dosha*. External factors such as

---

16 Shaik Anwar (2005) identifies the symptoms of *kaphonmada* as they are described in *Caraka Samhita*: lack of taste, loss of interest, vomiting, reduced activities, little desire for food, reduced talk, increased libido, desire for solitude, increased salivation and discharges from mouth and nose, disgusting appearance, aversion to cleanliness, increased sleep, swelling of the face, aggravation in the night and after taking food, remaining on one place, white and timid eyes, pale nails and skin, indigestion, cough, decrease in intellectual capacities, fondness for warm things, increased fatigue (Shaik Anwar 2004).

tension, bereavement, loss, or unavailability of a desired thing, guilty consciousness related to social norms, different forms of poison, or an incorrect
diet could trigger the disease. With regard to diet, food that is improperly
cooked, spoiled, or incompatible (such as fish and curd) and food that is
regarded as *rajasika* (of *rajas* quality) or *tamasika* (of *tamas* quality), such as
spicy food and meat, is understood to precipitate depression. Passions and
intense emotions such as sadness, grief, anger, lust, or the desire for material
goods that result from too much attachment, false sensory perceptions, or
faulty judgment also cause *kaphonmada*. In contrast to Western theories,
all intense emotions, passions, and desires are considered to be causative
factors of mental disorders. In order to develop *kaphonmada*, a certain
psychic predisposition or vulnerability expressed in the terminology of the
three *gunas* is required. In the words of Dr. Rasheed:

> *Sattva* is the healthy factor. If *sattva guna* is there, the mind will be strong,
> no mental disorder will occur. *Rajas* and *tamas* are the factors that are
> causing ill health for a mind. What may be reason, how many stress factors
> may have occurred, how many problems the patient has, if the mind of
> the person becomes *hina* [weak] – that means unhealthy – then only the
> mental disorder will occur. That is the principle in Ayurveda. Stress is
> for everyone. [...] Life is always stress. Only very few are getting mental
> disorders. And that is because of ill-mindedness, mental unhealthiness.
> This mental unhealthiness is caused by *rajas* and *tamas*. If the *tamas* or
> the *rajas* part is predominant in a person that person is vulnerable to a
> mental disorder. If the same stress occurs to a person who has *sattva guna*,
> mental disorder may not occur. *Sattva guna* will create mental strength.

In this sense, deficient *sattva* quality constitutes the predisposition for all
mental disorders, whereas an abundance of *sattva* (i.e. mental strength or
willpower), prevents them. Only in people with a weak sattva can certain
external factors give rise to a mental disease. The *dosha* that is predominant in the body at the time of its exposure to a triggering external factor
determines the manifestation of the disease as *vata*, *pitta*, or *kapha* forms
of mental illness.

Vitiated *doshas* may also lead to disrupted perception as I learnt from
teaching and MD theses at the Ayurveda College in Kottakkal. When the
mind-carrying channels are blocked by kapha, *manas* cannot flow freely
and function well, and this leads to a disruption of the chain of perception
between *artha* (sense objects), *indriya* (senses), *manas*, and *buddhi*. Proper
perception and knowledge results only if all elements in chain are connected

smoothly and united. Since the transmission from one element to the other is governed by *vata*, a vitiation of *vata* leads to disruption. Zimmermann (2014), based on his readings of Ayurvedic texts, argues that all causes of disease are recognised in Ayurveda as either of insufficient, perverted, or excessive union (*yogam*). As Dr. Sundaran (1993) writes,

> Mental diseases are born out of the excessive thinking, undesirable or unwanted thinking; and unreal thinking distorts the *indriya* which are working in unison with the mind. The union of the mind and *indriya* is jeopardized here. And this ill union ruins the *buddhi*. The excessive, insufficient or perverted union of the thinking process is of course an undesirable effect; it goes without saying.[17]

Vitiated *doshas* lead to a blockage in the mind-carrying channels (*manova-hashrotas*) that may disrupt the chain of perception. This disrupted union includes mind and emotions as well as morals and habitual behaviour. According to Dr. Nayar, disobeying social norms may be a sign of mental illness:

> These people lose discipline in their lives. They will not do what we tell them. They don't obey the rules of the society. If you tell a psychiatric patient, 'You should not speak' then they will not obey. They can hear our voices; they can see us. But something happens in their analysing mind. Their *buddhi*, their *manas* is getting deranged. *Manas* does not properly accept the sensory stimulus. They may hear but they do not listen. Our words are not being processed to their mental faculties.

As Dr. Nayar makes clear, the cognitive in Ayurvedic mental health is closely associated with the moral.

It is through the purifying and pacifying procedures and medications that I described above that the perverted union of the chain of perception produced by a blockage in the mind-carrying channels becomes normalised. "By making the body purified, the mind gets clear and good thoughts occur," Dr. John explained. This assumption – one shared by many Ayurvedic psychiatrists with whom I spoke – is based on the notion that mental illness hinders clear perception, correct morals, and good behaviour. Like a tainted mirror that cannot reflect its image clearly, depression and other forms of mental illness are seen as obstacles that hinder a person from perceiving

---

17   Translated from Malayalam to English by Babu Appat.

the world "as it is" and from behaving according to social norms. It is the disruption in the chain of perception that leads to wrong cognition, wrong conclusions, and wrong behaviour. In other words, depression is described as a state of ignorance.

Ayurvedic Psychotherapy

Developing mental strength is one of the main aims of *sattvavajaya*, which Ayurvedic psychiatrists often translated as "Ayurvedic psychotherapy". "*Sattvavajaya* is because medicine alone will not work in a mental problem. We also have to stimulate the patient with different aspects, morally, psychologically," said Dr. Mangalam, a teacher of Ayurvedic psychiatry at the college. The reconstruction of *sattvavajaya* as psychotherapy began in the 1980s and has found its way into the teaching and practice of Ayurvedic psychiatry in Kerala. The reconfiguration of *sattvavajaya* as Ayurvedic psychotherapy resembles the bifurcation of treatment into pharmacological therapy and psychotherapy in globalised psy regimes.[18]

In *sattvavajaya*, as Langford pointedly notes, "not only is an entire field of specialisation elaborated from one verse, but this field is also found to correspond to and anticipate a modern therapeutic technique" (Langford 2002, 244). This verse[19] lists *yuktivyapasraya* (rational treatment), *daivavyapasraya* (spiritual treatment), and *sattvavajaya* (psychotherapy) as the three types of therapy for mental disorders. In an English translation this verse reads: "There are three types of therapy; spiritual, rational and psychological. The spiritual therapy consists of recitation of mantras, wearing

18   Smith (2011) argues that in its original meaning, *sattvavajaya* was neither a technology of the self nor a kind of ancient psychotherapy, since the idea of self-care is a modern one and not anchored in the classic texts. According to Smith, the word "sattva" in *sattvavajaya* as it appears in the classical texts does not denote "mind", but rather refers to spirits. For Smith, *sattvavajaya* is "a form of ancient Indian therapeutic practice in which ritual possession was a probable component" (ibid., 23). According to this interpretation, *sattvavajaya* in the classical scriptures refers to non-Brahmanical healing forms involving the removal of spirit possession. *Sattvavajaya* would then not have been akin to psychotherapy but to practices that involved possession. This would, then, resemble the secularisation that gave rise to the discursive extrusion of *bhutas* as spirits from contemporary academic Ayurvedic discourse. My focus, however, is the way Ayurvedic psychiatrists *today* understand and practice *sattvavajaya*, and none of the Ayurvedic psychiatrists I spoke with related *sattvavajaya* to forms of possession. If Smith is correct and *sattvavajaya* was in previous times a form of exorcism, this meaning has been completely extruded from present-day understandings of *sattvavajaya*.
19   *Caraka Samhita Suthrastana* 11:54.

roots and gems, auspicious acts, offerings, gifts, oblations, following religious precepts, atonement, fasting, invoking blessings, falling on (the feet of) the gods, pilgrimage etc. The rational therapy consists of rational administration of diet and drugs. Psychological therapy (*sattvavajaya*) is restraint of mind from the unwholesome objects" (Sharma 1981, quoted in Langford 2002, 241). When I asked students and practitioners for a translation of *sattvavajaya*, the most frequent answer I received translated it as "defeating the mind", "controlling the mind", or "disciplining the mind". Other common translations included "winning the mind" and "attaining a *sattvika* [pure] state".

Although Ayurvedic psychiatrists stressed that the word "*sattva*" in *sattvavajaya* refers to the mind and not to the *sattva guna* (the quality of purity), *sattvavajaya* is closely related to the promotion of *sattva guna* and *sattvabalam* (mental strength, strength through *sattva*) as a predisposition and equivalent to mental health and protection against mental illness. Medical management mainly targets the *doshas*, doctors stressed, but *sattvavajaya* directly affects the *gunas* and therefore has a stronger moral element, but both the *doshas* and the *gunas* have physiological and psychological components. *Sattvavajaya* aims at increasing the proportion of *sattva* that is again related to local ideas of a good life and at decreasing *rajas* and *tamas* that are seen as responsible for passions, ignorance, and immoral behaviour. Enhancing these qualities and increasing the level of *sattva* (through change in thinking and behaviour patterns and through diet) is thus a key part of rehabilitation or preventive treatment once the acute problem has been addressed through purifying and pacifying therapeutic procedures.

Since *sattvavajaya*, conceptualised as helping the mind to refrain from unwholesome objects, is open to multiple interpretations, it is deployed in many ways. When I discussed *sattvavajaya* with Dr. Sundaran at the Government Ayurveda Mental Hospital, he began by defining it as "living according to the moral and religious rules of the society. These rules," he maintained, "are made aiming at good health." He enumerated examples including going to temples, lighting a religious lamp (*nilavilakku*), and associating with elders and wise persons. He further mentioned general advice such as controlling your emotions, telling the truth, and having compassion for every living being. Controlling thoughts and emotions is central to *sattvavajaya*, as it is to local moralities, physiologies, and psychologies in Kerala.

Sattvavajaya is a specific kind of technology of the self in an effort to monitor the mind and to use the mind properly. Rather than the self-explorative introspection of Western biodynamic psychotherapy with its aims of emancipation and autonomy of the self, in *sattvavajaya* the mind is brought into accordance with the social and cosmological order and streamlined according to moral norms and ideas of the good life. Rather than venting and expressing thoughts and emotions and making inner conflicts conscious as it is the aim in self-exploratory forms of psychotherapy, the aim of *sattvavajaya* is to suppress and replace unhealthy thoughts and emotions and to prevent them from moving into the conscious mind, keeping the mind and senses away from sense objects deemed unwholesome, thinking the right things, feeling at the right intensity. Whenever I heard Ayurvedic psychiatrists mentioning the unconscious mind they talked about it in terms of "purifying the subconscious mind", "eliminating bad thoughts and emotions", or "removing the subconscious mind". The unconscious of Ayurvedic psychiatry as I observed it in Kerala is something to be overcome, something epiphenomenal; its content to be replaced by more refined and morally superior contents in line with the socio-moral norms of the society.

Sattvavajaya is not only a psychological or moral process, but also a physiological one because thought and behavioural changes in accordance with local moralities transform the physiology of the body, and reciprocally, diet and daily regimes transform the gunas or qualities of the mind. Zimmermann (2014) is correct when he states that *sattva*, which he translates as "will-power" or "human agency", though designating the ethical dimension of health and disease, is materialised as a fluid in the body channels. Morals are closely interconnected with physiology in the Indian context, which is one of the reasons why Marriott (1976) in his ethnosociological attempt to understand India through Hindu categories, advocates giving up the Cartesian distinction between mind and body and describes South Asian notions of the self as bio-moral or physio-moral selves.

Sattvavajaya thus is a moral-physiological technology of the self with transformative power for both body and mind. It aims at restoring social harmony and social reintegration by means of controlling mental upheaval that arises within oneself as a result of passions and strong emotions (which are understood as causative of mental pathology and socially disruptive). Moral advice, dietary changes, and suggested daily regimes such as early wakening, exercises, bathing, and good dietary habits as forms of self-development and self-restraint are the most important techniques of *sattvavajaya*. Additionally, supportive techniques like reassurance and encouragement as well as social intervention are also common practices. Many doctors easily combined suggestions for cognitive, emotional, and behavioural changes with the consumption of ghee and milk when talking about improving the mental strength. A general Ayurvedic physician told me with regard to the treatment of mental illness: "We have to improve the *sattvabalam* [mental strength]. We have to apply daily *ghrta* and milk."

Sattvavajaya engages the mind as a physio-moral substance and cannot neatly be separated from more material interventions. Both medical substances *and* psychotherapy address minds, bodies and social relationships. Psychotherapy rebuilds and strengthens bodies as much as medicinal substances such as ghee pacify social relations and physiologies since they provoke insight and change behaviour (cf. Nichter 2002). Sattvavajaya as a physio-moral technique resonates with local physiologies and psychologies in Kerala that blur bodies, minds, social relations and larger social transformations.

Purifying Troubled Minds: The Case of Bindu

Dr. Rasheed referred Bindu, a woman in her late thirties from a rural middle class Hindu family, to me. He was one of the three consulting doctors at GAMH and had diagnosed Bindu with *kaphonmada*. Bindu's problems started after marriage around ten years back when she moved to her in-laws, who were much more orthodox than her birth family and very restrictive. She had to stop working as a tutor as she had done before her marriage and had to wear the more traditional saris rather than the more comfortable juridas. Gender and generational behaviour norms in Kerala, however, did not allow her to contradict or speak up in front of her father-in-law or other senior members of the family. Standing up for her well-being was the responsibility of her husband or his brothers. But even they were not supposed to speak against their parents. Bindu developed headache, had angry outbursts and several suicide attempts. Before coming to the GAMH, Bindu had been to a general hospital and had consulted several psychiatrists, a psychologist, and an astrologer and had been taken to Poonkudil Mana, a famous center where Namboodiri Brahmins combine Ayurveda and *mantravadam* (magic, sorcery) (Sax and Nair 2014).

Like most GAMH patients, Bindu was given *sarpagandha, a* "special powder", a mixture of powdered *sarpagandha* (Rauwolfia serpentina), *shankupushpa* (Clitoria ternatta), and *gokshura* (Tribulus terrestris) mixed with milk or honey. "All patients want this special powder," Dr. Sarasvati explained to me, "because the name itself suggests that it is something special, something specially powerful." *Sarpagandha* is used as a sedative, to induce sleep, and to control anger. *Shankupuspha* is a mind booster for the brain and is often given to children in Kerala to stimulate their intelligence.

Gokshura is a dehydrating and purifying diuretic that acts as an aphrodisiac and mind rejuvenating medicine. Taken together, the special powder has a calming effect that is seen as beneficial to the mental faculties. Bindu also had daily applications of *thalam* (oil application to the head) to counter the effects of *pittonmada* (*pitta*-related mental illness) and to induce sleep. She further received *dhumapanam* (medicinal smoking) each day. This is a treatment indicated for all diseases of the head, neck and mind, in which the patient inhales the smoke through a mixture of dried ingredients rolled together, usually through each nostril alternatively while exhaling through the other or through the mouth. The effect is described as eliminating *kapha* and pacifying *vata* and thus creates clarity of the mind and the sense organs and promotes a lightness of the head.

Doctors began Bindu's *shodana* (purification) treatment with *virechanam* (purging) to reduce symptoms, induce good sleep, improve calmness, and to make her more compliant. After virechanam, Bindu received fourteen days of *talapodichil*, literally "covering the head"); a medicated "mudpack" (Halliburton 2009) of Indian gooseberry (described in the canonical texts as rejuvenating) ground into a fine paste and soaked in whey or buttermilk overnight. Ayurvedic therapists apply it to the patient's head between the forehead and the top of the head, cover it with banana leaves, and leave it there for 45 minutes. They then remove and replace it by fresh paste and new leaves and kept in place for another 45 minutes. Finally, they remove the paste, and the patient bathes and washes the head with cold water. This treatment is not described in any of the canonical texts. Rather, it seems to be a part of folk medicine (*nadu marunnu*) in Kerala for "problems of the head" incorporated into the Ayurvedic treatment for mental diseases. A student once told me that there is a common joke in Kerala when somebody displays strange behaviour. People say: "It's time for *nellika thalam* [head application of Indian gooseberry]!"

Bindu told me that she liked *talapodichil* because it felt like it was cooling her mind and improved her sleep. It is cooling applications such as this that led Halliburton (2009) to argue that the Ayurvedic treatment for psycho-pathologies is perceived by patients as much more pleasant than mainstream psychiatric treatment, with its side-effect-heavy psychopharmaceuticals and unpleasant electroconvulsive therapy. Doctors at the GAMH applied *talapodichil* to all patients since it helped them maintain good hygiene because the procedure requires patients to wash their head and body daily. This in turn helps patients, they argue, to feel somewhat better. In this sense, doctors use *talapodichil* as a form of behavioural therapy. "It changes the behavioural pattern of the patients," Dr. Vidya said.

Following the *talapodichil* treatment and another day of purging, Bindu was given *snehapanam* (internal oleation), a preparatory procedure for further purification procedures. She had to drink daily doses of *ghrtam* (medicated ghee) starting with 50 mL and increasing daily by 50 mL up to a maximum of 300 mL per day. Doctors framed the effect of *snehapanam* in physiological terms as lubricating the *doshas* and toxins in the body in order to transport them into the gastrointestinal tract and stress the intelligence-boosting and brain nourishing qualities of the ghee.

Dr. Narayanan stressed the psychotherapeutic qualities of ghee. "If a person has a lot of anger and family quarrels, this ghee is very effective. It brings down the anger and helps the person to develop insight and to solve the problem." Similarly, Dr. Sarasvati: "If the quarrels in a family are the reason for the depression of a patient, counselling is not enough. You need some way of solving the problem in a pacifying way," she said referring not to psychotherapy or family counselling but to *snehapanam*. Rather than solving the problem in a purely psychological way, this approach favours addressing psychological and social problems on a physiological level (cf. Nichter 2002).

Snehapanam addresses key aspects of mental illness: embodied minds and social relations. It is interesting therefore to relate the Ayurvedic practice of *snehapanam* to a discussion of the Malayalam term *sneham* (care, affection, grease, unctuousness) (Halliburtion, this volume; Lang 2019). Osella and Osella (1996) use *sneham* to demonstrate how bodies and morals are intertwined in Kerala. *Sneham* denotes both a cooling lubricating fluid within the body and love and care for others. It can therefore be understood as a "bio-moral substance" (Osella and Osella 1996, 46), a quality both physiological and moral as a prerequisite of well-being. In both physiological and social contexts, a lack of *sneham* leads to *dosham* (problem, blockage) such as mental health problems, behavioural problems, lack of success in one's endeavours, or generally a difficult and frustrating life (ibid.). Although doctors did not talk explicitly about *snehapanam* in relation to this biomoral notion of *sneham*, they might be related and further studies are needed to explore the relationship of *snehapanam* to Malayali concepts of bodies, morals, care, and well being. The consumption of large quantities of ghee is difficult, and I suggest that these shared cultural assumptions regarding the beneficial effects of ghee and *sneham* for alleviating mental problems help patients to comply with this procedure. In Bindu's case, doctors had to stop the *snehapana* treatment because she had an aversion to it.

After a day of rest and another day of *svedana* (steam bath) to promote perspiration and further lubricate and purify the body channels, Bindu underwent *vamana* (therapeutic vomiting). She was given large quantities of milk and water along with medicine to induce intense vomiting. *Vamana* is applied to eliminate aggravated *kapha* from the body's channels, thereby purifying the mind (understood as a physiological substance). Doctors describe the effect of *vamana* as bringing clarity and calmness to the mind, brightening up the mind and cleansing the channels. Another effect is that *vamana* usually improves patient compliance for further treatment. Bindu was cooperative and did not resist treatment, but she found the *vamana* procedure very unpleasant, quite in contrast to the pleasant processes Halliburton describes. However, she told me that she felt calm afterward. In contrast to the Ayurvedic medical framing, many patients and their relatives understood *vamana* as a treatment for *kaivisham* (a local form of occult violence or sorcery), which they perceived as the cause of their problems. So doctors at GAMH do not only prescribe *vamana* for *kaphonmada* as per Ayurvedic theory. They also prescribe it for other patients with, as they express it, "a strong belief in *kaivisham*". For these patients and their families, the vomit is regarded as a sign that *kaivisham* has been expelled. This shows a significant difference between the way the treatments are conceptualised between practitioners and many of their patients (Lang 2018b).

Four days of observation followed, then Bindu was given two *thaila vastis* (oil enemas) and the day after, one *kashaya vasti* (enema with fermented decoction). There were two weeks remaining before the completion of her treatment and discharge from GAMH when I asked Bindu and her father Raman whether they felt the treatment was working. "Now she is 60 to 75 per cent cured, she is much better, we can feel it," said Raman. "80 per cent," Bindu corrected him. "What is the remaining 20 per cent?" I asked, engaging their quantitative estimation of Bindu's well-being. "Mentally I am very fine, but my body, I am fat," Bindu replied. After her treatment concluded, Bindu hoped to spend the holidays with her daughter and her parents and then go back to live with her husband. Her parents planned to visit regularly and take care of her.

Ayurvedic Psychiatry, Localisation and the Treatment Gap

Assembling local oral and textual and global bodies of knowledge and practice, Ayurvedic psychiatry provides treatment for a large number of patients in Kerala. Many Malayalis perceive Ayurveda as fitting their bodies and minds better than allopathic psychiatry that they perceive as powerful, efficacious, and quickly acting, yet also as weakening their bodies and imbued with side effects. The physio-moral approach to and the treatment of suffering embodied minds resonate with many Malayalis' ideas about embodied moral minds. While purifying treatments enable the mind conceptualised as subtle matter to flow smoothly, Ayurvedic psychotherapy aims to bring it in accordance with the moral order and streamline it according to local moral norms and ideas of the good life. Yet both are entangled and a purified physiology leads to healthy minds, as much as a morally sound life leads to a healthy physiological state.

The dynamic field of Ayurvedic psychiatry, described here with a focus on theorising and treating depression, transcends the binary between globalised Western psychiatry and local Ayurvedic psychiatry as radically different spaces and epistemologies. The case of Ayurvedic psychiatry shows how an indigenous medical field of knowing and treating mental health problems assembles parts of global psychiatry with local bodies and worlds while also resisting it. Ayurvedic psychiatrists incorporate and translate globalised psychiatry and psychology and at the same time frame Ayurveda as its alternative, stressing its epistemic difference, embodied alterity, and local appropriateness.[20]

Striving for globally scalable interventions – even if they are contingent universals (Bemme 2019) – has largely prevented the Movement for Global Mental Health from acknowledging the potential of indigenous medicinal knowledge and practices for local mental health care. The case of the well-established but highly dynamic field of Ayurvedic psychiatry shows how indigenous medicine engages global and local ways of knowing distressed minds, thereby escaping the strict designation as "local". Yet patients who seek Ayurvedic psychiatric care perceive Ayurveda as a traditional approach to mental health, fitting their distressed minds and suffering bodies better than allopathy. Although the hospital is not free from stigmatisation, patients in the Government Ayurveda Mental Hospital find the Ayurvedic treatment more pleasant, less intrusive and with lesser side effects than biopsychiatry. Ayurvedic psychiatrists in Kerala have formed an association to lobby for more state facilities and an increasing number of patients turn to Ayurvedic general physicians for signs and symptoms of depression. If the Movement aims at designing locally meaningful interventions, why not decisively promoting and investing in locally appropriate and even government-supported indigenous mental health care systems? With an increasing

---

20 This process happens without acknowledging that global psychiatry itself has become deeply suspicious of the validity of its own diagnostic categories (Frances 2013, Insel 2014) and forms of evidence-making through clinical trials (Healy 2004).

engagement of users of mental health services and established NGOs in the Movement there are already first signs of a slight turn of the tides when some South Asian members themselves are interested in traditional mental health care and local traditional approaches to mental health find their way into the publications (Patel et al. 2018) as complementary, rather than backward and human rights-violating.

References

Alter, Joseph S. 1999. "Heaps of Health, Metaphysical Fitness. Ayurveda and the Ontology of Good Health in Medical Anthropology." *Current Anthropology* 40 (Supplement): 43-66.

Anwar, Shaik. 2004. "A Study on Kaphonmada in Relation with Depressive Disorders." Doctor of Medicine (Ayurveda)." MD diss., P.S. Varier Ayurveda College Kottakkal.

Basu, Helene. 2014. "Davā and Duā. Negotiating Psychiatry and Ritual Healing of Madness." In *Asymmetrical Conversations. Contestations, Circumventions, and the Blurring of Therapeutic Boundaries*, edited by Harish Naraindas, Johannes Quack, and William S. Sax. New York, Oxford: Beghahn Books.

Bemme, Doerte. 2019. "Finding 'What Works': Theory of Change, Contingent Universals, and Virtuous Failure in Global Mental Health." *Culture, Medicine & Psychiatry* 43 (4): 574-95.

Chisholm, Dan, Kim Sweeny, Peter Sheehan, Bruce Rasmussen, Filip Smit, Pim Cuijpers, and Shekhar Saxena. 2016. "Scaling-Up Treatment of Depression and Anxiety: A Global Return on Investment Analysis." *The Lancet Psychiatry* 3 (5): 415-24.

Desjarlais, Robert. 1992. *Body and Emotion: The Aesthetics of Illness and Healing in the Nepal Himalayas*. Philadelphia: University of Pennsylvania Press.

Dumont, Louis. 1980. *Homo Hierarchicus. The Caste System and Its Implications*. Chicago & London: University of Chicago Press.

Ecks, Stefan. 2013. *Eating Drugs. Psychopharmaceutical Pluralism in South Asia Vol. 20*. New York: New York University Press.

Frances, Allen. 2013. *Saving Normal: An Insider's Revolt Against Out-Of-Control Psychiatric Diagnosis, DSM-5, Big Pharma, and the Medicalization of Ordinary Life*. New York: HarperCollins Publishers.

Giguère, Nadia. 2009. "Dosa, Satvabalam, Genes, and Pūjā. A God for Everything. An Ethnographic Study of a Government Ayurvedic Mental Hospital." In *Restoring Mental Health in India: Pluralistic Therapies and Concepts*, edited by Brigitte Sébastia, 48-70. Delhi: Oxford University Press.

Halliburton, Murphy. 2002. "Rethinking Anthropological Studies of the Body: Manas and Bodham in Kerala." *American Anthropologist* 104 (4): 1123-34.

—. 2009. *Mudpacks & Prozac. Experiencing Ayurvedic, Biomedical & Religious Healing*. Walnut Creek, CA: Left Coast Press.

Healy, David. 2004. *Let Them Eat Prozac: The Unhealthy Relationship Between the Pharmaceutical Industry and Depression (Medicine, Culture, and History)*. New York: New York University Press.

Insel, Thomas R. 2014. "The NIMH Research Domain Criteria (RDoC) Project: Precision Medicine for Psychiatry." *Am J Psychiatry* 171 (4): 395-97. doi: 10.1176/appi.ajp.2014.14020138.

Kohrt, Brandon A., and Ian Harper. 2008. "Navigating Diagnoses: Understanding Mind-Body Relations, Mental Health, and Stigma in Nepal." *Culture, Medicine & Psychiatry* 32: 462-91.

Lamb, Sarah. 2000. *White Saris and Sweet Mangoes. Aging, Gender, and Body in North India*. Berkeley, Los Angeles, London: University of California Press.

Lang, Claudia. 2018a. *Depression in Kerala. Ayurveda and Mental Health Care in 21st Century India, Routledge Studies in Health and Medical Anthropology*. Abingdon and New York: Routledge.

—. 2018b. "Translation and Purification: Ayurvedic Psychiatry, Allopathic Psychiatry, Spirits and Occult Violence in Kerala, South India." *Anthropology & Medicine* 25 (2): 141-161. doi: 10.1080/13648470.2017.1285001.

—. 2019. "Inspecting Mental Health. Depression, Surveillance and Care in Kerala, South India." *Culture, Medicine & Psychiatry* 43 (4): 596-612.

Lang, Claudia, and Eva Jansen. 2013. "Appropriating Depression: Biomedicalizing Ayurvedic Psychiatry in Kerala, India." *Medical Anthropology* 32 (1): 25-45.

Langford, Jean M. 2002. *Fluent Bodies. Ayurvedic Remedies for Postcolonial Imbalance*. Durham and London: Duke University Press.

Larson, Gerald James. 1969. *Classical Samkhya: An Interpretation of its History and Meaning*. Delhi: Motilal Banarsidass.

Marriott, McKim. 1976. "Hindu Transactions: Diversity Without Dualism." In *Transaction and Meaning: Directions in the Anthropology of Exchange and Symbolic Behaviour*, edited by Bruce Kapferer, 109-42. Philadelphia: Institute for the Study of Human Issues.

Marriott, McKim, and Ronald Inden. 1977. "Toward an Ethnosociology of South Asian Caste Systems." In *The New Wind. Changing Identities in South Asia*, edited by Kenneth David, 227-38. Berlin: Walter de Gruyter.

Mines, Mattison. 1994. *Public Faces, Private Voices. Community and Individuality in South India*. Berkeley: University of California Press.

Murray, Christopher J.L., and Alan D. Lopez, eds. 1996. *The Global Burden of Disease. A Comprehensive Assessment of Mortality and Disability from Diseases, Injuries, and Risk Factors in 1990 and Projected to 2020*. Geneva: World Health Organization.

Naraindas, Harish. 2014. "Nosopolitics. Epistemic Manging and the Creolization of Contemporary Ayurveda." In *Medical Pluralism and Homeopathy in India and Germany (1810-2010)*, edited by Martin Dinges, 105-36. Stuttgart: Franz Steiner Verlag.

Nichter, Mark. 2002. "The Political Ecology of Health in India: Indigestion as Sign and Symptom of Defective Modernization." In *Healing Powers and Modernity: Traditional Medicine, Shamanism, and Science in Asian Societies*, edited by L.H. Connor and G. Samuel, 85-106. Westport, CT: Bergin & Garvey.

Obeyesekere, Gananath. 1977. "The Theory and Practice of Psychological Medicine in the Ayurvedic Tradition." *Culture, Medicine, and Psychiatry* 1: 155-81.

Osella, Filippo, and Caroline Osella. 1996. "Articulation of Physical and Social Bodies in Kerala." *Contributions to Indian Sociology* 30 (1): 37-68.

Patel, Vikram, Shekhar Saxena, Crick Lund, Graham Thornicroft, Florence Baingana, Paul Bolton, Dan Chisholm, et al. 2018. "The Lancet Commission on Global Mental Health and Sustainable Development." *Lancet* 392 (10157): 1553-98. doi: 10.1016/S0140-6736(18)31612-X.

Patel, Vikram, and Graham Thornicroft. 2009. "Packages of Care for Mental, Neurological, and Substance Use Disorders in Low- and Middle-Income Countries: PLoS Medicine Series." *PLoS medicine* 6 (10): e1000160. doi: 10.1371/journal.pmed.1000160.

Rhodes, Lorna Amarasingham. 1980. "Movement Among Healers in Sri Lanka. A Case Study of a Sinhalese Patient." *Culture, Medicine, and Psychiatry* 4: 71-92.

Sax, William S. 2009. *God of Justice. Ritual Healing and Social Justice in the Central Himalayas.* New York: Oxford University Press.

Sax, William S., and Hari Kumar Bhaskaran Nair. 2014. "A Healing Practice in Kerala." In *Asymmetrical Conversations. Contestations, Circumventions, and the Blurring of Therapeutic Boundaries*, edited by Harish Naraindas, Johannes Quack, and William S. Sax, 200-36. New York, Oxford: Berghahn.

Sébastia, Brigitte. 2009. "Introduction. Restoring Mental Health in India. Pluralistic Therapies and Concepts." In *Restoring Mental Health in India. Pluralistic Therapies and Concepts*, edited by Brigitte Sébastia, 1-26. Delhi: Oxford University Press.

Smith, Frederick M. 2011. "Sattvāvajaya, Psychology, and Ritual Possession in India." *Asian Medicine* 6: 22-32.

Sundaran, K. 1993. *Manoroga Chikitsa Ayurvedathil (Treatment of Mental Diseases in Ayurveda)*. Unpublished Tranlation from Malayalam. Translated by Babu Appat. Kottakkal: Arya Vaidya Sala.

Zimmermann, Francis. 2014. "Medical Individualism and the Dividual Person." In *Asymmetrical Conversations. Contestations, Circumventions, and the Blurring of Therapeutic Boundaries*, edited by Harish Naraindas, Johannes Quack, and William S. Sax. New York, Oxford: Berghahn Books.

About the Author

CLAUDIA LANG is an associate professor (Heisenberg) of anthropology at University of Leipzig and research partner at the Max-Planck-Institute of Anthropology in Halle. Before, she was a postdoc at the ERC project "GLOBHELATH: From International Public Health to Global Health" in Paris, France. She works on the anthropology of health in India and has published on various topics, including traditional medicine, mental health, psychiatry, religion and ritual, health governance, and subjectivities. She is currently working on the digitization and proliferation of mental health and global psy in India's megacities, and on memories, traces, and genealogies of primary health care in Kerala. Her most recent publications include *Depression in Kerala: Ayurveda and Mental Health Care in India's 21st century* (2018) and a co-edited special issue of *Culture, Medicine and Psychiatry,* "Genealogies and Anthropologies of Global Mental Health" (2019).

9   Global Mental Therapy

William S. Sax

Abstract

There already exists a type of global mental therapy that has used by virtually everyone, in every culture and during all periods of human history: it is called 'ritual.' But this is not recognised by the MGHM, nor have the therapeutic aspects of ritual been adequately investigated by psychology and psychiatry, nor are these disciplines sufficiently aware of the degree to which their own practices are ritualised. Most advocates of Global Mental Health have an extremely limited understanding of what people throughout the world actually do when they experience extreme mental suffering: they perform rituals. What explains this lack of interest in what is likely the most ubiquitous type of global mental therapy? Why does the topic remain so woefully under-researched? Can "rituals" be effective in treating mental suffering, and if so, how? Drawing on several decades of ethnographic research on ritual healing in Asia, Africa, and Europe, I suggest a number of provisional answers to these questions.

Keywords: ritual, religion, science, medicine, traditional healing, exorcism, family

The Ubiquity of Ritual Healing

I write this chapter from the standpoint of a cultural anthropologist with a long-time interest in religion, ritual, and healing. Although traditional forms of healing for mental illness, including religion and ritual, are very widespread throughout the world, hardly any scientific studies have focused on them. The few studies that exist for India have concluded that around 80 per cent of the population makes use of religious healers for the treatment of mental health problems (Campion and Bhugra 1997; De Sousa and De Sousa 1984; Pakaslahti 1998; Quack 2012; Shah 1984). But pluralistic help-seeking

Sax, William, and Claudia Lang (eds), *The Movement for Global Mental Health: Critical Views from South and Southeast Asia.* Taylor & Francis Group, 2021
DOI: 10.5117/9789463721622_CH09

for mental disorders is by no means limited to India: around 25 per cent of psychiatric patients in the USA – including for example 43 per cent of patients with anxiety disorder (Bystritsky et al. 2012) and 53 per cent of patients with depression (Wu et al. 2007) – use Complementary or Alternative Medicine (CAM) to address their problems. A study from the UK found that 42 per cent of the people from the Indian subcontinent living in Britain seek help from a healer before coming into contact with mental health services (Singh et al. 2013). In the early 1990s, more than 30 per cent of 343 patients interviewed in Switzerland used ritual prayers and exorcism to counteract their diagnosed psychiatric problems (Pfeifer 1994); a similar study in the USA in the 1990s came up with a figure of 25 per cent (Eisenberg et al. 1993); other studies show a very high incidence of using religion for "coping" with mental illness (Kirov et al. 1998; Koenig et al. 1992; Tepper et al. 2001). A study published in *The Lancet* showed that "79% of the respondents believed that spiritual faith can help people recover from disease" (Sloan et al. 1999, 353, quoting from McNichol 1996). In another study of 157 hospitalised adults with moderate to high levels of pain, prayer was second only to medication (76 per cent vs. 82 per cent) as the most common self-reported means of controlling pain (Mueller et al. 2001). I could easily cite many more such studies.

Religious and/or ritual healing is quite possibly the most widespread – and probably the oldest – technique in the world for addressing mental problems, not only Asia but also in Europe and North America. Its ubiquity, along with evidence of its effectiveness (see below), raises a number of fascinating questions about the nature of mental illness, the relation of mind and body, and the use of non-scientific therapies. These are fundamental questions, and were they to be systematically pursued, they might lead to dramatic improvements in our understanding of mental disorders, and our therapies for them. But such questions are hardly addressed in the psychiatric literature.[1] Is it not obvious that a rational mental health policy, in India or elsewhere, should recognise the ubiquity of ritual and traditional healing and develop relevant policies concerning them? Perhaps, but this rarely occurs. On the contrary, both mainstream psychiatry and Departments of Health (along with the Global Mental Health movement) have been reluctant to conduct any research on traditional healing whatsoever, to say nothing of working with ritual healers in a mutually respectful manner or incorporating their methods.

---

1   They are certainly not addressed in the MGMH literature (e.g. Patel et al. 2014 and Sorel 2013). However, for exceptions within the psychiatric literature see Fallot 1998; Kaiser 2007; Koenig 2000, 2008; Muller et al. 2001; Pakaslahti 1998, 2009; Sax 2014 and Sloane et al. 2000.

Why is there such a lack of interest, and such a paucity of research, on this important topic? One reason is that the state and its public health apparatus, including those specialising in mental health, are structurally blind to the very existence of the myriad ritual healers in their midst. By "structurally blind" I mean that the epistemic practices of the state – the way it gathers and analyses information – prevent it from "seeing" (knowing, acknowledging) ritual healing. This first became clear to me when I visited Sri Lanka in 2002, and was discussing that country's health system with colleagues from the medical school. They boasted to me of how thorough their health statistics were, and told me that they had data on practically every visit to a doctor or a dentist throughout the country: the socio-cultural background of the patients, the reasons why they made these visits, the health outcomes, and so on. All of this was possible, they said, because they had inherited an excellent public health syste from the English, and Sri Lanka was after all a small island, relatively easy to administer. But when I asked them how many visits had been made to ritual healers, they shook their heads, puzzled that I would even ask such a question. Government departments of health don't count such things, even though individual psychologists and psychiatrists are more than capable of doing so (e.g. Kakar 1983; Pakaslahti 1998, 2009; Raguram et al. 2002).

In addition to the epistemological roots of the blindness of health authorities and of institutional psychiatry to ritual healing and its possible benefits, there are also philosophical grounds for neglecting these subjects. In the course of its development, modern medicine has adopted an increasingly materialist approach to its subject. This is as true of psychiatry – the branch of medicine that deals with diseases of the mind – as it is for any other medical sub-field. Roughly two centuries ago, European universities banished "soul" from the sciences, and "mind" is now emigrating to the Humanities faculties (where it can be safely ignored), leaving us only with a material "brain". Mainstream psychiatry has followed suit by transforming itself, in the final decades of the twentieth century, into a kind of "brain science" (Harrington 2019) whose methods depend on modern technologies of measurement. Armed with these methods, the medical sciences including psychiatry have been extraordinarily successful at uncovering the material and biological foundations of human life, but they have by the same token been rendered incapable of even posing questions about its meaning and significance. Psychiatry and psychology systematically subordinate hermeneutic, philosophical, and culture-historical inquiry to an overarching paradigm in which cognition, emotion, experience, and memory are understood as material, physiological, and above all *measurable* processes. Contemporary psychiatry seeks to stabilise a mechanistic and materialist model of human consciousness, and this involves the aggressive invasion of the human subject by sophisticated technologies of measurement, but never by means of religion or ritual. Such invasions are part of what the philosopher Ian Hacking (1995, 2002) calls the "looping effect": for psychology and psychiatry, this means the recursive and increasing use of testing, weighing, measuring, and medicating, which gradually leads human subjects to internalise the materialist model of consciousness upon which such methods are based, so that they increasingly come to understand themselves as machines with brains. Should we fully internalise this. model, what will happen to us? Will we become what Hacking calls a new "human kind"? The prospect is frightening.

But the state's inability to "see" the ritual practices of its citizens does not prevent medical scientists from speculating about them. The word "ritual" appears not infrequently in medical and psychiatric textbooks and scientific journals, where it is used to denote unreflective, habitual practices with no therapeutic value. The earliest such usage I have been able to find is from 1937, in an article entitled *Ritual Purgation in Modern Medicine*, published in *The Lancet* by L. J. Witts and his colleague, M. D. Manch, who argue that "much of the purging carried out by medical men to-day is rooted in archaic and primitive beliefs rather than physiology and pathology," and that doctors who perform purgation may be "exchanging the laboratory jacket of the twentieth century for the panoply of the witch doctor and the exorciser" (427). They conclude that "(t)he purgation of patients who are acutely ill or who are to undergo an operation is often a magic ritual rather than a rational treatment" (ibid.). Other, similar publications include that of Parker who argued in 1995 that many forms of infection control represent "ritual" rather than "reason", of Bolande who argued in the *New England Journal of Medicine* in 1969 that circumcision and tonsillectomy are both merely "ritualistic" and not truly therapeutic, and so on. Indeed, the meaning of the term "ritual" is so taken for granted by medical scientists, that it usually merits no discussion at all, appearing only in the titles of articles, as shorthand for an unscientific and ineffective practice that should be eliminated. Examples of such ostensibly useless practices include certain infection control procedures, shaving of the head completely before cranial surgery, "The Use of Random Biopsy Technique for Detecting Dysplasia in Patients with Colitis," "Lung Auscultation," the placing of a barrier between nursing supply bags and the tables on which they are placed, and the changing of Foley catheters on a regular basis in the absence of infection (Marion 2007; Schriger 2002; Russi 2005; Friedman and Rhinehart 2000).

In a 2002 article published in the *Journal of Advanced Nursing*, Philipin provides a useful chronological account of this literature in the field of nursing, pointing out that "the term [ritual] is often used in a pejorative sense and linked to unthinking, routinized action on the part of nurses" (144). Particularly influential here is Ford and Walsh's 1989 definition: "Ritual action implies carrying out a task without thinking it through in a problem-solving, logical way" (1989, ix, quoted at 145). Ford and Walsh later argue that both myths and rituals must be abandoned in order to progress to a "rational research-based footing" (ibid., 146). Elsewhere Walsh asserts that ritual consists of "traditions based on myths" which are "ritualistic and impractical" (ibid.). In their study of blood pressure measurement, O'Brien and Davison opine that ritual can be seen as "the antithesis of the problem-solving, holistic, research-based approach" (1994, 395, here cited 146). In this literature, the term "ritual" is not a topic of study or research, but only a pejorative term denoting practices considered by the author to be backward, archaic, unscientific etc. and therefore candidates for extirpation.

One might have expected psychiatry to show a more nuanced interest than other branches of medicine in the therapeutic use of non-scientific or traditional practices for relieving mental suffering: After all, they are widely used by their patients. But a search through the literature delivers slim pickings indeed. Anthropologists have compared psychoanalysis with ritual (Lévi-Strauss 2000 [1949]); Laderman 1988) but psychoanalysts have had surprisingly little to say about its therapeutic use. Ethnopsychiatrists (e.g. Devereaux and his followers) have been interested primarily in extending a Freudian approach outside of Europe, and those who went further by attempting to integrate rituals into their practice lost their professional standing, the best-known example being the French Ethnopsychiatrist Tobie Nathan (see Corin 1997).

Scientific discussion of the therapeutic use of ritual for mental illness has remained the provenance of anthropologists, and thus it is no surprise that psychiatrists who have made major contributions to this field have often been anthropologists as well, or have worked closely with anthropologists. The main contemporary examples would be Arthur Kleinman and his associates at Harvard University, Laurence Kirmayer and his colleagues in Montreal, and Sushrut Jadhav and Roland Littlewood and their circle in London. (Kirmayer and Jadhav are the editors, respectively, of the two journals where essays on this topic are most likely to appear these days: *Transcultural Psychiatry* and *Anthropology and Medicine*). Amongst public health psychiatrists, the leading figure is Joop de Jong from Amsterdam, founder and director of the Transcultural Psychosocial Organization (TPO), which has systematically made use of local healers in its provision of mental health and psychosocial services in more than twenty countries in Africa, Asia, and Europe.

Beyond this rather small circle of anthropologically-oriented psychiatrists is the great majority of their colleagues: health professionals who may well recognise that what they call "rituals" have some therapeutic value, perhaps as auxiliaries to mainstream (mostly psychopharmacological) treatment, but who would nevertheless be reluctant to explicitly recommend their use. This is true of the MGMH as well: Its advocates often claim that their movement is not about exporting Western therapies, but rather about providing "packages of care" developed in countries of the Global South. However, these "packages" always place the psychiatrist at the apex of the system, and none of them include the most prominent form of therapy in such countries: namely, religious rituals. Alternatives to psychopharmaceutical therapies are encouraged to a very limited extent, but nearly all of them originate within the disciplines of psychology and psychiatry, and virtually none are "indigenous." Local ideas are thought to consist of "metaphors and beliefs" rather than facts or knowledge, and the job of the mental health care worker is to ensure that those suffering from mental disorders comply with the psychiatric regime by "completing their homework" (Patel et al. 2018, 25).

When medical doctors and psychiatrists use the term "ritual" to denote unscientific and ineffective practices, they reiterate one the most widespread meanings of the term in German and English (and probably in other languages, too). In both languages, rituals are often described as "empty" or "meaningless," forms of habitual or prescribed action that have lost whatever significance they might once have had. A typical example is the German Chancellor Angela Merkel's remark that German-French relations have to do, "not with ritual, but rather with deep conviction".[2] In short, one popular meaning of the word "ritual" is "ineffective action," that is, action that is merely expressive and not instrumental, where the logical relation between means and ends is somehow problematic or unclear.

Anthropologists, too, tend to identify rituals in this way. Johannes Quack (personal communication) has noted that they normally identify a certain action or set of actions as "ritual" because of a hidden criterion, which is nothing other than the fact that the action in question seems somehow irrational, that it requires an explanation or an interpretation because it

2   "Es geht hier nicht um ein Ritual, sondern um die tiefe Überzeugung". (http://www.ta-gesschau.de/aktuell/meldungen/0,1185,OID4983142_TYP1_NAV_REF1,00.html), (http://www.sueddeutsche.de/deutschland/artikel/961/64897/print.html)

does not correspond to the anthropologist's ideas about cause and effect, or about the proper relation between means and ends. This is the great puzzle of ritual, and it is precisely what fascinates us: How can the natives believe that dancing makes it rain? Foucault defined the modern episteme as the conditions of possibility for what counts as scientific, and I am arguing that "ritual" is precisely the *negation* of this modern, scientific episteme – which is why psychiatrists find themselves unable to include rituals in their therapeutic regimes.

A similar point was made by Goody (1977) and by Lukes (1975), both of whom pointed out that in practice, the scholar of ritual recognises his object when he sees certain actions that seem disproportionate to their ostensible ends. In other words, when we see certain kinds of activities and beliefs that strike us as irrational, we label them "ritual" (ibid., 290). We do not say that driving an automobile or playing football or taking an examination are "rituals," even though they involve highly formal, rule-bound behaviour – we only refer to activities as "rituals" when the means they employ and the ends to which they are directed do not quite match up, when they do not correspond to our criteria of rationality, or better yet, of efficacy. It is precisely the assumed ineffectiveness of certain kinds of actions that make us regard them as rituals in the first place. In this sense, the definition of ritual found in medical journals is rather similar to that used (often implicitly) by anthropologists and others interested in the topic. The difference is that scholars of rituals regard them as fit objects of investigation; but they also tend to assume, like medical scientists, that rituals cannot be truly effective, and so their intellectual task consists in trying to find out rituals' hidden logic, their deeper meaning, which must certainly be other than the meaning reported by the natives, because *that* meaning strikes the scholars as irrational.

Such a dismissal of ritual by is thoroughly modern, in the way described so eloquently by Latour (2012), who shows how science constitutes itself precisely by means of identifying its own ritualistic, non-modern and non-rational practices, so that it can eliminate them. It searches out and destroys the markers of its own context, its cultural origins, its very history, thereby constituting itself as ahistorical, culture-free, and fundamentally rational. This is what Latour calls the "work of purification," and in this sense, the contributors to and editors of the medical journals are exemplary modernist "purifiers." This is not an easy job, since the rituals of medicine are, by definition, difficult to recognise. Shaving the heads of cranial surgery patients, placing a plastic bag underneath the visiting nurse's equipment bag, changing Foley catheters on a regular basis, and requiring birthing women to lay on their backs, are not seen as rituals but rather as rational techniques, at least until their non-rationality is exposed. The same is true of those other "natives" whose rituals we study in the jungles of New Guinea or amongst the peaks of the Himalayas. For them, the practices we call "rituals" are usually consistent with a cosmology, in terms of which they are logical and rational. And that is why "the natives," be they doctors or peasants, typically do not refer to such activities as "rituals," but rather as dancing, or healing, or technique, or simply as "work," as Raymond Firth (1967) pointed out in his classic ethnography of ritual, *The Work of the Gods in Tikopia*. To put it in a nutshell: what *we* see as ritual, *they* see as technique. That is because the term "ritual" is *our* term, not theirs, and it reflects *our* problem – how to classify a certain set of apparently irrational and/or ineffective practices. When we label something "ritual," we are making at the same time an ideological and an ontological claim, distinguishing "us" (modern and scientific) from "them" (non-modern and non-rational).

But What If ...

But what if the techniques that we label "rituals" do, in fact, work? One cannot easily respond this question without a definition of "ritual", and yet I have argued that there is no single "thing" that is denoted by the term "ritual" in standard English and German (and no doubt other languages as well); that what outsiders call "ritual" is often seen by insiders as "technique"; and that healing rituals in particular are normally defined negatively, in terms of what they are not: not modern, not scientific, and above all not efficacious, so that questions about their efficacy are self-contradictory. A further problem in defining "ritual" is that the actions for which we use the term are so various. Some so-called "rituals" are quite simple (a pinch of salt thrown over the shoulder), others are mind-bendingly complex (the elaborate offerings of the Balinese). Some are only momentary (bowing one's head or folding one's hands while passing a temple or shrine), others last a very long time (the presumably fictive 100-year-long rituals described in certain Hindu texts). Some take place regularly (five times a day, on Fridays, on Sundays, once a year) and others only occasionally (life-cycle rituals of birth, marriage, death). Rituals vary tremendously, not only along the dimensions of complexity, duration, and regularity, but also according to the gender, caste and class of the performer and the officiant, the resources available to perform them, and of course their purpose. For all these reasons and more, anthropologists and other scholars specialising in ritual studies have never been able to agree on definition of "ritual", even though they apparently know a ritual when they see one. And what they "see" is, to repeat, something irrational, ineffective, expressive but not instrumental, something where the means seem inappropriate to the ends. As Foucault might put it, "rituals" are understood as pre-modern and thus incompatible with the epistéme of the modern age, which has to do with the conditions of scientific truth.

But even though anthropologists can't agree on a definition of ritual, this doesn't stop them from explaining or interpreting what they regard as "rituals," usually in terms of "symbolic" meaning or social function. As we have already seen, this drive to decode the hidden meaning or function of ritual is a consequence of something more basic, which is the fact that a certain practice is identified as a ritual in the first place because the means it employs seem inadequate for the ends it pursues. Dancing can't make it rain, and praying can't cure disease. Or more likely, "the natives" can provide no reason for their actions, other than to say "We have always done it this way" – a typical response that drives the anthropologist into an interpretive frenzy. In other words, for those engaged in ritual studies, ritual raises the problems associated with the so-called "rationality debate" (Hollis and Lukes 1982). This debate takes different forms in disciplines as various as economics, cognitive science, and philosophy, and it lies at the heart of cultural anthropology, where I would frame the central question like this: "How does one explain the apparently irrational beliefs and actions of other cultures without asserting that they are primitive, or ignorant, or both?" Or like this: "Is rationality a single, universal thing, or do different cultures have different forms of rationality?"

The relevant issues emerge with startling clarity in the study of medicine and psychiatry where, by defining ritual explicitly as "non-effective action," mainstream scientists lead us straight to the problem of rationality and the apparent misfit between means and ends: Praying, they say, might make you feel better, but it cannot cure cholera. Exorcism is based on irrational superstition, and cannot cure schizophrenia. As I have shown above, a defini-tion of ritual as "non-effective technique," which pervades the medical and psychiatric literature, has the advantage of being reflexive: the "others" have their shamans and prayers; we have our head shavings, Foley catheters, and circumcisions. Once more: my argument is that in much scientific usage, and especially within medicine and psychiatry, the term *ritual* has no content. It only points to what these practices are *not*: not modern, not rational, not effective. Were we to take a truly anthropological perspective, and ask what these so-called "ritual" practices *are*, then we would have to stop using the term, not only because in most cases it has no translation equivalent, but also because we would discover that our term ritual points to so many things: attempts to influence the outer world (curing and healing, rain dancing); formal and public ceremonies confirming certain relationships (marriage, adulthood) or statuses (convicted, elected); methods for communicating with unseen beings (ancestors, gods); techniques for elevating one's own consciousness (meditation); and much more.

But let us return to what are called "rituals" of healing and ask: What if they do what the natives say they do? What if they truly heal... at least sometimes? The very few epidemiological studies of this topic conducted in India and elsewhere suggest that non-scientific, traditional or religious healing may indeed have therapeutic value, and they point to the urgent need for further research (Somasundaram 1973; Finkler 1985; Frank and Frank 1993; Jilek 1994; Kleinman 1980; Kleinman and Gale 1982; WHO 2002; Shields et al. 2016). Studies of what is called "ritual healing" throughout the world have been conducted by anthropologists for over a century, and provide rich anecdotal evidence for the claim that non-scientific, traditional or religious healing can sometimes be therapeutically effective. Many of these studies have been carried out in India (Basu 2009; Bellamy 2011; Flueckiger 2006; Kakar 1983; Sax 2015, 2014, 2009, 2004; Sax, Weinhold, and Schweitzer 2010; Sax and Quack 2010; Sax, Quack, and Weinhold 2010; Skultans 1987), but because they are almost exclusively qualitative and not epidemiological/quantitative, they have had little effect on mental health policy or on mainstream psychiatry.

The problem is not that we have no evidence that "rituals" heal: actually we have abundant evidence for that. Rather, the problem is that we have no plausible or acceptable theory for *how* they heal, because we have no shared agreement about what rituals *are*, and in the absence of such a theory, "ritual healing" has the same fate as homeopathy, or placebo: a scientific outcast shunned by most researchers, about which little research is done. In fact, the evidence suggests that many of the vast number of therapeutic techniques that we call "ritual" are indeed effective, but we have very little idea of how they work. Is it the herbs and other substances that the client/patient is required to ingest that do the healing? Has it to do with the body-mind's capacity to heal itself? Does it depend on the patient's faith and trust in the healer? Or perhaps on the healer's confidence in her own techniques? Do "rituals" heal because of the way they order and reorder worlds? My hunch is that all of these factors (and many more as well) play a role in the efficacy of various forms of what we call ritual healing, but because so little research has been done on this topic, it remains a hunch.

I can, however, offer rather more than a hunch with regard to my own research. In what follows, I describe two separate healing techniques, about each of which I conducted research for many years: healing through reconciliation in the Western Himalayas of North India, and healing through exorcism among Muslims in South Asia, North Africa, and the United Kingdom. In most of the cases, both Hindu and Muslim, someone was motivated by envy to engage a sorcerer to harm his enemy. Over the course of my research, I was disturbed to learn that this malevolent "someone" was usually from the same family as the victim. Despite constant and public professions of family unity and solidarity, despite the deep-seated belief that cursing others or employing sorcery against them is a terrible sin resulting in hellish punishments after death, and despite the fact that directing such black magic against family members is an even *more* heinous crime, nevertheless I was regularly told (by victims, sorcerers, priests, clerics, and healers) that most such attacks did indeed originate within the family. And after roughly twenty years of research on the topic, I have come to see that this is true.

Healing through Reconciliation in the Western Himalayas

For more than ten years I investigated a cult of ritual healing in the Western Himalayas of North India (Sax 2002, 2004, 2009a, 2009b, 2009c; Sax, Weinhold, and Schweitzer 2010).[3] In this cult, diagnosis and healing are clearly distinguished: When someone has an illness that cannot be medically diagnosed or cured, s/he typically visits an oracle to find out the cause of the problem, and the oracle may advise him or her to seek out a healer. Typical afflictions include fever, stomach ache, lack of energy, sleeplessness, sexual problems, and behavioural disturbances like involuntary possession, bouts of fear and panic, or excessive strife within the family. People also turn to local oracles for information about runaway children or stolen property, for help with problems connected to livestock (cows that do not give milk, barren sheep or goats, etc.), because of economic difficulties, or simply from a persistent run of bad luck. Already, we see an important difference between modern medicine and such forms of traditional or ritual healing, which often deal with all facets of the person, and not just somatic problems. In other words, the medicalisation of human suffering has only partially taken hold in the Western Himalayas. The oracles, most of who

3   The research was financed by the German Research Council.somesome

have undergone an initiatory illness,[4] are the vehicles of local deities, and answer clients' questions while in trance.

Clients are often impressed by the accuracy of the oracles, who seem to have intimate knowledge of their lives, which could only be obtained by supernatural means. But when I carefully examined transcripts of oracular consultations, it became clear that the oracles were *eliciting* information from clients, who were usually not aware that this was occurring. I believe that the oracles, too, were unaware of it, and that they did not consciously exploit the credulity of their patients, but rather perceived themselves to be vessels of the god or goddess, engaged in a conversation with the client; a mutual attempt to discover the causes of suffering.[5] Oracular consultation rests on the assumption that it is only the body of the oracle that is present, his "self" or "personality" having been temporarily replaced by that of the possessing agent. Elsewhere I have called this the "ideology of absence" (Sax 2015) and without it, the entire edifice would crumble. But clients are not so naive or incredulous as one might think: most believe that such diagnoses are never 100 per cent reliable, and so they typically "triangulate" them by consulting more than one oracle. Only when the client consistently receives a specific explanation for his troubles from multiple oracles does he take the next step, and seek out a healer. These healers are called *guru*s, not because they are spiritual masters, but rather because they are masters of the spirits. By dint of certain magical and liturgical practices, they are able to control and pacify afflicting spirits and deities, or transform them into deities or allies.

In most of the cases I documented – around 70 per cent – the oracle located the cause of affliction in episodes of strife within the family: The client had quarrelled with someone and been cursed by them; or perhaps it was a parent, an uncle or aunt, or even the grandparents or their antagonists who had quarrelled and uttered the curse. Cursing took a standard form, in which one's personal deity was asked to "take care of" the victim, usually by making them ill. Clients often denied having cursed anyone, or insisted that their parents or grandparents were not involved in such bitter quarrels. But the fact is that in the Western Himalayas, as elsewhere in the world,

---

4   The term "initiatory illness" refers to the extensively documented fact that many shamans and other ritual healers (and all of the oracles whom I studied) are inducted into this vocation only after they themselves have undergone ritual healing.

5   For an explicit discussion of this issue, see Sax 2009a, Chapter 3. Compare Levi-Strauss' classic discussion (1963, 175-85) of the Kwakiutl shaman Quesalid who, despite his self-conscious use of various techniques to "trick" patients and thereby increase their faith in his methods, nevertheless retained a strong belief in the efficaciousness of shamanism.

harsh words and threats of violence are rather common. Tension and strife within the family lead to physical and psychological affliction. Quarrels over land, jealousy at another's success, abuse and exploitation of young wives, conflict between the generations, pressure on young people to do well in school, demands that newly-married couples produce children – such forms of intra-familial tension were regularly identified during oracular consultations as the root *causes* of affliction, because they led one family member to curse another, whose subsequent illness and misfortune was attributed to the curse. Intra-familial tension was also understood to be a *symptom* of affliction: many clients complained of family disharmony, and visited an oracle precisely in order to discover its underlying causes.

Because the family was the locus of so much conflict, one of the very first questions asked by an oracle was, "Is the family united?" If the client answered "No", then the oracle could reasonably infer that the affliction had something to do with family discord, so that the next question was likely to be, "*Can* the family be united?" If the client still said "No", then the oracle could be fairly certain that there was serious conflict within the family. Such cases were usually associated with deep intransigence on the part of the quarrelling parties and with the practice of sorcery and black magic. If the quarrelling parties would or could not reconcile, then these dark practices proliferated, and often ended in tragedy and death. On the other hand, if the client replied that the family could indeed be united, the oracle would usually prescribe what can, for purposes of description, be called a "ritual" (a *puja*, literally a "worshipping" or "honouring" of the afflicting deity)[6] obliging relatives to pull together and cooperate closely. Funds had to be collected, the *guru* summoned, ritual articles like lamps and oil and coloured powder purchased, along with sacrificial animals and rare plants. Animals and insects had to be collected from the forest or the river, the house cleaned, and food and drink prepared, along with a hundred other tasks, large and small. Everyone contributed in a way that was appropriate to his or her gender, age, and position within the family. Close kin who had been absent for months or even years returned to the village, while nearby friends and relatives gathered to participate in the ritual and the feast with which it concluded. Family unity was emphasised, strengthened, and created anew in preparations for, as well as the performance of, the ritual, which involved numerous collective acts, for example tying the family together with a grass rope in order to demonstrate its unity. I am convinced that

6   See Witzel's comments at http://list.indology.info/pipermail/indology_list.indology.info/2001-December/026580.html.

in the very act of cooperating and working together to perform a ritual, families began a process of self-healing (Sax 2009a, Chapter 5, 2009b; Sax, Weinhold, and Schweitzer 2010). Family unity was thus not only a diagnostic principle: it was also a ritual principle, a therapeutic principle, and a moral principle. As a diagnostic principle, the presence or absence of family unity helped indicated a state of affliction. As a ritual principle, family unity was a necessary condition for conducting the ritual in the first place, and was embodied and performed at several points during the proceedings. As a therapeutic principle, it was taken to be the result of a successful healing ritual, and a sign of health. Finally, family unity was a moral principle, the violation of which could have deadly effects. In my 2009 monograph on this healing cult, I provided numerous examples of how symptoms were reduced or eliminated following such ritually mediated forms of what one might call "intra-familial *rapprochement*." Here is one such example, an abbreviated version of a much longer version found in the book:

> Mathura Lal was the younger of two brothers. His elder brother died, leaving behind two widows and five children. Three children were the offspring of the deceased elder brother's senior wife, and two were the offspring of his junior wife. After the senior wife died, the junior wife took good care of her own two children, but she didn't pay much attention to the three children of her deceased senior co-wife. One day Mathura Lal pointed this out to her. She became furious and called upon her god, saying, "God, my brother, you alone must look after me!" Fourteen years later, the god "seized" Sapna, the daughter of Mathura Lal's son, Makkhan Lal. The eight-year-old had agonising stomach pains, so bad that Makkhan Lal "thought that she would die", but the doctors could find nothing wrong with her. Her parents consulted many oracles, but received contradictory diagnoses of the causes of Sapna's problem. Finally, an oracle said that the curse of Mathura Lal's sister-in-law, fourteen years earlier, was the root cause of the girl's suffering. Makkhan Lal made a small offering to the god and vowed to worship him if he removed the affliction, and the girl's symptoms went away for three months. But Makkhan Lal was a poor man with insufficient money for the ritual, and the girl's pains returned. When I first met Makkhan Lal, he was planning to finally complete the ritual, and I was invited to observe (and contribute to the costs). Makkhan Lal had already had several oracular consultations, and had been told that in order to cure Sapna of her affliction he had to erect a shrine to the afflicting god in his house. A priest was summoned to conduct the ritual, during the course of which the ghost of the deceased junior wife – the one who

had uttered the curse – possessed Makkhan Lal's wife (Sapna's mother). The ghost kissed and hugged the children of the family, and reconciled herself with all of them, before she was exorcised Later the shrine of the god was built, the ritual was brought to a successful conclusion, and Sapna's symptoms disappeared, never to return.

This is all reminiscent of the standard anthropological argument that rituals re-establish, underline, and strengthen the social order. But while my argument does indeed resemble this argument, there is an important difference, which is that in this case, the ritual not only "strengthened the social order" by confirming the unity of the family; at the same time it *healed the patient*. How can we account for this? My central argument in *God of Justice* was that stress, tension, and unresolved conflicts continue to resonate within the family; that they have not only psychological effects but also physical ones, which tend to effect particular persons. In Family Therapy as practiced in Germany, such persons are called "index persons," and there are numerous similarities between Family Therapy and Garhwali oracular healing (see Sax, Weinhold, and Schweitzer 2010). Such persons absorb the negative consequences of conflicts that have not been resolved; perhaps not even recognised. Such repercussions – in this case, Sapna's stomach aches – are a kind of somatisation of conflicts that may have happened years or even decades previously. Ritual in this case heals a broken world/family by naming the conflict, settling it through a process of reconciliation, and re-establishing normative relationships.

Muslim Healing

From 2012 to 2015 I conducted research on Muslim Healing in the United Kingdom, with short research trips in India, Tunis, Sri Lanka and Bangladesh. I use the term "Muslim Healing" rather than "Islamic Healing" because, while there is no doubt that those amongst whom I conducted research were Muslims, the question whether the practices I documented are "Islamic" is controversial. Many Muslim reformers insist that certain practices (for example the use of amulets and the making of alliances with jinn) contravene the tenets of Islam, and campaign for their abolition.

In practice, Muslim healing amounts to exorcising malevolent jinn, battling against black magic, and counteracting the evil eye. The latter consists in the capacity to do harm by gazing enviously at another person, his property, wife, and so on, even though the person who envies another does not consciously intend any harm. Ideas about the damaging effects of envy are very widespread in all the Muslim cultures I know, along with practices to protect oneself from them. When one feels a twinge of envy, for example, one should mutter *mashallah* ("God willing") to protect the objects of one's envy from possible harm. One should also mutter the phrase before one eats, lest someone be affected by one's own envy – perhaps someone who has obtained a larger portion!

For pious Muslims there is no room for scepticism regarding the existence of jinn, since they are frequently mentioned in the Koran (the 72nd Sura is called *surat al-jinn*) as one of the three kinds of sentient beings created by Allah: angels from light, jinn from "smokeless fire," and human beings from clay. Like humans but unlike angels, the jinn possess free will. They have their own society, and are divided into communities of Hindus, Christians, Jews and Muslims. For humans, the most problematic aspect of the jinn is that although they are all around us and can see us, we cannot see them. The existence of black magic (*sihr*) is also uncontroversial and indeed, the Prophet himself is said in some reliable Hadiths to have been a victim of it (e.g. Bukhari 3175 and 5765).

Muslim healers exhibit great diversity in their attitudes toward the jinn. In Bradford, UK (often referred to by its Muslim residents as "Bradistan" because of its large Muslim population) I got to know a part-time bus driver who had educated himself regarding the jinn and become a modestly successful healer. He seemed to accept every report of jinn possession that reached his ears, without the tiniest shred of criticism or scepticism; asking himself neither if the person involved might be mentally disturbed, nor if he or she might have a medical problem. My patience for this healer finally ran out when I found myself sitting on the floor of my fancy hotel room along with him, his assistant, and the client, whose face he was continuously spraying with an atomiser containing holy water. This was meant to force the jinn to appear in the body of the client, but he was showing no signs of possession. His entire upper body was soaked with water, and the healer was blaming this lack of response on the duplicity of the jinn, when suddenly there was a knock at the door by a member of the hotel staff, who wanted to know what all the noise was about. What to do?

This (rather unsophisticated) healer's attitude was in stark contrast to that of the Koranic scholar living in Birmingham, who hailed from Egypt and had a modest healing practice to supplement his income from teaching Arabic at a local mosque. Perhaps the most learned of all the healers I met, he had obtained a degree in exorcism from the prestigious Al-Azhar University in Cairo. He told me that many of his cases did not involve jinn affliction, but rather social and familial problems: difficulties in school, or in marriage, or with the family. Just the previous week, he had been summoned to heal a new bride in the Bangladeshi family, but quickly realised that she was not suffering from jinn affliction at all, but rather from the most typical conflict in North Indian and Bangladeshi families: tension between daughter-in-law and mother-in-law. The exorcist ordered the family to leave the room and then spoke privately with the young woman, telling her that that he knew she was dissimulating. But when the family returned, he went through the exorcism anyway, because he knew from experience that this would help everyone to regain a sense of harmony and security. He told me that 90 per cent of his cases did not involve jinn possession at all, but rather social and familial problems of various kinds. (He promised however to let me know when he encountered a case belonging to the other 10 per cent.)

My point is that even among the healers, there is a wide range of attitudes regarding the jinn. The chief cleric of a Sufi mosque in a large city in Northern England said repeatedly that although, as a pious Muslim, he accepted the real existence of the jinn, nevertheless he had never seen a case of "true" jinn possession in his life. He repeated several times that he was a scientist like me – he had an undergraduate degree in psychology – and that those claiming to be affected by jinn or by black magic were simply suffering from "stress." (Later on, I discovered that he was in great demand as a practitioner of *jhadna* or "sweeping", a ubiquitous practice in North India and Pakistan where invisible, negative influences are "swept" from the body with a feather, while reciting powerful mantras or verses from the Koran.)

In September 2014 I visited a healer in a Muslim slum in the city of Pune, near Mumbai in Western India. He was a Hafiz, someone who had learned the Koran by heart, and the disciple of a Pir, a holy man of the Chishtiyya order of Sufis. Twice a week, the Hafiz would conduct healing sessions in a large first-floor room in the slum. Clients would tell him their problems and he would meditate until he "saw" what needed to be done. They complained of various kinds of sickness, chronic pain lasting for years, headache, backache, pain in the feet, sleeplessness, and other afflictions, and he would give them advice that was often rather pedestrian: They should see a doctor, they were not victims of witchcraft, they should sit and talk with the relatives with whom they were quarrelling. He also dispensed powerful amulets or *tawiz* that had been drawn by his spiritual guide, the Pir. After some time, when people began to go into trance and gyrate, call out, writhe on the floor, and so on, he would exorcise the jinn that were afflicting them by invoking the name of his Pir and commanding them to leave. Sometimes he would even "hang" the jinn with a tiny length of string twisted into the shape of a noose. I was struck by how often, following some particularly dramatic incident of possession or trance, he would "shift gears" as it were, and continue with the most mundane kinds of treatments: giving herbal remedies and distributing the amulets like candy. Were his treatments successful? Although I observed temporary relief of symptoms in these gatherings; I did not do the kind of follow-up study that would be necessary to demonstrate long-term recovery. Most members of the public seemed to regard him as an effective healer, judging from the size of the congregation. At the very least, one can say that he effectively met their needs: for healing, for solace, for companionship, for hope.

His gentle manner can be compared with that of Shaykh Ben Halima Abderraouf, whom I visited in 2014 at his healing centre in Tunis, along with my colleague Naz Hussain from the UK. The Shaykh has an international reputation, partly because of his sophisticated website and partly because he has developed a new form of exorcism, popularly known as "jinn catching," that appeals to many modern, urban Muslims. Normally, an exorcist has to struggle to compel a jinn to speak, and the entire process can be physically painful and emotionally draining for the patient. But in the Shaykh's new method the patient is passive and merely observes, while a Hafiz recites the Koran, and the catcher "catches"– one might say that he or she "channels" – the jinn. During my visit I noticed that nearly all the jinn "caught" by the Shaykh and his coterie of jinn-catchers were Christians, Jews, and Hindus. He said that this was only to be expected, since proper Muslim jinn would not harm anyone. Typically, the Shaykh interviewed the client, paying particular attention to their dreams, before the séance began. Once the jinn was "caught," he invited it to convert, which it could do by reciting (through the mouth of the "catcher") the Shahada, a verse affirming belief in Islam. At first the jinn would do so hesitantly and incorrectly, and its body, said Ben Halima, would be black and heavy. But as it continued, it would manage to recite the Shahada correctly, and its body would grow lighter, and whiter. But if it refused to convert, the Shaykh beheaded it by "chopping" its neck with short, gentle karate-like strokes. He would then "chop" its body into pieces and summon a number of (invisible) hellhounds to consume its corpse, so that it could never trouble anyone again.

The great majority of the Shaykh's clients came from Tunis or from neighbouring Algeria and Libya, although some came from Europe as well. Here are four examples of presenting symptoms, selected from the dozens of cases I observed in Tunis:

1   A man from England, mid-thirties, who was staying several weeks at the Shaykh's establishment. A history of drug abuse along with his

brother, he had strayed from religion but wished to be more observant and conquer his compulsive masturbation.

2   Married woman, 40 years of age, chronic bodily pain, vomiting, headache, and the feeling that someone was grabbing her feet and attacking her in her sleep. She reported that she awoke with scratches and wounds on her body, and a feeling of dizziness. She had suffered from stomach problems and a weak heart her whole life, and her prayers were disturbed on Saturdays and Sundays, but not on the holy day of Friday. She suffered from memory loss, heard voices, and had an "up and down" relationship with her husband. She likened them to "two different countries" and said that he was very disrespectful to her and their two children. She was afraid for the son, who was "always crying and cold, and continuously banged his head on the wall." He had done this since he was twelve years old, when he moved to the house where they live now, and fell down while sleeping. The son often found money in the house and told her, but the money would always disappear. People would come in her dream and strike her. She was often very angry. She thought about death while praying, and asked Allah to take her. She felt that her life was useless.

3   An unmarried working woman perhaps thirty years old suffered from chronic fatigue and nightmares. She dreamt that she was running but could not scream. There were animals in her dreams, snakes and cats, but also the Koran. She would see herself in the toilet, but the jinn would not leave her body. She also saw water in her dreams. She would be standing on the seashore with a Tsunami coming, but did not fall. She said that she got angry a lot. Recently she had suffered from lack of energy and did not want to go to work. She thought a lot about death. She was unmarried because several suitors never completed their respective contracts. Money "did not stay with her." She reported pain and migraine headaches, that half of her face was always tired, and that she had low blood pressure, occasional heart pains, stomach pains, frequent vomiting, and that every third menstrual period was painful.

4   A married couple, the man perhaps 30 years old, the woman early twenties. She had been plagued by fears since she was twelve years old. She was brilliant at school, but began waking at night with panic. She could not read any more, could not concentrate. She stopped school for a year and then began again, but she was not such a good student as before, and only went for the exams. Three or four times a year she would get very ill. She reported stomach pain, stabbing pains in her heart, menstrual

period pain, pain in her legs, and severe foot pain, sometimes so intense that she would weep. In her dreams, she was sometimes wearing a wedding dress and running. She dreamt of tigers, water, blood, toilets. Occasionally she had sexual dreams, or saw her own teeth "coming down." She said that she had a very bad temper. She was studying English literature and civilisation and passing, but was bored and "couldn't be bothered" with her studies. She tried not to think about death, since the topic frightened her. But thoughts of death kept returning and she would weep and scream, sometimes day and night. When the Shaykh asked about her marital status, she began to weep, and reported that it was not working out. She had problems, and took anti-depressants. The woman's English was self-taught. At the age of twelve she had prayed a lot, and made many visits to hospital, took different anti-depressants. She had not seen her mother from the age of one-and-a-half until she was fourteen. The mother had rejected Islam, was officially Catholic and said that she believed in God, but in the girl's view she didn't. When the girl was young, her mother had given her books on magic, and she thought that this was intended to wean her away from Islam. The Shaykh said that this was probably the point where the jinn were sent to afflict her.

I was struck by the profound similarities between these two types of healing, one from the Muslim world and another found amongst West Himalayan Hindu peasants. Although both Hindus and Muslims believe that supernatural beings sometimes choose their victims for personal reasons (e.g. because the victim offended them by treading on their shrines or otherwise polluting them, or perhaps just out of spite), nevertheless such cases are rare. It is much more common for a human enemy to attack his victim by sending a jinn, demon, or other spirit to afflict him, even though this is regarded as a highly immoral act. But in either case, the immediate and primary cause of the patient's suffering is an external agent: a jinn, a ghost, a demon. This agent is an "other" to the patient, and the healing is effected by blocking, pacifying, or simply killing it, although of course this does not eliminate the enmity that lies behind the jinn attack. The idea of an external and hostile agent makes of the patient a victim, with all of the moral implications associated with that role, and if this hostile agent has been sent by a human enemy or even a relative, then the patient's victimhood is even more strongly emphasised. Such a constellation is very common in traditional healing, and clearly has its uses: As anthropologists have often noted, it relieves the patient from personal responsibility for his suffering, which s/he instead projects onto a supernatural "other."

But similarities between Hindu and Muslim healing go only so far, and there are important differences as well. While the Muslim healers tend to kill (by hanging, beheading, chopping into pieces) the afflicting jinn, Indian Hindus are more likely to pacify it with offerings and gifts, or transform it into a benevolent spirit or ancestor. My colleague Annette Hornbacher suggests that in Bali there is yet another variation on this model: There, when one is afflicted by black magic, the typical response is neither to annihilate the spirit nor to "fight back" with counter-magic, but rather to try and understand what one has done in the first place to make oneself vulnerable. In other words, the illness is seen as an opportunity to lead a more pure, spiritual, and "moral" life. The Balinese say that this is a practical way to proceed, since one has little influence over the actions of an attacker, even if he or she is from one's own family.[7]

Amongst all the groups mentioned – West Himalayan Hindu peasants, British Muslims, South Asian Sufis, North African Muslims, and Balinese Hindus – one particular contradiction kept emerging. On the one hand, most traditional families from these regions are intensely solidary, and family members support each other as much as they can. All those stories about the eldest brother working at a terrible job so that the youngest brother can go to college, or people making tremendous sacrifices so that one of their family members can have an important operation, are not "fake news". No, these are real people making real sacrifices. In many if not most traditional societies, the family is indeed one's greatest and most reliable source of moral and material support. But the family is also associated with a reservoir of repressed feelings: envy, anger, resentment and so on. If you make colossal sacrifices for your younger sibling out of a sense of duty, but secretly feel that you were the worthier recipient of support, then your anger and resentment may be great. If the person whom you helped later betrays you or fails to help you in your time of need, you may be tempted to take revenge.

And so, embroiled in such negative emotions and moral contradictions, clients visit the healer. They reveal their physical and mental sufferings, hoping and praying to be healed. Are they suffering from mental disorders? The answer to that question depends entirely on how one defines the term. How often are their sufferings relieved by the healer? I cannot say, because I have not conducted any follow-up studies. But certainly such healers represent a very widely used resource, and it behooves us, not only to better

7   See Hornbacher's (2010) description of the Balinese reaction to the Islamist attack of 2002, which has inspired my interpretation of ritual healing.

understand their techniques, but also to investigate the degree to which they are effective in reducing suffering.

Rituals of Medicine

The theory and practice of modern medicine is based on a set of mechanistic and materialist assumptions that are quite different from those of traditional healing. The "machine" of the body may be damaged or weakened by external agents like viruses or bacteria, or it may be defective because of heredity, or it may have been damaged by an accident, or by external conditions like malnutrition or an extreme climate, but in all these cases, the cause of illness is to be understood in material and not moral terms. For mainstream psychiatry as well, mental illness is a kind of "brain disease" that may have a number of causes – heredity, an accident, the influence of toxic substances, etc. – and the proper response is to try and re-establish the chemical balance of the brain, usually with drugs (Moncrieff 2008).

Sophisticated approaches to the aetiology of mental illness recognise that it is caused by a mix of biological and environmental factors related to lifestyle, relationships, support networks and so on, but even such a "mixed" aetiology pays little attention to the moral subjectivities of those suffering from mental disorders, and research on this topic is dwarfed by neuropsychiatric (read: mechanistic and materialist) approaches. Morality – by which I mean judgements of right and wrong, good and evil – plays a minor role in mainstream medicine and psychiatry; and unseen agents like ghosts, demons, and jinn play no role at all, except as elements of a non-or pre-scientific worldview based upon mistaken ideas of causation. Similarly, the non-scientific therapies that we call "rituals" are thought to be helpful only insofar as they help the patient relax, increase his confidence, and so on.

But perhaps the moral and affective qualities of one's relationships play a much larger role in healing than we realise, and perhaps this is also true of conventional medicine and psychiatry. Perhaps envy, cursing, black magic, and the like really can be causal vectors of physical and mental illness. Such ideas are strongly supported by research on placebos and the "placebo effect". Indeed, placebo is like ritual in several senses: both terms refer to something that is thought to be inherently non-effective, even though there is much evidence showing that both placebos and "rituals" (non-scientific, often religious, therapies) are in fact quite powerful, sometimes even more powerful than mainstream biomedical techniques and medications. The medical anthropologist Daniel Moermann has written a wonderful, short book on the topic entitled *Meaning, Medicine, and the Placebo Effect* (2002) in which he has assembled evidence from dozens of rigorous experimental trials that show precisely this. He summarises the literature on a large number of such cases, and comes to the conclusion that we should avoid term "placebo" altogether, just as I argued above that we should avoid the term "ritual." Why? Because although both terms refer to something that is not effective, the evidence shows that they are highly effective: Indeed, placebos are often more effective than the medications themselves. Moermann argues that we should therefore replace the word "placebo" with the term "meaning effect". In other words, he argues that the meaningful, social aspects of healing, and above all the patient's faith in the therapy, accounts for a significant proportion of all medical cures. Perhaps one could add "ritual healings" as well.

Moermann's book is full of fascinating examples, but to me the most interesting of all was the experiment performed on a group of dentists who thought that they were participating in a study of placebos, and did not know that they themselves were the objects of the study. The experiment had to do with painkillers administered after the patients' wisdom teeth had been removed. During the first trial, dentists believed that they were administering only placebos, and in the second trial, they believed they were administering a mix of placebo and real medication. In fact, in both trials both kinds of drugs where being administered, so that all four possibilities were tested: administering the "real" painkiller while thinking it was "real"; administering the "false" painkiller while thinking it was "real"; administering the "false" painkiller while thinking it was "real"; and administering the "false" painkiller while thinking it was "false". The experiment clearly showed that the doctors' own beliefs regarding whether or not they were administering placebos was a highly significant factor in the efficacy of the treatment. Somehow, this belief was communicated to the patient, who then experienced more effective pain relief as a result. But the placebo effect has received very little attention by psychiatric research, despite its clear effectiveness. Harrington cites one highly-regarded study which showed that 75 per cent of the improvement shown by patients taking the active medication against depression could be attributed to the so-called "placebo effect" (2019, 262-64). Moermann concludes that the self-healing properties of the human body are much greater than we previously realised, and that these are somehow triggered by the healer's confidence in his or her therapeutic technique. I think that this has important implications for the study of ritual healing. Clearly, much of it is intended to inspire the patient with confidence, not only in Asia but also in our own hospitals with their healing rituals: the special costumes, the ritualised language, the position of the body, and so on.

What has all this to do with the Movement for Global Mental Health? First of all, let me be very clear: I am not advocating that mental health workers in South Asia or anywhere else begin practicing jinn exorcism or establishing shrines for local deities. My intention is rather twofold: (1) to show that there is a chasm between what the MGMH would have people do when they experience "mental disorders" and what they really do; and (2) to suggest that in developing its diagnostic and therapeutic programs, the MGMH should consider drawing upon paradigms that originate within South Asia rather than, in perfectly neocolonial fashion, taking all its theories and therapies from "the West." Is it possible to conceptualise mental health interventions that truly take local ideas and experiences into account, and to do so in an ethical and scientifically responsible way? Until now, the gestures of the MGMH in this direction have been superficial at best.

Medical knowledge and practice changes and develops over time, and it would be irrational to claim that medical scientists have learned everything there is to know about health, illness, and their causes. Bloodletting was once regarded as rational and scientific, but has now fallen into disfavour, while new theories and discoveries such as those of Pasteur took some time to be accepted by the scientific and medical communities. Inevitably, many therapies in use today will one day be looked back upon as irrational "rituals." Many aspects of current obstetrical practice (for example, the horizontal position of the birthing mother, the use of stirrups, the over-use of Caesarean sections) are already widely regarded as techniques that served social purposes, but not medical ones. On the other hand, we may one day understand why it is that going on a pilgrimage, worshipping one's ancestors, exorcising the presumptive external agent of disease, or reconciling the family by means of ritual helps to reduce mental suffering. There are already some fascinating moves in this direction: various studies of the poorly-understood and misleadingly-named "placebo effect"; the effects of dramatic rituals on human cognition (Whitehouse 2004); research on mirror neurons, which shows how the body reorganises itself according to experience. What all of these studies point to is the close dependence of human health on all aspects of our experience, psychological and social as well as somatic. They suggest that a truly empirical psychiatry must reject a radical separation of nature from culture, and of mind from body. Modern science has devoted enormous amounts of intellectual energy and physical resources to prying them apart. It is time to take up the challenging task of stitching them back together. Global Mental Health would be a good place to start.

References

Basu, Helene. 2009. "Contested Practices of Control: Psychiatric and Religious Mental Health Care in India." *Curare* 32 (1+2): 28-39.

Bell, Catherine. 1992. *Ritual Theory, Ritual Practice.* New York: Oxford University Press.

Bellamy, Carla. 2011. *The Powerful Ephemeral: Everyday Healing in an Ambiguously Islamic Place.* Berkeley: University of California Press.

Bolande, Robert P. 1969. "Ritualistic Surgery: Circumcision and Tonsillectomy." *New England Journal of Medicine* 280 (11): 591-96.

Bystritsky, Alexander, Sarit Hovav, Cathy Sherbourne, Murray B. Stein,, Raphael D. Rose, Laura Campbell-Sills, Daniela Golinelli, et al. 2012. "Use of Complementary and Alternative Medicine in a Large Sample of Anxiety Patients." *Psychosomatics* 53 (3): 266-72. doi: 10.1016/j.psym.2011.11.009.

Campion, Jonathan and Dinesh Bhugra. 1997. "Experiences of Religious Healing in Psychiatric Patients in South India." *Social Psychiatry and Psychiatric Epidemiology* 32 (4): 215-21.

Corin, Ellen. 1997. "Playing with Limits: Tobie Nathan's Evolving Paradigm in Ethnopsychiatry." *Transcultural Psychiatry* 34 (3): 345-58.

De Sousa, Alan, and D. A. De Sousa. 1984. "My India, our India." In *Psychiatry in India*, edited by Alan De Sousa and D.A. De Sousa, 1-12. Bombay: Bhalani.

Eisenberg, David M., Ronald C. Kessler, Cindy Foster, Frances E. Norlock, David R. Calkins, and Thomas L. Delbanco. 1993. "Unconventional Medicine in the United States: Prevalence, Costs, and Patterns of Use." *New England Journal of Medicine* 328 (4): 246-52.

Fallot, Roger D. 1998. "The Place of Spirituality and Religion in Mental Health Services." *New Directions for Mental Health Services* 1998 (80): 3-12.

Finkler, Kaja. 1985. *Spiritualist Healers in Mexico.* New York: Praeger Publishers.

Firth, Raymond. 1967. *The Work of the Gods in Tikopia.* London: The Athlone Press.

Flueckiger, Joyce B. 2006. *In Amma's Healing Room. Gender and Vernacular Islam in South India.* Bloomington: Indiana University Press.

Ford, Pauline, and Mike Walsh. 1989. *Nursing Rituals, Research and Rational Actions.* Oxford: Butterworth-Heinemann.

Frank, Jerome D., and Julia R. Frank. 1993. *Persuasion and Healing. A Comparative Study of Psychotherapy.* Baltimore, MD: John Hopkins University Press.

Friedman, Mary M., and Emily Rhinehart. 2000. "Improving Infection Control in Home Care: From Ritual to Science-Based Practice." *Home Healthcare Now* 18 (2): 99-105.

Goody, Jack. 1977. "Against Ritual: Loosely Structured Thoughts on a Loosely Defined Topic." In *Secular ritual,* edited by Sally Falk Moore and Barbara G. Myerhoff. Assen/Amsterdam: Van Gorcum.

Hacking, Ian. 1995. "The Looping Effect of Human Kinds." In *Causal Cognition: A Multidisciplinary Debate*, edited by Dan Sperber, David Premack, and Ann James Premack. New York: Oxford University Press.

—. 2002. *Historical Ontology*. Cambridge, MA: Harvard University Press.

Harrington, Anne. 2019. *Mind Fixers: Psychiatry's Troubled Search for the Biology of Mental Illness*. New York: W.W. Norton & Company.

Hollis, Martin, and Steven Lukes. 1982. *Rationality and Relativism*. Cambridge, MA: MIT Press

Jilek, Wolfgang G. 1994. "Traditional Healing in the Prevention and Treatment of Alcohol and Drug Abuse." *Transcultural Psychiatric Research Review* 31 (3): 219-58.

Kaiser, Peter. 2007. *Religion in der Psychiatrie: Eine (un)bewusste Verdrängung?* Göttingen, Germany: V&R unipress.

Kakar, Sudhir. 1983. *Shamans, Mystics and Healers. A Psychological Enquiry into India and Its Healing Traditions*. Oxford: Oxford University Press.

Kirov, George, Roisin Kemp, Kiril Kirov and Anthony S. David. 1998. "Religious Faith after Psychotic Illness." *Psychopathology* 31 (5): 234-45.

Kleinman, Arthur. 1980. *Patients and Healers in the Context of Culture*. Berkeley: University of California Press.

Kleinman, Arthur and James L. Gale. 1982. "Patients Treated by Physicians and Folk Healers: A Comparative Outcome Study in Taiwan." *Culture, Medicine and Psychiatry* 6 (4): 405-20.

Koenig, Harold G., Harvey J. Cohen, Dan G. Blazer, Carl Pieper, Keith G. Meador, Frank Shelp, Veeraindar Goli, and Bob DiPasquale. 1992. "Religious Coping and Depression among Elderly, Hospitalized Medically Ill Men." *American Journal of Psychiatry* 149 (12): 1693-700.

Koenig, Harold G. 2008. "Religion and Mental Health: What Should Psychiatrists Do?" *Psychiatric Bulletin* 32 (6): 201-03.

Laderman, Carol. 1988. "Wayward Winds: Malay Archetypes, and Theory of Personality in the Context of Shamanism." *Social Science & Medicine* 27 (8): 799-810.

Latour, Bruno. 2012. *We Have Never Been Modern*. Cambridge, MA: Harvard University Press.

Lévi-Strauss, Claude. 2000 [1949]. "The Effectiveness of Symbols." In: *Cultural Psychiatry and Medical Anthropology: An Introduction and Reader*, edited by Roland Littlewood and Simon Dein, 162-178. London: The Athlone Press.

Lukes, Steven. 1975. "Political Ritual and Social Integration." *Sociology* 9 (2): 289-308.

Marion, James F. 2007. "An Expensive and Empty Ritual: The Continued Use of Random Biopsy Technique for Detecting Dysplasia in Patients with Colitis." *Inflammatory Bowel Diseases* 13 (10): 1271-72.

McNichol, Tom. 1996. "The New Faith in Medicine." *USA Today Weekend*, 5-7 April 1996.

Moncrieff, Joanna. 2008. *The Myth of the Chemical Cure: A Critique of Psychiatric Drug Treatment.* London: Palgrave Macmillan.

Moerman, Daniel E. 2002. *Meaning, Medicine, and the "Placebo Effect".* Cambridge: Cambridge University Press.

Mueller, Paul S., David J. Plevak and Teresa A. Rummans. 2001. "Religious Involvement, Spirituality, and Medicine: Implications for Clinical Practice." *Mayo Clinic Proceedings* 76 (12): 1225-35.

O'Brien, Daniel and Maria Davison. 1994. "Blood Pressure Measurement: Rational and Ritual Actions." *British Journal of Nursing* 3 (8): 393-96.

Pakaslahti, Antti. 1998. "Family Centered Treatment of Mental Health Problems at the Balaji Temple in Rajasthan." In *Changing Patterns of Family and Kinship in South Asia: Proceedings of an International Symposium on the Occasion of the 50th Anniversary of India's Independence Held at the University of Helsinki,* 6 May 1998, edited by Asko S. Parpola and Sirpa Tenhumen, 129-68. Helsinki: Finnish Oriental Society.

Pakaslahti, Antti. 2009. "Health-Seeking Behaviour for Psychiatric Disorders in North-India." In *Psychiatrists and Traditional Healers: Unwitting Partners in Global Mental Health,* edited by Mario Incayawar, Ronald Wintrob, and Lise Bouchard, 149-66. Oxford, UK: Wiley-Blackwell.

Parker, Lynn. 1999. "Infection Control: Ritual or Reason?" *Nursing Times* 95 (20): 60-63.

Patel, Vikram, Harry Minas, Alex Cohen, and Martin Prince. 2013. *Global Mental Health: Principles and Practice.* Oxford: Oxford University Press.

Patel, Vikram, Shekhar Saxena, Crick Lund, Graham Thornicroft, Florence Baigana, Paul Bolton, Dan Chisholm, Pamela Y. Collins, et al. 2018. "The Lancet Commission on Global Mental Health and Sustainable Development." *The Lancet* 392 (10157): 1553-98.

Pfeifer Samuel. 1994. "Belief in Demons and Exorcism in Psychiatric Patients in Switzerland." *British Journal of Medical Psychology* 67 (3): 247-58.

Philipin, Susan M. 2002. "Rituals and Nursing: A Critical Commentary." *Journal of Advanced Nursing* 38 (2): 144-51.

Quack, Johannes. 2012. "Ignorance and Utilization: Mental Health Care outside the Purview of the Indian State." *Anthropology & Medicine* 9 (3): 277-90.

Raguram, Ramanathan, A. Venkateswaran, Jayashree Ramakrishna, and Mitchell G. Weiss. 2002. "Traditional community resources for mental health: A report of temple healing from India." *British Medical Journal,* 325 (7354): 38-40.

Russi, Erich W. 2005. "Lung Auscultation – a Useless Ritual?" *Swiss Medical Weekly* 135 (35/36): 513-14.

Sax, William S. 2002. "Heilungsrituale: Ein kritischer performativer Ansatz." *Paragrana* 12 (1-2): 385-404.

—. 2004. "Healing Rituals: A Critical Performative Approach." *Anthropology and Medicine* 11 (3): 293-306.

—. 2009a. *God of Justice: Ritual Healing in the Central Himalaya.* New York: Oxford University Press.

—. 2009b. "'I Have No One!' Ritual Healing and Family Relationships in Garhwal." In *Divins Remèdes. Médecine et Religion en Asie du Sud,* edited by Caterina Guenzi, and Ines Zupanov, 359. Éditions de l'École des Hautes Études en Sciences Sociales.

—. 2009c. "Performing God's Body." *Paragrana* 18 (1): 165-87.

—. 2014. "Ritual Healing and Mental Health in India." *Transcultural Psychiatry* 51 (6): 829-49.

—. 2015. "Gods of Justice." In *The Law of Possession: Ritual, Healing, and the Secular State,* edited by William S. Sax and Helene Basu, 227-48. New York: Oxford University Press.

Sax, William S., and Johannes Quack. 2010. "Introduction: The Efficacy of Rituals." *The Journal of Ritual Studies* 24 (1): 5-12.

Sax, William S., Johannes Quack, and Jan Weinhold, eds. 2010. *The Problem of Ritual Efficacy.* New York: Oxford University Press.

Sax, William S., Jan Weinhold, and Jochen Schweitzer. 2010. "Ritual Healing East and West: A Comparison of Ritual Healing in the Garhwal Himalayas and Family Constellation in Germany." *The Journal of Ritual Studies* 24 (1): 61-77.

Sax, William S., and Helen Basu, eds. 2015. *The Law of Possession: Ritual, Healing, and the Secular State.* New York: Oxford University Press.

Schriger, David L. 2002. "Problems with Current Methods of Data Analysis and Reporting, and Suggestions for Moving beyond Incorrect Ritual." *European Journal of Emergency Medicine* 9 (2): 203-07.

Shah, V.D. 1984. "Mental Health Service in India." In *Psychiatry in India*, edited by Alan De Sousa and D.A. De Sousa, 733-56. Bombay: Bhalani.

Shields, Laura, Ajay Chauhan, Ravindra Bakre, Milesh Hamlai, Durwin Lynch, Joske Bunders. 2016. "How Can Mental Health and Faith-Based Practitioners Work Together? a Case Study of Collaborative Mental Health in Gujarat, India." *Transcultural Psychiatry* 53 (3): 368-91.

Skultans, Vieda, 1987. "The Management of Mental Illness among Maharashtrian Families: A Case Study of a Mahanubhav Healing Temple." *Man* 22 (4): 661-79.

Sloan, Richard P., Emilia Bagiella, and Tia Powell. 1999. "Religion, Spirituality, and Medicine." *The Lancet* 353 (9153): 664-67.

Sloan, Richard P., Emilia Bagiella, Larry VandeCreek, Margot Hover, Carlo Casalone, Trudi J. Hirsch, Yusuf Hasan, and Ralph Kreger. 2000. "Should Physicians Prescribe Religious Activities?" *New England Journal of Medicine* 342 (25): 1913-16.

Somasundaram, O. 1973. "Religious Treatment of Mental Illness in Tamil Nadu." *Indian Journal of Psychiatry* 15:38-48.

Sorel, Eliot. 2013. *21st Century Global Mental Health*. Burlington, MA: Jones & Bartlett Learning.

Tepper, Leslie, Steven A. Rogers, Esther M. Coleman, and H. Newton Malony. 2001. "The Prevalence of Religious Coping among Persons with Persistent Mental Illness." *Psychiatric Service* 52 (5): 660-65.

Whitehouse, Harvey. 2004. *Modes of Religiosity: A Cognitive Theory of Religious Transmission*. Lanham, MD: AltaMira Press.

World Health Organization. Programme on Traditional Medicine. 2002. *WHO Traditional Medicine Strategy 2002-2005*. Geneva: World Health Organization. https://apps.who.int/iris/handle/10665/67163.

Witts, Leslie J. 1937. "Ritual Purgation in Modern Medicine." *The Lancet* 229 (5921): 427-31.

Wu, Ping, Cordelia Fuller, Xinhua Liu, Hsin Chien Lee, Bin Fan, Christina W. Hoven, Donald Mandell, Christine Wade, and Fredi Kronenberg. 2007. "Use of Complementary and Alternative Medicine among Women with Depression: Results of a National Survey." *Psychiatric Services* 58 (3): 349-56.

About the Author

WILLIAM S. ("BO") SAX studied at Banaras Hindu University, the University of Wisconsin, and the University of Washington (Seattle), and the University of Chicago, where he earned his PhD in Anthropology in 1987. From 1987 to 1989 he was lecturer in Anthropology at Harvard University, and postdoctoral fellow in the Harvard Academy. After that, he taught Hinduism in the Department of Philosophy and Religious studies at the University of Canterbury in Christchurch, New Zealand, for eleven years. In 2000 he took up the Chair of Anthropology at the South Asia Institute in Heidelberg. He has published extensively on pilgrimage, gender, theatre, aesthetics, ritual healing, and medical anthropology. His major works (all published by Oxford University Press, New York) include *Mountain Goddess: Gender and Politics in a Central Himalayan Pilgrimage* (1991); *The Gods at Play: Lila in South Asia* (1995); *Dancing the Self: Personhood and Performance in the Pandav Lila of Garhwal* (2002); *God of Justice: Ritual Healing and Social Justice in the Central Himalayas* (2008); *The Problem of Ritual Efficacy* (with Johannes Quack and Jan Weinhold, 2010); and *The Law of Possession: Ritual, Healing, and the Secular State* (with Heléne Basu, 2015). He is currently working on a book about archaic polities in the Western Himalayas, tentatively entitled *In the Valley of the Kauravas: From Subject to Citizen in the Western Himalayas*. His 1991 book *Mountain Goddess* has been translated into Hindi under the title *Himalaya ki Nanda Devi* (Dehra Dun: Wimsar).

Afterwords

10   Global Mental Health

Love and Justice

Johannes Quack

This volume brings together various arguments and authors from across the world, spanning different methods and disciplines, from anthropology, sociology, and history to public health and clinical psychiatry. Such diversity allows for different levels of argumentation – empirical, methodological, moral, epistemological, ontological, and political – as well as varied styles: from radical to moderate, from polemical to sober, from overviews to detailed analyses. It goes without saying that not all of these arguments are consistent with each other; some abide by and some argue against a division of labour in academia, some assume and some question radical alterity, some teach the importance of learning, and there are arguments for both diversity and universality, love and justice.

The papers nevertheless share a common thread: they all take issue with the Movement for Global Mental Health (henceforth MGMH). The MGMH consists of those psychiatrists and psychologists, academic and government agencies, public health professionals and policy makers that jointly and explicitly aim at closing "the treatment gap for people living with mental disorders worldwide" (Patel et al. 2011). No representatives or advocates of this movement are included in the volume. Rather, its authors examine the main aims of the MGMH, as well as its justifications, from a social science perspective. And they often do so in ways that question the very nature of this movement as one primarily concerned with global mental health.

This afterword recapitulates some of the respective arguments by setting a question mark behind all three terms of the movement's designation (Global? Mental? Health?) as well as its main justification (Treatment Gap?). Against this background, it further discusses more fundamental issues at stake, issues that are located in the philosophy of science and related to distinctive political agendas and the division of labour between academic disciplines and the relationship between diversity and universality, love and justice.

Sax, William, and Claudia Lang (eds), *The Movement for Global Mental Health: Critical Views from South and Southeast Asia*. Taylor & Francis Group, 2021
DOI: 10.5117/9789463721622_CH10

Global?

In what sense is the MGMH global? Many papers in this volume argue
that the interventions and therapies the MGMH proposes originate in
the disciplines of psychology and psychiatry. The introduction speaks
of a "reflexive and self-confirming loop" where mental disorders are "defined primarily in terms of western psychiatric nosology, for which only
biomedical, or biomedically-approved, therapies are considered" (xxx).
Moreover, it is argued that representatives of elite institutions based in the
North Atlantic world dominate the discussions and interventions. In other
words, the MGMH does not consist of people situated around the world
who are concerned with the wide range of different global therapeutic
practices (e.g. therapeutic practices that are labelled "complementary"
and "alternative" if one takes the perspective of the dominant biomedical
paradigm, or "indigenous" if one does not take into account the indigeneity
of biomedicine). The Global North is the "tacit if not the explicit point of
reference" (Naraindas, this volume xxx) according to which the alleged
treatment gap of those in other parts of the world are measured. While
MGMH representatives contend that "all countries can be thought of as
developing countries in the context of mental health" (Patel et al. 2018, 1),
their proposed interventions – justified by the "treatment gap" argument –
focus almost exclusively on the Global South: "In practice, MGMH focuses
on lower and middle-income countries, where the gap is deepest between
what MGMH advocates think should be done and what is actually done"
(Ecks, this volume xxx).

In what sense, then, is the MGMH global? The answers this volume offers
indicate that it aims at globalising local therapeutic traditions. Das and
Rao (this volume, with references to Mills 2014, Watters 2010, and Bemme
and D'Souza 2012) hold that the MGMH is part of an "imperialistic form of
globalisation", that it is "deeply neo-imperial", and that "it carries forward
the neo-colonial psychiatrization of the majority world". Moreover, these
contributions illustrate it as a "top-down, imperial project that exports
Western illness categories and treatments that would ultimately replace
diverse cultural environments for interpreting mental health". It is exactly
this Western centrism that some contributors take issue with. As Sax (this
volume, xxx) adds: "the MGMH should consider drawing upon paradigms
that originate within South Asia rather than, in perfectly neo-colonial
fashion, taking all its theories and therapies from 'the West'".

In this perspective, the MGMH is not global in the sense of being equally
spread across the world or in the sense of trying to do justice to the different

therapeutic practices that can be found in various countries or in the sense of other recent trends to add "global" to a disciplinary tradition (for a discussion see e.g. Hanafi 2019). Instead, it is an intervention from the so-called North (or West or high income countries) in the so-called South (or East or low and middle income countries) that does not give further investigation to whether and to what degree the proposed interventions are applicable and beneficial for global actors, since the universality of its workings and positive outcomes are presupposed. Ironically, however, this volume highlights the degree to which some of the therapeutic practices the MGMH ignores or denigrates can be seen as truly global. Sax, for example, illustrates the importance of rituals for human beings across time and space, that is, in high- as well as low-income countries. To this end, Naraindas depicts the asymmetrical standards at play in the respective assessments. On the one hand, séances, which anthropologists and other scholars refer to as "possession", can be quite similar to the séances of *Familienaufstellung* that take place, for example, in a psychosomatic department at the University of Heidelberg Hospital (Sax and Weinhold, 2010). On the other hand, the first is labelled a pathology in psychiatry while the latter is referred to as a variation of psychodrama and group psychotherapy as randomized controlled trials study its efficacy and the German *Beihilfe* pays for such therapies. On this basis, Naraindas's study of various therapeutic practices in Germany raises important questions: "How have we come to such an impasse? And what does it mean for that movement called Global Mental Health?"

> Why does "mental health" in the Global South appear to revolve around the material substance of the psychopharmaceutical, while the quiddity called psychosomatic medicine, which in the German context is a separate discipline divorced from psychiatry, is normatively built on eschewing psycho-pharmaceuticals. Why in the Global South is "mental health" built on the distinction between superstition (past lives, trance, possession, in short, "rituals" invoking the spirits and the dead) and science (psychiatry, rational diagnosis, asylums, drugs,), while in Germany (exemplary of the Global North?) the two are often fused. (this volume, xxx)

Thus, several contributors to this volume stress that the MGMH's logic implies that so-called "alternative" forms of healing may never be seen as universal even if they are global, while it tries to globalise certain local forms of therapy.

Mental?

To what degree is the MGMH movement concerned with the mind? Several authors question the assumption that mental disorders can be clearly identified, even within a biomedical framework. They point to the problems of psychiatric disease classifications and of singling out individuals from larger social relationships, modes of belonging, and socio-political structures. Such interjections underscore "the fundamental problems of validity and the reliability of symptom classifications" (Ecks, this volume xxx) and contribute to debates about whether a symptoms-based diagnosis should be superseded by a focus on biomarkers.

A further point of concern is how the MGMH tries to assess mental illnesses. While there are some references by MGMH representatives that take social determinants of mental health into consideration, their critics see this as mere lip service, particularly as the MGMH seemingly favours biomedical models of health care in its emphasis on the concept of disability as assessed in the Disability Adjusted Life Years (DALY) metric. Moreover, the papers in this volume almost unanimously point to a lack of engagement with social determinants of mental suffering, such as class, race, wealth, and inequality, as well as with larger social, economic, and political contexts that significantly shape, for instance, "local biologies" and ecologies of well-being and suffering (see Lock and Ngyyen 2010).

Although several of the chapters in this volume accordingly discuss alternatives to this focus on the minds of individual patients, here I focus on three. Das and Rao illustrate how the framework for global mental health could be appropriately and fruitfully broadened by emphasising the political economy of mental illness. Halliburton's chapter highlights not only generalised social support structures but also provides detailed examples of the moral and affective qualities of social relationships, "how people attend to and care for others" not the least because of the importance of love in processes of healing and therapy. Linking "biomedicine's continued failures to address certain types of suffering" (xxx) – such as those labelled "mass hysteria" – to its exclusive focus on the mind of individuals rather than the social context in which the problem arose, Mukharji raises the counter example of ordinary believing Muslims. Representatives of modern and corporate spaces like schools and factories (the "proletarian mumin", in his terminology) have often been diagnosed with "mass hysteria", independent of each other, which seemingly contradicts the focus on the mental health of individual (xxx).

Health?

Probably the most provocative question this volume raises is whether the MGMH actually fosters health or whether it is itself counterproductive to its stipulated aims. In addition to the problems of medicalisation and depoliticisation of mental illness briefly indicated above (and well discussed in the literature), Lang and Sax underscore in the introduction that the MGMH's "rejection of non-psychiatric ontologies of suffering is a form of epistemic violence" (xxx). Moreover, Ecks argues that the global "scaling up" of interventions seems to scale up the suffering as well. He sees this as one of the key paradoxes of mental health in the world today and speculates that the promised economic investment gained via the MGMH also may lead to a "*worsening* of mental health" (xxx, emphasis in original). The MGMH thereby "runs the risk of epistemically disregarding, if not actively pathologising, vernacular forms of healing, especially those that labour under the epithet of faith and religion", as Naraindas contends in his chapter (xxx). He further extrapolates that "the risk of extirpating the vernacular" can be seen as part of "a trajectory of ontological genocide that eviscerates other ways of being in the world" (xxx).

While some papers question the movement's impact on the improvement of health and well-being, others agree that it will certainly have an impact on big pharma's profit. As the introduction to this volume spells out: "pharmaceuticalisation creates markets for the pharmaceutical industry, either by depoliticising and silencing social inequality, marginalisation, and suffering or by providing an idiom of critique and a powerful tool for mobilising care and social inclusion" (Sax and Lang xxx; Kitanaka 2012; Lang 2019).

Treatment Gap?

And what about MGMH's main justification for intervention, the treatment gap? Here, the question seems to be whether there is even such a thing. The proposition that people with mental health problems have nowhere to go, given the lack of hospitals, psychiatrists, and so on in the so-called Global South, has already been contested. For example, the Indian psychiatrist Neki estimated in 1973 that around 80 per cent of the Indian population approaches "alternative" practitioners for the treatment of mental health problems and this figure has been subsequently corroborated by various other studies (see Campion and Bhugra 1997, 215; Shah 1984, 737; De Sousa and De Sousa 1984, 6; Quack 2012). The Finnish psychiatrist Pakaslahti generalised this observation:

> Most developing countries have a network of non-Western traditional health practitioners operating outside the modern official health care system, often unknown to health professionals. In fact, such local healing systems provide the vast majority of care and support for those who suffer from mental health and substance dependence problems (1998, 129).

The contributors to this volume largely share this scepticism about the very existence of a "treatment gap". Hence, the introduction proposes that "treatment difference" ought to be acknowledged rather than postulating a "treatment gap". The ways in which most advocates of the MGMH gather and analyse data about MH are "structurally blind" (Sax, this volume, xxx) to alternatives outside the public biomedical sector. As Ecks contends:

> When GMH calculates treatment gaps for countries of the global South, private sector pharmaceutical prescriptions and private practitioners providing mental health care are "entirely excluded" and this produces "a skewed picture of treatment gaps in countries of the South". (this volume, xxx)

Even within a biomedical framework it is important to note – as several contributors to this volume do, particularly Halliburton – that World Health Organization studies have concluded that some countries of the Global South, such as Nigeria and India, in fact have better rates of recovery from some severe forms of mental illness when compared with their European and American counterparts (WHO 1973, 1979; Sartorius et al. 1986, 1996; Hopper et al., eds. 2007).

Division of Labour?

All such arguments invite us to reconsider the movement's terms and aims (global? mental? health?) as well as its central justification (treatment gap?). Implicitly they also raise the question: Who is to assess the MGMH and on what basis? It is not difficult to imagine the ways in which MGMH representatives would react to the arguments outlined above. It is likely, for example, they would underscore that many of the "alternative" therapeutic offers their critics list are in fact more harmful than therapeutic and that it is the expertise and duty of psychiatry and psychology, not the social sciences and humanities, to make such assessments. Underlying such disagreements seem to be more fundamental debates about the different ways in which therapeutic practices can and are to be assessed, the philosophy of science, the role and implications of distinctive political agendas and, on this basis, in what ways there is and should be a division of labour between academic disciplines.

What are the relationships and hierarchies between the different academic disciplines represented and addressed in this volume? Would it be possible and desirable to incorporate social science models into the theory and practice of global mental health, as Das and Rao (this volume) propose? Or are the respective approaches and concerns fundamentally at odds, as Naraindas' (this volume) distinction between Life and Culture (the provenance of all the non-scientific disciplines including anthropology) and Non-life and Nature (the provenance of science) may imply? The thrust of Naraindas' chapter further highlights the ways in which the respective politics of life/non-life are also politics of "us" versus "them", the politics between an alleged rational, secular West/North as opposed to a supposedly backward (not only due to the "treatment gap"), religious East/South, where the "evangelical" MGMH "appears to be predicated on redeeming the millions of 'under-diagnosed' and 'misdiagnosed' patients through psychiatry and the psychopharmaceutical". Only in the Global North "the redemption for a large class of mental problems seems to be eschewing psychopharmaceuticals and practices that blur, if not altogether abrogates, the distinction between human/non-human and life/non-life" thereby upholding, however, the distinction between "us/West/North" and "them/East/South" (this volume, xxx).

Is there a place for religious and mystical concerns within the MGMH, science and academia at large or are religion and ritual fundamentally at odds with the modern medical and scientific episteme? What are the respective hierarchies, power relations, "works of purification" (Sax, this volume, xxx) and "ontopolitics" (Mukharji, this volume, xxx)? Are there universal human bodies and disease patterns that affect people in societies all around the world in similar ways and therefore should be treated similarly? Hornbacher's contribution, by contrast, assumes the existence of, and distinguishes different ways to engage with, "radical alterity". How should such forms of "radical alterity" (if there are any) be dealt with? Are there different ways to consider someone to be cured of madness? Are we dealing with political attempts to "normalise" radical alterity by treating it as a pathological individual deviance that must be corrected by the modern disciplinary society (as prominently argued by Michel Foucault and Thomas Szasz, among others)? Academics familiar with debates of the last decades will recognise well-known and frequently discussed themes in these questions: secularisation, medicalisation, normalisation, scientism, positivism, reductionism, instrumentalism, modernisation, relativism, emancipation, critique, othering, and above all, ethnocentrism ("the anthropologist's severest term of moral abuse", Geertz 1973, 24).

What would alternatives look like? Lang highlights the possibility of moving "beyond the usual dichotomy of global psychiatry and local traditional healing by showing how a (re)invented tradition assembles local bio-moral embodied minds, classic texts, vernacular practices, and globalised psychiatric knowledge to recognise and treat distressed, embodied minds" (this volume, xxx). Naraindas' paper also investigates the "queer spaces" in the West/North that call into question usual dichotomies (nature vs. culture, body vs. mind, real vs. symbolic, inanimate vs. animate, us vs. them). Such a focus on the intricate messiness of actual therapeutic practices in the East/South as well as in the West/North is often seen as one of sociocultural anthropology's key contributions to such debates. A second key contribution, also frequently highlighted in this volume, is anthropology's self-depiction as learning from, rather than preaching, teaching, or treating, others. As Hornbacher puts it: "anthropology tries to understand the alterity of sociocultural realities in its own terms and by analysing the internal logic of radically different human lifeworlds" (this volume, xxx).

Based on this self-depiction, it is possible to raise polemic questions: What might anthropologists learn from another "radical other" – the psychiatrists – rather than teaching them about learning and about the true nature of their beliefs and practices? How would such a volume look like if advocates of the MGMH were included? What would happen if anthropologists "imagine themselves in the psychiatrists' shoes"? How could they try to grasp what it means to be "on the other side" so as to make the psychiatrists' allegedly "inadequate" and "odd" behaviour understandable "in terms of a coherent, if unfamiliar, set of beliefs and desires – as opposed to explaining this behaviour with terms like stupidity, madness, baseness or sin"?

I do intend to deliberate these questions, however, only indirectly (in the next section – which features references to the quotes in the paragraph above) and not directly here for three reasons. First, there are, of course, anthropological studies trying to understrand the psychiatrtrists' (as "natives") point(s) of view (e.g. Luhrmann 2011). Second, this would require an extensive discussion of the different power structures at stake in these examples and the intricate distribution of ethical commitments (or forms of neutrality) when "studying up" (those with more power, authority, wealth, etc.) as opposed to "down" (the disempowered, disenfranchised, exploited, etc.). Third, while representatives of psychiatry and related disciplines would probably reject the assertion that they merely try to "normalise" behavioural, cognitive and emotional alterity in the favour of the pharmaceutical industry, they are likely to admit and defend that they aim for universal scientific generalisations and, on this basis, therapeutic interventions. Such differences between psychiatry and anthropology (and related disciplines on both sides) raise an important question: Are we dealing with a "division of labour" where proponents of each side engage in incommensurable projects, based on different epistemic, ontological and political concerns? Or is a "division of labour" in itself how psychiatry would see the respective concerns of psychiatry and anthropology? Should we rather contrast anthropology's way of seeing the (more or less) whole, versus psychiatry's way of seeing, again, the (more or less) whole? And should we see global human well-being as a shared and collaborative concern?

Love and Justice?

To conclude this afterword, it might be helpful to look at one famous predecessor of such debates. In the "drunken Indian debate" between Clifford Geertz and Richard Rorty, both address questions of therapeutic practices, disciplinary boundaries, and ethnocentrism on the basis of a story of an alcoholic "American Indian" who against the advice of doctors did not curb his drinking habit but continued treatment on one of the rare and in-demand kidney machines. Both Geertz and Rorty discuss how one should react to such "inadequate" behaviour of a "racial other" in a liberal society. On one hand, Geertz deplores that there was "a failure to grasp, on either side, what it was to be on the other, other, and thus what it was to be on one's own" (1986, 117). Like most contributors to this volume (though not all), he suggests that the doctors should become more like anthropologists, try to understand "radical difference". Rorty, on the other hand, wonders to what degree one should expect doctors to understand and accommodate other ways of life. He distinguishes between anthropologists as "connoisseurs of diversity" and "agents of love" and doctors (as well as lawyers and teachers) as "guardians of universality" and "agents of justice" (1986, 528). Anthropologists are, according to Rorty, "the people who are expected and empowered to extend the range of society's imagination, thereby opening the doors of procedural justice to people on whom they had been closed".

That is, they explain "odd behaviour in terms of a coherent, if unfamiliar, set of beliefs and desires – as opposed to explaining this behaviour with terms like stupidity, madness, baseness or sin" (1986, 529). Doctors, by contrast, should not imagine themselves in their patients' shoes. A society built around procedural justice needs both kinds of agents, agents of love and agents of justice: those who make "odd behaviour" understandable in coherent terms (presumably this means in most cases in biomedical terms) and those "who do not look too closely at such matters" but get their job done by, for example, operating a kidney machine (1986, 529) or administering a movement for global mental health.

Some arguments in this volume are based on assumptions of radical alterity while others assume a common humanity. Some accept the division of labour between academic disciplines and formulate correctives to the MGMH from a social science and humanities perspective. Others propose that this division of labour is the source and sign of the "impasse" (Naraindas, this volume) of biomedicine because it reproduces the asymmetries that lead to the conquest of death over life, that place the natural sciences over the social sciences and humanities, that privilege drugs over talking, rituals, seances, and other non-material(istic) forms of therapy, and that thereby deepen the alleged "gap" between us (the developed West/North) and them (the developing East/South).

This volume gives no general answers, but it invites us to ask: Can we acknowledge such asymmetries while upholding a fruitful and collaborative division of labour? When is the time to understand and to learn from, and when is to the time to teach and to treat the (radical) other? Should and can we always care about both diversity and universality, love and justice?

References

Bemme, Doerte, and Nicole A. D'souza. 2014. "Global Mental Health and Its Discontents: An Inquiry into the Making of Global and Local Scale." *Transcultural Psychiatry* 51 (6): 850-74.

Campion, Jane, and Dinesh Bhugra. 1997. "Experiences of Religious Healing in Psychiatric Patients in South India." *Social Psychiatry and Psychiatric Epidemiology* 32 (4): 215-21.

De Sousa, Alan, and D. A. De Sousa. 1984. "My India, Our India." In *Psychiatry in India*, edited by Alan De Sousa, and D.A. De Sousa, 1-12. Bombay: Bhalani.

Geertz, Clifford. 1973. *The Interpretation of Cultures*. New York: Basic Books.

—. 1986. "The Uses of Diversity." In *Tanner Lectures on Human Values, Vol. 7.* edited by Sterling M. McMurrin, 251-75. Cambridge and Salt Lake City: Cambridge University Press.

Hanafi, Sari. 2020. "Global Sociology Revisited: Toward New Directions." *Current Sociology* 68 (1): 3-21.

Hopper, Kim, Glynn Harrison, Aleksandar Janca, and Norman Sartorius, eds. 2007. *Recovery from Schizophrenia: An International Perspective: A Report from the WHO Collaborative Project, the International Study of Schizophrenia.* New York: Oxford University Press.

Kitanaka, Junko. 2012. *Depression in Japan: Psychiatric Cures for a Society in Distress.* Princeton and Oxford: Princeton University Press.

Lang, Claudia. 2019. "Inspecting Mental Health: Depression, Surveillance and Care in Kerala, South India." *Culture, Medicine & Psychiatry* 43 (4): 596-612.

Lock, Margaret and Vinh-Kim Ngyyen. 2010. *An Anthropology of Biomedicine.* Oxford: Wiley-Blackwell.

Luhrmann, Tanya M. 2011. *Of two minds: An Anthropologist Looks at American Psychiatry.* New York: Vintage.

Mills, China. 2014. *Decolonizing Global Mental Health: The Psychiatrization of the Majority World.* Hove and New York: Routledge.

Pakaslahti, Antti. 1998. "Family Centered Treatment of Mental Health Problems at the Balaji Temple in Rajasthan." In *Changing Patterns of Family and Kinship in South Asia: Proceedings of an International Symposium on the Occasion of the 50th Anniversary of India's Independence Held at the University of Helsinki,* edited by Asko S. Parpola and Sirpa Tenhume, 129-68. Helsinki: Finnish Oriental Society.

Patel, Vikram, Pamela Y. Collins, John Copeland, Ritsuko Kakuma, Sylvester Katontoka, Jagannath Lamichhane, Smita Naik, and Sarah Skeen. 2011. "The Movement for Global Mental Health." *British Journal of Psychiatry* 198 (2): 88-90.

Patel, Vikram, Shekhar Saxena, Crick Lund, Graham Thornicroft, Florence Baingana, Paul Bolton, Dan Chisholm, Pamela Y Collins, Janice L Cooper, Julian Eaton, et al. 2018. "The Lancet Commission on Global Mental Health and Sustainable Development." *Lancet* 392 (10157): 1553-98.

Quack, Johannes. 2012. "Ignorance and Utilization: Mental Health Care outside the Purview of the Indian State." *Anthropology & Medicine* 19 (3): 277-90.

Rorty, Richard. 1986. "On Ethnocentrism: A Reply to Clifford Geertz." *Michigan Quarterly Review* 25 (3): 525-34.

Sartorius, Norman, Assen Jablensky, Alisa E. Korten, Gunila Ernberg, Martha Anker, John E. Cooper, and Robert Day. 1986. "Early Manifestations and First-Contact Incidence of Schizophrenia in Different Cultures." *Psychological Medicine* 16 (4): 909-28.

Sartorius, Norman, Walter H. Gulbinat, Glynn Harrison, Eugene M. Laska, and
    Carole Siegel. 1996. "Long-Term Follow-Up of Schizophrenia in 16 Countries:
    A Description of the International Study of Schizophrenia Conducted by the
    World Health Organization." *Social Psychiatry and Psychiatric Epidemiology*
    31 (5): 249-58.
Sax, William, Jan Weinhold, and Jochen Schweitzer. 2010. "Ritual Healing East and
    West: A Comparison of Ritual Healing in the Garhwal Himalayas and 'Family
    Constellation' in Germany." *Journal of Ritual Studies* 24 (1): 61-77.
Shah, V. D. 1984. "Mental Health Service in India." In *Psychiatry in India*, edited by
    Alan De Sousa and D.A. De Sousa, 733-56. Bombay: Bhalani.
Watters, Ethan. 2010. *Crazy like Us: The Globalization of the American Psyche*. New
    York: Simon and Schuster.
World Health Organization. 1973. *The International Pilot Study of Schizophrenia*.
    New York: Wiley and Sons.
—. 1979. *Schizophrenia: An International Follow-up Study*. New York: Wiley and Sons.

About the Author

JOHANNES QUACK is Assistant Professor of Social Anthropology at the
University of Zurich. He has conducted ethnographic research on medicine,
ethics, and religion (secularity and non-religion) in India and elsewhere.
Quack is the author of *Disenchanting India: Organized Rationalism and
Criticism of Religion in India* (Oxford University Press, 2012). He co-edited
the volumes *The Problem of Ritual Efficacy* (Oxford University Press, 2010),
Religion und Kritik in der Moderne (LIT, 2012), *Asymmetrical Conversations:
Contestations, Circumventions and the Blurring of Therapeutic Boundaries*
(Berghahn, 2014), *Religious Indifference* (Springer, 2017), and *The Diversity
of Nonreligion* (Routledge, 2020), and he co-edits the book series *Religion
and Its Others: Studies in Religion, Nonreligion, and Secularity* (De Gruyter).

11 "Treatment" and Why We Need Alternatives

An Autoethnographic Reflection on Psychiatric Incarceration in India

Anonymous

"The Sick Woman is all of the 'dysfunctional', 'dangerous', and 'in danger', 'badly behaved', 'crazy', 'incurable', 'traumatised', 'disordered', 'diseased', 'chronic', 'uninsurable', 'wretched', 'undesirable' and altogether 'dysfunctional' bodies... who have been historically pathologised, hospitalised, institutionalised, brutalised, rendered 'unmanageable', and therefore made culturally illegitimate and politically invisible."
– Johanna Hedva, *Sick Woman Theory*

Part 1

treatment

that was treatment
those hands crawling on your body
the poison injected
as you are stripped
dragged along the corridor,
the faint smell of formaldehyde
and phenyl

that was treatment
the laughing of nurses
the condescension of doctors

Sax, William, and Claudia Lang (eds), *The Movement for Global Mental Health: Critical Views from South and Southeast Asia.*Taylor & Francis Group, 2021
DOI: 10.5117/9789463721622_CH11

the asking of the same questions
until you utter the words they want to hear

      that was treatment
      that was treatment
      that was treatment

in a hospital with walled windows
in a hospital with more guards
than doctors

      that was treatment
      the waking up
      to odours of stale food
      the laughter of guards
      the ringing of their cell phones
      in your cell

that was treatment
befriending of rajan, tour guide from ajmer
who spoke of love, loss and longing,
drooling, his feet in shackles,
his eyes telling me a hundred stories

      that was treatment
      taking a mother from her sons,
      that was treatment

and when they strip every last bit of human dignity
along with your clothes, the skin on your bones,
the laughter in your eyes, and the sun upon your tongue

      they walk with their heads held high
      they are doctors, you see
      treatment is the name of the game
      and that was treatment

             * * *

The police roughly pull me off the jeep. *Chalo, chalo*, they say. *We have other work to do*. I am taken into an entrance labelled EMERGENCY. The police have a brief discussion with a group of people who appear to be expecting me, then they leave.

A large room with doctors and nurses in white are milling around me. There is a counter, like a Reception, a woman in a starched nursing uniform standing behind it. They take my purse and mobile phone from me and ask me to lie down on a bed covered with a dirty floral sheet. I protest, I don't want to lie down. There are daisies printed on the sheet, I note distractedly.

"Why am I here? Surely, I am allowed one phone to call my family?"

"No phone calls allowed," they inform me, smiling. Panic rises like a wave in my throat and I can't swallow.

And then I see him. He is advancing towards me with a huge injection. In my peripheral vision, I am aware of a cage in the corner of the room, painted dark green. It is the sort in which an animal might be locked, or perhaps a mad woman? My eyes shift to his pocket, the words, 'Dr Rakesh' monogrammed on a white coat in red. The injection is coming closer and, as if mesmerised, I watch as he pulls my sleeve up.

The sting of the syringe in my forearm. My throat starts to close up. After that, nothing.

Minutes later, hours later, I don't know which, a wheelchair rolls me through a dark and narrow corridor. Blue walls close in on me. A chemical haze, my body unable to move, or speak. Where are they taking me? I want to scream or walk, but can't. They push me along, chattering and whistling. Steps. The wheelchair at a frightening angle – I am being carried up. My throat feels like it is full of warm cotton wool.

Grey shiny steps move and white walls close in. I'm petrified I'm going to fall. I'm scared of heights. I feel like I'm falling, I am falling… and they still keep carrying me higher and higher. Flat ground again – such a relief, and a blue door is pushed open. A small room, too brightly lit, a single bed against a wall, a small window. The men lift me out of the wheelchair and I sink into a pillow. My limbs are heavy, so heavy.

I can't move.

I can't speak.

Cotton wool clouds. Shining white light. It's so bright and it's so heavy. Can't keep my eyes open. I sink into the clouds.

* * *

"I want to make a phone call," I say. I hear my own voice shaking, quavering and sounding higher than normal.

"Sorry, the phone is busy." Sister does not even look up. Weird. The telephone is lying on her desk, unused and obviously available. Black and solid, spiral cord connecting the handset to the main telephone.

"It's okay, I'll wait." I lean against the wall.

"No, no, go back to your room. I'll send word for you when you can use the phone. Who will you call, anyway?" Then she laughs, as though she has told a joke. The indifferent nurse looks at me and then at Aparna and Reshma, who have followed me here.

Minutes pass dismally slow. I stay leaning against the damp and dirty wall, shifting my weight from my legs to the wall.

Sister picks up the phone and makes some calls. She places her hand on the receiver and says, "Can't you see, the phone is busy?"

"It's fine. It's not like I have anything to do. I'll just sit here quietly on the floor." I sit down, cross-legged, on the floor. The floor is cool, the grey mosaic shiny. There is a faint smell of formaldehyde and phenyl in the air. In the General Ward, I hear voices and some chairs being moved. Sister is starting to get flustered and I decide to keep sitting patiently, wordlessly. There's no law against waiting, right?

She angrily punches a few numbers into the phone and then rings a bell. Two orderlies appear. She nods in my direction and they walk over to me. I look up at them and suddenly I feel one of them yank my arms, holding my forearms. The other one is just following. The walls shift and my hair hurts as it gets trapped under me. My arms hurt and feel like they will be pulled out of their joints.

I am being dragged on the floor like a unclaimed corpse being moved off the streets by the police.

I feel my kurta rising, feel the shame of my exposed midriff, my bra probably showing. But my hands are over my head and the orderly keeps dragging me. The floor is smooth and hard under me, very cold. I hear Aparna and Reshma laugh a little and say something to Sister. Sister laughs loudly. All I can smell is the formaldehyde and the phenyl. I see the side of my bed and we are in my room. Number 16. The other orderly picks up my feet and I am dumped on the bed. A nurse appears, pulls down my pants and I feel the cool swab of spirit, the hot sting of an injection.

The door closes. As I swim into unconsciousness – it seems to me this is what rape feels like – this utter powerlessness, this being violated, my body not my own any more, just a piece of meat for anyone to do anything to it that they wish.

* * *

At eight o'clock after dinner, like clockwork, Dr Sethi appears after a quick rap on the door. A minion follows holding a clipboard, a pen tucked into the left pocket of his shirt. Today, Dr Sethi is wearing a blue shirt, chocolate – brown slacks and the same black pointy shoes. I don't trust men with pointy shoes. He smiles but the smile does not reach his eyes. Aparna and Reshma stand up in his presence like he is some God they must revere.

I hate him more with each passing day.

"So, Deepali, you had a good day?"

I want to scream, "No, I did not, thank you very much!" I want to shout my outrage at being dragged on the floor. I want to tell him that I have never felt so violated in my life. I want to cry and protest and ask for justice. But something tells me he will gloat. They are winning and I must not let him see that.

Instead I smile. "Yes." I look directly at him, willing him to refute my good day. He must know something. But he does not engage.

"Good, good," he says distractedly. He looks at Aparna.

"Appetite okay?"

"Yes, Doctor."

"So, Deepali, do you feel guilty yet?"

Every day he comes in at 8 pm, every day he asks me the same question.

Guilty for what? I have done nothing wrong. I have been a good wife. Does he mean I was guilty of making a fuss at Abacus Hospital? Are they the ones who have locked me up for life? Guilty of being a bad daughter? Going public with my story when I felt persecuted? But no, I have done nothing wrong. Who has asked him to ask me this and what should I be feeling guilty for?

I try to figure out this question. Why does he ask me this every day?

* * *

The therapy room is dingy and painted grey. The desk is cluttered with files with curling edges – ignored and irrelevant like me – getting older and gathering dust. Behind it sits Dr Anuradha, who is a young woman in her late twenties. She briefly looks up at me when I am brought in, then waves at me to sit down while she keeps speaking with someone on the phone. Aparna and Reshma leave me alone with her for a twenty-minute session.

"So, Deepali, I have been told you have bipolar disorder."

"So the doctors tell me. But how do they know? I have never been tested. They just injected me when I was brought here."

"Well, it says in your case notes you do. So let's talk about how you feel."

"I am confused why I am here. I don't know where my family is. Will I be here forever?"

Dr Anuradha smiles a secretive smile.

"I'm not at liberty to discuss those things. Let's talk about you. Let's talk about your symptoms. How do you feel? How do you think you could improve?"

I don't feel like answering. I look out of the window. Its glass panes have been painted with white paint, presumably to save on the cost of curtains while giving the room's inhabitants a sense of privacy. The white paint is peeling in places showing me a view of the corridor outside, glimpses of people walking by and a spot of green from a tree. I come back to Dr Anuradha, who has been speaking all this time.

"I want you to walk every morning and pump your arms, like this." She makes a boxing movement in front. "You think you could do that?"

I nod. I want to tell her I walk already and practice yoga in the park with the balding grass. But I don't feel like talking with her. There is something of an I-Know-It-All demeanour about her.

"How is your appetite?"

"Fine."

She gets another phone call and takes it. She laughs and says "I can't speak now" to the person on the phone, but keeps listening, smiling coyly, laughing, twirling a strand of long hair in her fingers. She holds her palm up, as if to tell me to wait and continues to listen on the phone. Meanwhile, the clock on the wall continues to tick and soon our time is over. She hangs up the phone and looks at me.

"So, same time on Friday. I will see you twice a week." It is not a question and she does not check whether I wanted to see her. It was simply her decision and my choice was irrelevant – a prisoner who is only allowed to obey. She rings the bell and Aparna and Reshma come in and escort me out.

* * *

Evening is approaching. Marigolds bloom with thick spindly stems along the wall that lines this garden. There is a driveway that curves away from the garden and beyond it, the gate through which they brought me in. What will happen if I break into a run and try and scale the gate? I am sure it will not be pretty and I will be dragged back and injected again. This time maybe the ECT machine will be used on me. Successfully. Was brought to my room last night.

I had been asleep; it was midnight, maybe. Suddenly the room was awash with light and there was a junior doctor standing there with two male orderlies. I was groggy and disoriented. Sister stood present and there was a machine with electrodes and a display looking like a fridge voltage regulator. I knew I was in danger. I screamed.

"Don't worry. We only want to measure your blood pressure. This is just a better machine to check."

"You call my family! If you want to give me electric shocks, then do it when my parents are here. Get my husband! Bring my children! I need someone with me."

"Come now, don't make a fuss."

I screamed even louder and they looked at each other. In the next room, another patient woke up. I heard the sound of a glass being knocked over and footsteps shuffling. As if speaking some secret language, they turned around and left. In the morning, I wondered if it had all been a dream.

I look again at Mr Agarwal and Vinod and wonder if we will all get ECT at some point. Maybe we will become zombies, or do they call them cyborgs now, as they did in that book, *The Stepford Wives*? Maybe we will all become robots and go back to our previous lives – improved, enhanced, perfect.

* * *

A young woman has just been brought into the room across from me. She is emaciated and her hair is in dreadlocks. Aparna tells me she used to be a famous model.

"You know, she was in all the top fashion shows. *Lakme, India Week*, the cover of *Femina*, everything. Then she went crazy and started living on the streets."

How do seemingly successful people go crazy? Is it, as the doctors have been telling me here, a chemical imbalance in the brain? Is it something else? Some trauma or abuse? I know that sexual predators exist in the world of modelling. I used to be a model in my early twenties. Not big, but I dabbled enough to know the creepy men who offer to get you gigs for "favours." So I decided modelling was not for me, it would be better to study Mathematics and do something else.

"I think she started doing drugs as well. Then her mother came to know. Her mother lives in the US you know. Came back and found her living on a bench in Hauz Khas. Got her picked up and brought her here to get clean."

Alka is continuing her story in conspiratorial whispers. "All the famous people get Dr Sethi. Like you." And she nods knowingly.

Am I famous? I don't think so. But my father is. Maybe the fact that I am married to a white man? Is Dr Sethi a celebrity doctor? So many riddles. And if lucky, a lifetime to decipher them. Because getting out seems an impossible dream.

"Let's go for a walk. Maybe this new girl, Suzanne, also wants tea."

I step out into the corridor and knock gently on Room 10, across from me.

"Come in." A soft voice.

"Suzanne? I'm going down for a walk and some *chai*. Want to come?"

* * *

BUTTON

Persuaded to try medication,
"very few side effects, no problem,"

Dr Rakesh smiles at your husband.
You are just a possession, a car

to service, a house to maintain.
He proudly leads you home,

10 mg of this and that,
and a brand new wife.

Your voice does not matter,
the thickening tongue,

the diminishing libido.
Your body not your own,

your limbs swim in treacle,
your mind, anaesthetised,

your smile pasted.
The new, improved Wife,

Model 101 – will last
Repaired, and without complaint.

Just press the button.

* * *

It is Day 14, I think. I have been in solitary since I came in. I learn this is a term for when they keep you secluded or away from your family.

Because it appears my family indeed knows I am here.

It is just after breakfast. I am sitting on the green checked bedspread reading the newspaper. I have devised several plans for staying busy. I read the paper for a long time. I tear out bits of interest to me. I read the advertisements and the obituaries. I read about society people and I read about crime. I read the *Letters to the Editor*. Just as I am tearing out another article I may like to read again, there is a knock on my door and without my saying, "Come in," the door opens. Robert is standing in the doorway. He is thinner, looks weaker, but he is really there – and he is smiling at me.

I run to him and hug him.

"Oh, thank goodness! I kept asking them and they would not tell me call you! How did you find out I was here? Can we go home now? Aparna, Reshma: See, this is my husband! I told you I would get out of here."

They are smiling, a little sadly, more pityingly.

"No, you can't come home yet, hon." Robert's voice is low and soft. "You're not well and you need to get better."

"But I will be fine at home. I will be good. I will eat these awful medicines if you want me to."

"Let's see. For now, you need to stay here and get better."

"Did you know I was here all this time? I thought you were dying. I went to the Embassy. But no one helped me."

"You're really not well, babe. The hospital here thought it was best to keep you sedated but I came and saw you a few times. Plus your father has been sleeping in the hospital here in the family area – those are the rules. We were not allowed to meet you, the hospital thought it was best we stayed away for two weeks."

Best for whom?

What will they get by lying to me, not telling me my family had locked me up?

All this time I was wondering how I had ended up locked up in a psych ward, and it really had been my parents and husband. They had conspired to lock me up, just like Mr Agarwal's family, and Vinod's.

Like *everyone* else here.

I feel strangely deflated.

All the excitement of seeing Robert falls from me like a discarded party dress, once so bright but then used, worn – and thrown into the laundry.

* * *

Therapy Day. Dr Anuradha's room, as if time stood still. Files sit untouched and dusty on her desk. The air is still and quiet and nothing seems to have moved since our last session. The only thing she seems to care about is her phone and she is constantly checking it every few minutes, even our session.

"You know, Deepali, bipolar disorder is one of the toughest conditions. After schizophrenia, it's the next most difficult thing to live with. You will have to really be constant with your medication and therapy. It can never be cured."

I hang my head. What can I even say to this?

"So let's talk about diet. Are you eating fruit?"

"Well, they only serve bananas here. At home, I eat a lot of fruit. But I don't know when I'll go home."

"OK, when you go home, make sure you eat a lot of fruit and salad. It all helps. Now, let's talk about the problem in your relationship with your husband.

What would you like him to do?

What seems to be missing?"

I think of Robert, the unwanted sex, the bleeding from my vagina, from my anus, the vomiting, the claustrophobia.

I think of my four children.

Maybe I can still fix this.

"Maybe if there is romance, it will get easier to have sex with him. Maybe he could call me a few times a day from work?" Even to me, my words sound weak.

A weak woman pleading for a few scraps of her busy husband's time.

"OK, I am going to mention this to him. You know, everyone at home is very keen to have you recover. They want you to understand the things you are doing wrong so you can go home soon. They have been in to see me and I'm a professional, I know this. So it is all in your hands how soon you start making these changes and recover. Of course, you will be on medication forever, but hopefully, therapy will also help you to change your behaviour."

Her phone buzzes again and she looks at it. I look at the clock ticking, her hands as she holds the phone. Pearly pink nail polish, a coral ring from an astrologer. She looks at me and speaks again.

"Anything you want to ask me about bipolar disorder? Anything else you want to know?"

I shake my head.

"I have three books on it in my room. Let me read them and understand. I'll be sure to ask you if I have any questions."

"OK then, see you in a few days – take care, Deepali!"

I rise and leave her room. These visits to the therapist in Sanctuary always make me feel unsettled, like they are trying to mould me into someone else. What exactly is this Sanctuary place designed to do?

* * *

The pain is intense. Cramps in my legs and my back feels like it's on fire. I struggle to open my eyes. I'm still in Sanctuary. It's the middle of the night I think. The chairs where Aparna and Reshma sit are empty.

What is this new pain? I can't breathe, it's that bad. My legs seem to be locking and cramping. Turning over, I try to see if I can get comfortable or breathe. It's no good. Maybe I am having a stroke. Maybe it's some terrible side effect of the pills. I need the doctor.

Turning on the light, I hobble to the Nursing Station. Tonight, luckily, it's the young and pretty nurse on duty; the older one who had me dragged on the floor is not here. She looks up from the book she is reading. The time on the clock above her head says 1:25 am.

"What is it? Can't sleep?" She is not smiling or looking happy at being disturbed.

"Pain. So much pain. Doctor?" I gasp, pointing at my legs. I wonder which doctor may be on duty and what is wrong with me.

"So much trouble you all are! All of you are crazy, you mad people. And we have to look after you. Makes us all go crazy as a result." She angrily pushes aside her chair and it topples over. I take a step back.

"Go and lie down. I am coming in two minutes."

"But..."

"Go. Don't wake up the other patients. See, everyone is sleeping."

The ward is completely quiet at this time. I've never seen it this way. So orderly, so quiet. But then, I'm always asleep or sedated at this time. I wonder where Aparna and Reshma and the other attendants sleep. No sign of them anywhere. I somehow hobble back to my bed. The pain is getting more intense. I bite my lip in order to stay quiet. Gulping a glass of water, I wait. And then the door opens.

Sister Neetu, that's her name, is there with a tray holding a large injection. She motions me to lie down and without even taking my pyjama bottoms down or asking me to, she injects me in my bottom through the fabric. I feel the sting and then nothing. She roughly pushes me to the centre of the bed and then she is gone.

My eyes burn with tears. But my body starts to relax with the injection soon and the pain starts melting to waves of slight discomfort and then it is gone. I fall asleep with the lights still on, Sister having come and gone in a flash of injection rape.

* * *

Three years earlier

I feel his hands on my back. I try to keep my breathing even, so he will think I am asleep. His hands grow more insistent and I feel his fingers on my nipples, trying to arouse me. As I lie still, his hands wander into the warm space between my legs and I know he will not stop or be able to sleep without sex. I roll over and let him begin to kiss me. His kisses are so wet and repulse me. He's wet and disgusting, slobbering in my ear. His belly is soft, and lower, my hands fondle his limp penis. I know what's next. It is always this way. I get up and go down on him, trying to moan the way he likes, trying to let my mouth do what my mind was protesting against. He keeps fondling my breast. I feel myself sighing.

He pushes me on all fours and enters me. I let him have his way, using my body the way he wants. The way he needs to so he can sleep. This way, it'll be over sooner. The clock face gleaming in the dark bedroom shows 2 a.m. I am now wide awake.

And he moves, grunting, his hand on my right breast. And in my head, I am planning the next day's tiffins for the boys. Should it be grilled cheese sandwiches or the leftover banana cake and some fruit? He is still moving, he is still not done. I can't breathe. All I feel is wetness and his weight. I want it to be over. I want to go wash up. He moans, stops moving and reaches for tissue. I kiss him, relieved that it is over.

"Love you, honey," he says, rolling over.

"Love you." My automatic response. "Go to sleep."

"Goodnight." He voice is sleepy. "That was great, wasn't it?"

"Mmmm."

In the guest bathroom, I retch violently. I gargle with Listerine. I hate throwing up. Do I hate it more than the sex? And then the tears come, mixed with a feeling I can't understand. A feeling of claustrophobia, a feeling that I have to run away, a feeling I can't breathe. Pushing the bathroom window open, I try to inhale huge gusts of air. The tears are warm, thick, salty, mixed with snot. I feel them trickling down my face. The tap is running, the tears are flowing, and I need to escape. But to where?

The bathroom cabinet is so full. All the mini shampoos, the conditioners, the lotions from various hotels and conferences, all the things I bring back never to use, the nail files, the nail polishes, the pumice stones. I organise, stack, clean, discard. The tears start to stop. The breathing gets more even. I am wide awake and going back to bed is not even an option.

I walk into the study, turn on my computer, and go into the kitchen to make some tea while the computer starts up. As if on autopilot, I add ginger and cardamom and let the water simmer as I start unloading the dishwasher and use a dishtowel to dry the tiffins for the morning, just a few hours away. Greedy for this 'me time', I pour my tea into a blue mug with flowers and take it into the study. I start writing a post on my blog. The hours pass. As I start yawning, finally, I look at the time. 5:30 am. Almost time to wake up the boys. Knowing I can't sleep now, I wander into the kitchen to make another cup of tea and some toast for breakfast. I am so sleepy but force myself to stay awake. Maybe I can sleep after dropping the boys at school.

* * *

Violence is doors being slammed. Violence is the sound of silence – or loud noises or voices shouting at me. Violence is staying away from the bedroom and reading late into the night. Violence is laughing on the phone with someone else and stony silence again. There are many shades of violence and Robert knew them all. Violence spread on my skin like a purpling bruise no one ever saw. I felt violence on my chest, suffocating me while I slept. I felt violence on my thighs, being forced open while my mind screamed, "No!" I felt violence on my arms, being twisted till my eyes watered. I felt violence like a door slammed on my face. I felt violence like a wet and heavy shaggy dog, the smell of wet dog pervading everywhere, robbing the lightness of my very being.

And yet, as I spritzed some perfume behind my ears as I got dressed up to go out, his hand on the curve of my back, he opened doors for me, always the gentleman, always so solicitous.

Darling, another glass of wine? Pulling out my chair at restaurants. An arm at my waist, gently supportive. Who would believe me if I told them that I couldn't breathe? That his pouting at home and sulking for sex was driving me crazy? That there was no physical beating, but I hurt everywhere.

Even if I said anything, I would be considered crazy indeed to find fault with such a perfect husband.

And so it continued. And I broke again and again as I offered my body, like a peace offering, a white flag. There are many routes to becoming crazy and this was mine. Telling myself to ignore what my body was saying. Shutting my ears to the screaming in my head. Closing my nostrils as I struggled to breathe when I was taking him into my mouth. Suppressing the urge to vomit because this is what good wives do. Cringing from his kisses. Making lists in my head while he was moving on me, in me, over me. Disassociating from my body.

And what a disastrous mistake it turned out to be.

* * *

A personal reflection, eight years later

As I write this memoir and work critically and reflexively – vomiting out the rape and the drugs, I realise that you, dear reader, may wonder what I had done to "feel guilty" about. In truth, it was nothing at all because all I had done was to try and be a "good wife". However, the sexual trauma, perhaps coupled with emotional neglect from my parents in childhood, created in me low self-esteem and a distress so physical that it took a toll on my health. I became a dysfunctional wife and mother; and in my parents' and husband's opinion, someone who needed to be locked away, someone who needed to be "fixed".

This pathologisation of suffering, especially in the context of marriage and the roles expected of women, is unfortunately all too commonplace. It is also a commentary on how women are raised, perhaps more so in cultures like India, where we are raised to be compliant, to be "good", even if our bodies and minds are screaming in pain. At the time of my being locked up, my ex-husband was being treated for a fever in hospital and I was having a panic attack because I thought he might die. I was pacing the walls of the hospital and sitting in corridors chanting religious mantras for the health of my husband. These were my ways of dealing with the stress at the time and everyone should be allowed to manage their stress their way, but perhaps, as this was alien to my family, they thought this would be a good time to have me put away.

Although it was never discussed explicitly, by piecing together the pieces later, I believe my parents were instrumental in organising the police and the hospital, where I was taken for "treatment" after my ex-husband signed some forms. There are humane ways of dealing with a wife who is having a panic attack, but using ten police officers to have her committed, in the absence of her family, is not one of them. It is also important to mention that I had been undergoing talking therapy for the previous eight months because, at the time, I was desperate to save my marriage. All of these factors led to me being the "problem" figure, unable to function as per patriarchal expectations.

This was what the doctor in the Sanctuary perhaps referred to, when he kept asking whether I felt guilty yet. Unfortunately, this is common as many women, especially in India, are routinely put away for these inabilities to conform to patriarchal standards and I was just another one of them. In my case, aligning with feminism, using writing to reclaim my own self, and aligning with advocacy helped me towards recovery, and this is what the second part of this chapter describes.

* * *

Part 2

When we think of labels people are given, the ones that come to mind are ones like "disabled", "bipolar", "queer", "black", "white" and so many others. Perhaps "human" is now the most underused and neglected baggage tag.

Menzies (2018) criticises the clinical psychology industry for abandoning its links to anthropology, sociology, and philosophy, and she argues that pain that is a human suffering are being ignored. If we used these more, the suffering and pain that being human brings with it would not lead to so much pathologising; it would be accepted as a part of the human experience.

That is one of the problems with the movement for global mental health (MGMH) and the way it pays insufficient attention to sociopolitical occurrences like war, economic deprivation, environmental factors, and so on. Kirmayer and Pedersen state that war, trauma, and ongoing forms of regional violence clearly contribute to mental distress (Kirmayer 2012). Pathare adds to this conversation by saying that "treatment" carries a medical connotation and implies biomedical treatment of mental illness, and he suggests treatment should be expanded to look at psychosocial needs (Pathare et al, 2018). Although suicides among farmers are cited time and again by proponents of the MGMH (Patel et al. 2012), this should be the responsibility of government and not psychiatry. It has been suggested by scholars that state interventions to stabilise prices of cash crops and relieve farmers in debt may be effective at reducing suicide rates in India (Kennedy 2014).

Domestic violence, including sexual violence, affects 34 per cent of women in India (2005-2006) and can result in psychological trauma including mental disorders. India, like many other countries, lacks mental health practitioners with competencies in psychosocial trauma-focused assessment, trauma-focused psychosocial interventions, and trauma-informed professionalism (Suman 2015). In my own case, sexual trauma caused temporary mental health distress which was completely ignored in the "treatment" I received, which became another traumatic event to heal from.

Common treatments for mood disorders target current symptoms rather than the core transdiagnostic variables that drive mental health disorders. If only the symptoms are suppressed or treated, and the root cause is not explored, can true recovery or healing take place? Perhaps this is the reason for the revolving door in mental health (Iverach et al. 2014). In addition, the illness model itself is problematic as it implies something is wrong with the person, whereas one might instead ask what is wrong with the environment around her. It is the difference between asking "What is wrong with you?" and asking, "What happened to you?" (Sweeney 2018).

It is interesting how, from time immemorial, women have been considered to be a problem that needs fixing. External sources like sexual abuse, financial worries, and the like, are not taken into account. Childhood neglect or abuse is not considered. The woman acting irrationally becomes the malfunctioning part of a patriarchal system.

The labelling begins. Along with the "treatment". There is a vast literature – feminist literature in particular – on the topic of women and mental illness, including the pathologisation of women and critiques of psychiatry, psychology, and psychoanalysis. From Phyllis Chesler to Kate Millett, along with many others, much has been written about the pathologising of women's unhappiness and the use of psychiatry as a means to control them (Wright 2001) and the fact that psychiatry is patriarchal and oppressive (Wiener 2005).

In her memoir, *The Loony Bin Trip* (1990), Millett writes about psychiatry as "a terrifying form of social control" after her own relatives twice put her into a mental health hospital (as mine did to me). Throughout the book, she questions her family and friends, feeling "betrayed" by them for obeying psychiatrists blindly. Chesler (2005) considers Greek mythology, using Demeter and her four daughters to explore and reveal the relationships between the female condition and madness.

A memoir is a literary text, consisting of words that have been "artfully arranged" with authenticity at their core, according to Joyce Carol Oates, author of more than one hundred books. Memoir is different from novels and auto-fiction, which may be inspired by real life but plug in fictional elements for readability. Memoir is a kind of life writing that demands truth: as Morrison (2019) says, "any whiff of fiction breeds doubt". Leslie Jamison (2010), author and memoirist, claims that confessional memoir creates dialogue, gives rise to responses and creates a chorus. My memoir is my story, sufficiently removed from the time it happened to allow for objectivity, hopes for response, and chorus, as Jamison writes. Why are our stories important and why do they matter? And can the MGMH learn from them?

Memoirs are an important way of bringing marginalised voices into the mainstream. As Phillips (2001) writes, "even our most personal stories are always a far broader cultural and political affair." Memoir "can serve to help us escape from the strictly personal, to contemplate the bigger picture" (Miller 2000). For instance, with the continued upsurge in feminist consciousness, which bloomed through the 1960s and beyond, and is indeed blooming today in the #MeToo movement, Segal (2009) notes a new form of writing that emerged via the solidarity and support of other women, which gave rise to slogans such as "the personal is political". Furthermore, Marion Roach Smith (2011) writes on the importance of memoirs, saying that, without them, "We would not know about the lives of the disenfranchised. That awareness alone is worth real study". Building upon this, Liz Stanley (1992) discusses the term "intellectual autobiography" as she describes how writers can use their own life experiences to make their position explicit by showing their experiences in a way that elicits thought. I hope that my own memoir will inform readers and scholars about trauma, patriarchy, class, race, psychiatry, and its intersections.

The medicalisation and psychiatrisation of women also strips women of agency. My memoir depicts Indian psychiatric institutions that are still run in a patriarchal, paternalistic manner – and perhaps, also reflects Indian culture in general.

Ann's husband put her here, Mary's in-laws, Margaret's own mother. And the visits of the culprits, are cherished, awaited, loved, hated, feared (Millett, The Loony Bin Trip, 19: 217)

Indeed, from the earliest times to the present, this practice continues: "As early as the sixteenth century, women were 'shut up' in madhouses by their husbands" (Chesler 93, 2005). Although more men are also seeking psychiatric help now, it is more prevalent to find women seeking "help" for their problems, according to Chesler. The patriarchal nature of psychiatric institutions has been explored in the works of Foucault, Szasz, Goffman, Sceff, and many others (ibid. 2005). According to Hodges (2003), psychiatry's claims to help people who are a "danger to themselves or others" and to be for "their own good" are in fact coercive. She claims that since women still make up the majority of psychiatric patients, treating them will reunite them (albeit in their new, improved, functional role as wife and mother) with their male partners and children, which therefore serves patriarchal societal structures. Hodges herself is a survivor of the mental health system. Chesler writes, "Clinicians all too often treat their patients, most of whom are women, as 'wives' and 'daughters'" (ibid.: xxi).

My work provides an Indian context where scholars may not have considered these facts as rigorously, especially the idea that psychiatry is controlling and paternalistic. At the Centre for Mental Health Law and Policy in Pune, India, I was giving a talk on Gender and Mental Health to an international group of young psychiatrists, social workers, and activists from around the world, and mentioned precisely this on one of my slides. Some of the Indian male psychiatrists in the workshop were very offended. It was obvious they had not even considered the patriarchal dimensions of psychiatry. Clearly, there is much work to be done in this regard in India.

Psychiatry can also be re-traumatising for the very people it professes to help. The snapshots in Part 1 – being dragged on the floor, restrained by shackles on the feet, forcibly injected, and stripped of agency – depict modes of treatment designed to discipline and punish, rather than to cure. Perhaps mental patients are less "human" than medical patients or criminals "because they have been abandoned by their own families and have no one to tell what is happening to them" (Chesler 2005). In May 2001, 26 patients who had been kept chained in a religious asylum in Erwadi died when the building caught fire. Be it religious asylums or the more "organised" medical institutions, there are "violations within psychiatric institutions" in India and mentally ill people face stigmatisation and discrimination because there are misconceptions about the nature of mental illness (Trivedi 2007). I was quoted in a 2014 report by Human Rights Watch as follows:

The nurses would make us have the medications in front of them. If I complained that there were too many tablets, the nurse would sometimes forcefully put the pills in my mouth and stroke my throat to send them down, the way I feed my dogs... I woke up one night and I couldn't move;

my body was in intense physical pain. A nurse came and jabbed an injection into my body, without even taking off my clothes. You are treated worse than animals; it's an alternate reality. – *Deepali*, a 46-year-old woman with a perceived psychosocial disability, Delhi, August 25, 2013. (Sharma for HRW 2014)

If psychiatry is the apex form of treatment for MGMH, we need to closely examine what psychiatric therapy entails. From re-traumatising already disturbed and traumatised people to furthering the agenda of Big Pharma (Beder 2003), Psychiatry continues to be paternalistic and patriarchal, insisting that its therapies are "good for" the people it treats. The MGMH wishes to avoid these methods of treatment and that is why memoirs, and other documentation, are vital to see where change is needed. It is also important to be aware of other forms of healing and recovery, like writing, aligning with feminist consciousness raising, and advocacy, which can exist alongside the MGMH, leading to more holistic ways of living with trauma and distress. Of course, some of the initiatives of the MGMH should be lauded, like the practice of creating laypeople for counselling, making therapy more accessible, and so on.

My interest in the trauma-informed approach led me to examine the types of interventions used in mental health distress in India that still use indigenous, religious and classical means of healing including *ayurveda, dargahs, jad phuk*, and religious asylums (Biswal 2017). On the one hand, Sax (2014) argues that ritual healing can be therapeutic, in many cases looking more holistically at "healing", considering the whole person, his family, the environment, and more, whereas modern medicine and psychiatry continues to look only at symptoms. On the other hand, some indigenous systems of healing suffer from power imbalances similar to psychiatry, but sometimes, especially if the person affected chooses these methods, they can be less invasive. However, indigenous forms of healing are difficult to replicate and scale up, and perhaps that is why they do not find a home in the MGMH.

It is very important to ask whether treatment is voluntary or involuntary. A feeling of individual agency, of being in control, is important for healing and recovery, and so the question of whether a patient has chosen a particular hospital or institution, or been forcibly put there. Person-centred care including shared decision-making has been shown to give better results in long term recovery (Dixon et al. 2016). Unfortunately, India and the MGMH are still some distance from Open Dialogue and similar systems of care.

One reason I advocate "alternatives" to the biomedical approach is to give affected persons more choice. In my work as a poet, activist, and founder of a mental health charity in India, I use Creative Writing as an important tool for helping people heal from trauma, or perhaps make more sense of living with their distress, or learn to cope. In prison settings, classroom settings, or workshop settings, I have used these sessions with varying results, mostly positive and powerful.

As a young male service-user in a British secure unit claimed, "I don't know what it is, but I feel so much better after writing!" I think that poetry in particular helps one to make sense of grief and trauma. It opens a door to light. In the 1990s, James W. Pennebaker (1993) began publishing results from clinical trials he had conducted, in laboratory conditions, on the connections between health markers and expressive writing. He found that subjects who wrote on distress or trauma showed significant improvements in their health levels over the next six months. Although the connection between personal expression and improved mental wellbeing is widely understood, Pennebaker's trials followed a scientific protocol, so that his work was accepted as "scientific".

In his book *The Body Keeps The Score*, psychiatrist Bessel van der Kolk (2014) drew on his own thirty years of experience to argue that trauma and the effects of stress cause physiological changes in the body and brain that predispose us to diseases like diabetes, heart disease, or cancer. Of course, the first place trauma manifests is often the psyche, but when a person does not feel heard, problems shift to the body.

Van der Kolk drew on hundreds of studies to show how the effects of neglect, sexual abuse, domestic violence, and other adverse childhood effects create adults who may have abnormalities in the ratios of their immune cells as compared to non-traumatised people, further exposing them to autoimmune diseases. He suggests bodywork like yoga, massage, kung fu, and other body-based therapies as well as creative prescriptions like poetry and art.

When I was regarded as *"crazy"* all those years ago, I remember feeling ashamed and angry when people would ask me how I was. We would be at a party or a picnic, and then an acquaintance, someone I barely knew, perhaps a colleague of my ex-husband, would come and ask, with a sorrowful and serious face, "How are you?" And if I replied, "Fine," they would look at me as if I was hiding something, as if they knew the *"secret"*. When you have been diagnosed with mental illness, the world keeps on turning and people discuss your condition behind your back, and then when you appear, they offer you space but only if you play your part as the "sick woman". Even now, after many years, some things make me angry.

Recently, I was at my mother's friends' home for dinner; a lot of mutual acquaintances were present. I was discussing weight loss and lamenting my inability to lose weight when Usha Auntie, my mother's friend, mentioned how she had recently taken some supplements and pills and lost weight. When I said, "I don't like to take chemicals and pills," she laughed and said, "Yes, some things never change!" She was of course referring to the time, many years ago, when my mother would say to her friends, "Deepali is crazy, she won't take her medication, poor us," and so on.

Having survived such experiences, I can now see how much work we need to do to change the world so that rights, agency, and personal choice matters, trauma is acknowledged, and the perpetrator is not let off scot free – in my own case, the husband who committed sexual and domestic violence, and kidnapped my children without court orders, was not punished and lives a free life with my children, some whom I have not seen for eight years. I hope that my writings and my activism may change the Usha Auntie's of the world and will lead to some policy changes that will improve the ways treatment is carried out in India and elsewhere. I am aware that the MGMH does not envisage the kind of treatment I, or several other survivors have experienced, especially in closed psychiatry, and I am certain that, if they were to encourage the alternatives that a lot of us are working on, it would be a step in the right direction.

References

Beder, Sharon, Richard Gosden, and Loren R. Mosher 2003. "Pig Pharma: Psychiatric Agenda Setting by Drug Companies." In *Family Therapy as an Alternative to Medication: An Appraisal of Pharmland*, edited by Phoebe S. Prosky, and David V. Keith, 193-208. New York: Brunner-Routledge.

Becker-Blease, Kathryn A. 2017. "As the World Becomes Trauma-informed, Work To Do." *Journal of Trauma & Dissociation* 18 (2): 131-38. DOI: 10.1080/15299732.2017.1253401.

Biswal Ramakrishna, Chittaranjan Subudhi, and Sanjay Kumar Acharya. 2017. "Healers and Healing Practices of Mental Illness in India: The Role of Proposed Eclectic Healing Model." *Journal Health Research and Reviews* 4 (3): 89-95.

Bunton, Robin, and Alan R. Petersen. 1997. *Foucault, Health and Medicine*. London: Routledge. https://doi.org/10.4324/9780203005347.

Chavan B. S., and Jitender Aneja. 2016. "Global Mental Health Movement Has Not Helped in Reducing Global Burden of Psychiatric Disorders." *Indian Journal of Social Psychiatry* 32 (3): 261-66.

Chesler, Phyllis. 2005. *Women and Madness*. New York: Palgrave Macmillan.

Crenshaw, Kimberlé. 2017. "Kimberlé Crenshaw on Intersectionality, More than Two Decades Later." Interview by Columbia Law School, posted on 8 June 2017. https://www.law.columbia.edu/pt-br/news/2017/06/kimberle-crenshaw-intersectionality.

Das, Anindya. 2011. "Farmers' Suicide in India: Implications for Public Mental Health." *International Journal of Social Psychiatry* 57 (1): 21-29. https://doi.org/10.1177/0020764009103645.

Dixon, Lisa B., Yael Holoshitz, and Ilana Nossel. 2016. "Treatment Engagement of Individuals Experiencing Mental Illness: Review and Update." *World Psychiatry* 15 (1): 13-20. doi:10.1002/wps.20306.

Hedva, Johanna. 2015. "My Body Is a Prison of Pain so I Want to Leave It Like a Mystic But I Also Love It and Want It to Matter Politically." Lecture, Human Resources, Los Angeles, 7 October 2015.

Hodges, Katherine 2003. "The Invisible Crisis: Women and Psychiatric Oppression." *Off Our Backs* 33 (7/8): 12-15. Retrieved from http://search.ebscohost.com/login.aspx?direct=true&db=agh&AN=10368097&site=ehost-live.

Humphreys, Cathy, and Ravi Thiara. 2003. "Mental Health and Domestic Violence: 'I Call it Symptoms of Abuse.'" *British Journal of Social Work* 33 (2): 209-26.

Iverach, Lisa, Ross G. Menzies, and Rachel E. Menzies 2014. "Death Anxiety and its Role in Psychopathology: Reviewing the Status of a Transdiagnostic Construct." *Clinical Psychology Review* 34 (7): 580-93.

Kennedy, Jonathan, and Lawrence King. 2014. "The Political Economy of Farmers' Suicides in India: Indebted Cash-crop Farmers with Marginal Landholdings Explain State-level Variation in Suicide Rates." *Global Health* 10 (1): 16. doi:10.1186/1744-8603-10-16.

Kirmayer, Laurence J., and Duncan Pedersen. 2014. "Toward a New Architecture for Global Mental Health." *Transcultural Psychiatry* 51 (6): 759-76.

Kumar, Camille. 2018. "Fault Lines: Black Feminists' Intersectional Practice Working to End Violence against Women and Girls (VAWG)." In *Intersectionality in Social Work*, edited by Rachel Robbins, and Suryia Nayak, 184-98. Oxford: Routledge.

Lakeman, Richard. 2014. "The Finnish Open Dialogue Approach to Crisis Intervention in Psychosis: A Review." *Psychotherapy in Australia* 20 (3): 26-33.

Mann, Susan Archer, and Douglas J. Huffman. 2005. "The Decentering of Second Wave Feminism and the Rise of the Third Wave." *Science & Society* 69 (1): 56-91. http://www.jstor.org/stable/40404229.

Menzies, Rachel E. 2018. "Impermanence and the Human Dilemma: Observations Across the Ages." In *Curing the Dread of Death: Theory, Research and Practice*, edited by Rachel E. Menzies, Ross G. Menzies, and Lisa Iverach, 3-19. Samford, Queensland: Australian Academic Press.

Miller, Nancy K. 2000. "But Enough About Me, What Do You Think of My Memoir?" *The Yale Journal of Criticism* 13 (2): 421-36.

Millett, Kate. 1990. *The Loony Bin Trip.* Champaign, IL: University of Illinois Press.

Morrison, Blake. 2019. "The Naked Truth: How to Write a Memoir." *The Guardian,* 14 December 2019. https://www.theguardian.com/books/2019/dec/14/the-naked-truth-how-to-write-a-memoir.

Patel, Vikram, Chinthanie Ramasundarahettige, Lakshmi Vijayakumar, J. S. Thakur, Vendhan Gajalakshmi, Gopalkrishna Gururaj, Wilson Suraweera, and Prabhat Jha. 2012. "Suicide Mortality in India: A Nationally Representative Survey." *Lancet* 379 (9834): 2343-51. 10.1016/S0140-6736(12)60606-0.

Pathare, S., A. Brazinova, and I. Levav. 2018. "Care Gap: A Comprehensive Measure to Quantify Unmet Needs in Mental Health." Epidemiology and Psychiatric Sciences 27 (5): 463-67. doi: 10.1017/S2045796018000100.

Phillips, Adam. 2001. *Promises, Promises: Essays On Psychoanalysis And Literature.* New York: Basic Books.

Pennebaker, James W. 1993. "Putting Stress into Words: Health, Linguistic, and Therapeutic Implications." *Behaviour Research and Therapy* 31 (6): 539-48. https://www.sciencedirect.com/science/article/pii/0005796793901054?via%3Dihub.

Sax, William S. 2014. "Ritual healing and mental health in India." *Transcultural Psychiatry* 51 (6): 829-49. https://doi.org/10.1177/1363461514524472.

Segal, Lynne. 2009. "Who Do You Think You Are? Feminist Memoir Writing." *New Formations* 67:120-33. Retrieved from https://search.proquest.com/docview/211548512?accountid=17233.

Sharma, Kriti. 2014. "'Treated Worse than Animals': Abuses against Women and Girls with Psychosocial or Intellectual Disabilities in Institutions in India." *Human Rights* Watch, 3 December 2014, https://www.hrw.org/report/2014/12/03/treated-worse-animals/abuses-against-women-and-girls-psychosocial-or-intellectual.

Smith, Marion Roach. 2011. *The Memoir Project: A Thoroughly Non-Standardized Text for Writing and Life.* Grand Central Publishing.

Suman L. N. 2015. "Domestic Violence, Psychological Trauma and Mental Health of Women: A View from India." *Women Health Open Journal* 1 (1): e1-e2. doi: 10.17140/WHOJ-1-e001.

Stanley, Liz. 1992. *The Auto/Biographical I, the Theory and Practice of Feminist Auto/Biography.* Manchester University Press.

Sweeney, Angela, Beth Filson, Angela Kennedy, Lucie Collinson, and Steve Gillard. 2018. "A Paradigm Shift: Relationships in Trauma-informed Mental Health Services." *BJPsych Advances* 24 (5): 319-33. doi:10.1192/bja.2018.29.

Trivedi, J. K., Puneet Narang, and Mohan Dhyani. 2007. "Mental Health Legislation in South Asia with Special Reference to India: Shortcomings and Solutions." *Mental Health Review Journal* 12 (3): 22-29.

Van der Kolk, Bessel A. 2014. *The Body Keeps the Score: Brain, Mind, and Body in the Healing of Trauma*. New York: Viking.

Wiener, Diane. 2005. "Antipsychiatric Activism and Feminism: The Use of Film and Text to Question Biomedicine." *Journal of Public Mental Health* 4 (3): 42-47. https://doi.org/10.1108/17465729200500023.

Wright, Nicola, and Sara Owen. 2001. "Feminist Conceptualizations of Women's Madness: A Review of the Literature." *Journal of Advanced Nursing* 36 (1): 143-50. doi:10.1046/j.1365-2648.2001.01951.

About the Author

ANONYMOUS is a poet, writer and activist. She is the founder of an Indian charity that is active in mental health advocacy. She advocates "Poetry as Therapy" and is working on a few initiatives, both in the UK and India, intended to introduce this into prisons and hospitals. She works on gender, mental health, and trauma and has published two books. The snapshots in Part 1 of this chapter are part of her forthcoming memoir. This bio has been anonymised to protect the identities of the people described in her chapter.

Contributors

ANONYMOUS is a poet, writer and activist. She is the founder of an Indian charity that is active in mental health advocacy. She advocates "Poetry as Therapy" and is working on a few initiatives, both in the UK and India, intended to introduce this into prisons and hospitals. She works on gender, mental health, and trauma and has published two books. The snapshots in Part 1 of this chapter are part of her forthcoming memoir. This bio has been anonymised to protect the identities of the people described in her chapter.

ANINDYA DAS is currently Consultant Psychiatrist and Associate Professor of Psychiatry at All India Institute of Medical Sciences, Rishikesh, India. He has an MD in Psychiatry from Central Institute of Psychiatry, Ranchi, and a Master's in Public Health from Jawaharlal Nehru University. He is a full time clinician responsible for training graduate medical students and postgraduate residents of psychiatry. He has established and manages a tele-training psychiatry service. He has a particular interest in community and social psychiatry, and is working with the state government to establish a community mental health programme at the local level.

STEFAN ECKS co-founded Edinburgh University's Medical Anthropology programme. He teaches social anthropology and directs postgraduate teaching in the School of Social and Political Sciences. He has conducted ethnographic fieldwork in India, Nepal, and the UK. Recent work explores value in global pharmaceutical markets, changing ideas of mental health in South Asia, poverty and access to health care, as well as multimorbidity. His publications include *Eating Drugs: Psychopharmaceutical Pluralism in India* (New York, 2013) and *Living Worth: Value and Values in Global Pharmaceutical Markets* (forthcoming), as well as numerous journal articles on the intersections between health and economics.

ANNETTE HORNBACHER is professor of Cultural Anthropology at the University of Heidelberg. She received her PhD in philosophy (University of Tübingen) with a thesis on Friedrich Hölderlin's concept of poetic language as "higher enlightenment", and her *Habilitation* in Cultural Anthropology with a book on Balinese ritual dance as an alternative to modern Western paradigms of representation. She has conducted extensive fieldwork in Indonesia, particularly in Bali, where she worked on ritual dance drama as a kinaesthetic embodiment of cosmological knowledge. She has led several research projects: on *Religious Dynamics* in Post-Suharto Indonesia (funded by the German Ministry for Education and Research), on *Local Traditions and World Religions* (funded by the German Research Council), and on *Waterscapes* as interrelated nature-culture landscapes in Bali and Komodo (Heidelberg, Cluster of Excellence). In this context, she began working on competing concepts of ecology and human-animal relationships in the marine reserve of Komodo. Currently, she leads a research project on esoteric Balinese manuscripts in an interdisciplinary research area titled *"Material Textcultures"* (SFB933), and is conducting a comparative research project together with Prof. William Sax on tantric text practices in Bali and India.

MURPHY HALLIBURTON studied anthropology at Stanford University and the City University of New York (CUNY) Graduate Center, where he earned his PhD in 2000. Currently he is Professor in Anthropology at Queens College and the Graduate Center of CUNY. Since the 1990s, he has been conducting research on mental health and illness in Kerala, India. His first book, *Mudpacks and Prozac* (Routledge, 2009), compared ayurvedic, biomedical, and ritual forms of healing for mental illness and related problems, and he recently completed a Fulbright-Nehru-funded study of recovery from schizophrenia in Kerala. He has also conducted research on the struggle between Indian pharmaceutical companies and global big pharma over patent rights and concerns about biopiracy of ayurvedic knowledge, which is the subject of his book *India and the Patent Wars* (Cornell University Press, 2017). He is currently investigating the history of eugenic research at Stanford University and the role of biological determinism in American culture.

CLAUDIA LANG is an associate professor (Heisenberg) of anthropology at University of Leipzig and research partner at the Max-Planck-Institute of Anthropology in Halle. Before, she was a postdoc at the ERC project "GLOBHELATH: From International Public Health to Global Health" in Paris, France. She works on the anthropology of health in India and has published on various topics, including traditional medicine, mental health, psychiatry, religion and ritual, health governance, and subjectivities. She is currently working on the digitization and proliferation of mental health and global psy in India's megacities, and on memories, traces, and genealogies of primary health care in Kerala. Her most recent publications include *Depression in Kerala: Ayurveda and Mental Health Care in India's 21st century* (2018) and a co-edited special issue of *Culture, Medicine and Psychiatry*, "Genealogies and Anthropologies of Global Mental Health" (2019).

PROJIT BIHARI MUKHARJI is an Associate Professor at the University of Pennsylvania. He was educated at the Presidency College, Calcutta, Jawaharlal Nehru University, New Delhi, and the School of Oriental and African Studies, London. He is the author of *Nationalizing the Body: The Medical Market, Print and Daktari Medicine* (London, 2009) and *Doctoring Traditions: Ayurveda, Small Technologies and Braided Sciences* (Chicago, 2016). He is also the Editor-in-Chief of *History Compass,* Associate Editor of *South Asian History & Culture* and Book Review Editor of *Isis.*

HARISH NARAINDAS is currently professor of sociology at Jawaharlal Nehru University, and honorary professor at the Alfred Deakin Institute, Faculty of Arts and Education, Deakin University. He works on the history and sociology of science and medicine and has published on a range of topics, including an epistemological history of tropical medicine, a comparative history of smallpox from the eighteenth to the twentieth century, and work on the creolisation of contemporary Ayurveda, spa medicine in Germany, pregnancy and childbirth within the context of competing medical epistemes, and recently, how anthropology attempts to explain the non-human. He is currently working on AyurGenomics and P4 medicine, past-life aetiologies and therapeutic trance in German psychosomatic medicine, and a multi-sited study of perinatal loss and bereavement in the Anglophone world. His most recent publication was a co-edited special issue of *Anthropology and Medicine* called "The Fragile Medical: The Slippery Terrain between Medicine, Anthropology and Societies" (2017).

JOHANNES QUACK is Assistant Professor of Social Anthropology at the University of Zurich. He has conducted ethnographic research on medicine, ethics, and religion (secularity and non-religion) in India and elsewhere. Quack is the author of *Disenchanting India: Organized Rationalism and Criticism of Religion in India* (Oxford University Press, 2012). He co-edited the volumes *The Problem of Ritual Efficacy* (Oxford University Press, 2010), *Religion und Kritik in der Moderne* (LIT, 2012), *Asymmetrical Conversations: Contestations, Circumventions and the Blurring of Therapeutic Boundaries* (Berghahn, 2014), *Religious Indifference* (Springer, 2017), and *The Diversity of Nonreligion* (Routledge, 2020), and he co-edits the book series *Religion and Its Others: Studies in Religion, Nonreligion, and Secularity* (De Gruyter).

MOHAN RAO was, till recently, a Professor at the Centre of Social Medicine and Community Health (CSMCH), School of Social Sciences, Jawaharlal Nehru University, New Delhi. A medical doctor specialising in public health, he has written extensively on health and population policy, and on the history and politics of health and family planning. He is the author of *From Population Control to Reproductive Health: Malthusian Arithmetic* (Sage, 2004) and has edited *Disinvesting in Health: The World Bank's Health Prescriptions* (Sage, 1999) and *The Unheard Scream: Reproductive Health and Women's Lives in India* (Zubaan/Kali for Women, 2004). He has edited, with Sarah Sexton of Cornerhouse, UK, the volume *Markets and Malthus: Population, Gender and Health in Neoliberal Times* (Sage, 2010); and with Sarah Hodges, *Public Health and Private Wealth: Stem Cells, Surrogacy and Other Strategic Bodies* (Oxford University Press, 2016). His latest work is the edited volume *The Lineaments of Population Policy in India: Women and Family Planning* (Routledge, 2018). He has been a member of the National Population Commission, as well as several Working Groups of the National Rural Health Mission of the Government of India. He has worked on the Committee established by the National Human Rights Commission to examine the two-child norm in population policy, and is a member of the Executive Committee of the Centre for Women's Development Studies. He is also actively involved in the Jan Swasthya Abhiyan (People's Health Movement).

WILLIAM S. ("BO") SAX studied at Banaras Hindu University, the University of Wisconsin, and the University of Washington (Seattle), and the University of Chicago, where he earned his PhD in Anthropology in 1987. From 1987 to 1989 he was lecturer in Anthropology at Harvard University, and post-doctoral fellow in the Harvard Academy. After that, he taught Hinduism in the Department of Philosophy and Religious studies at the University of Canterbury in Christchurch, New Zealand, for eleven years. In 2000 he took up the Chair of Anthropology at the South Asia Institute in Heidelberg. He has published extensively on pilgrimage, gender, theatre, aesthetics, ritual healing, and medical anthropology. His major works (all published by Oxford University Press, New York) include *Mountain Goddess: Gender and Politics in a Central Himalayan Pilgrimage* (1991); *The Gods at Play: Lila in South Asia* (1995); *Dancing the Self: Personhood and Performance in the Pandav Lila of Garhwal* (2002); *God of Justice: Ritual Healing and Social Justice in the Central Himalayas* (2008); *The Problem of Ritual Efficacy* (with Johannes Quack and Jan Weinhold, 2010); and *The Law of Possession: Ritual, Healing, and the Secular State* (with Heléne Basu, 2015). He is currently working on a book about archaic polities in the Western Himalayas, tentatively entitled *In the Valley of the Kauravas: From Subject to Citizen in the Western Himalayas*. His 1991 book *Mountain Goddess* has been translated into Hindi under the title *Himalaya ki Nanda Devi* (Dehra Dun: Wimsar).

Index

For Product Safety Concerns and Information please contact our EU
representative GPSR@taylorandfrancis.com
Taylor & Francis Verlag GmbH, Kaufingerstraße 24, 80331 München, Germany

www.ingramcontent.com/pod-product-compliance
Lightning Source LLC
Chambersburg PA
CBHW060808220326
41598CB00022B/2563

9 7 8 1 0 4 1 1 8 8 5 2 0